an outline text

Human

Gross

Anatomy

by

Robert J. Leonard, Ph.D.

New York   Oxford
OXFORD UNIVERSITY PRESS
1995

Oxford University Press

Oxford   New York
Athens   Auckland   Bangkok   Bombay
Calcutta   Cape Town   Dar es Salaam   Delhi
Florence   Hong Kong   Istanbul   Karachi
Kuala Lumpur   Madras   Madrid   Melbourne
Mexico City   Nairobi   Paris   Singapore
Taipei   Tokyo   Toronto

and associated companies in
Berlin   Ibadan

Library of Congress Cataloging-in-Publication Data

Leonard, Robert J.
Human gross anatomy : an outline text / by Robert J. Leonard.
p. cm.   Includes index.
ISBN 0-19-509003-9
1. Human anatomy—Outlines, syllabi, etc.   I. Title.
[DNLM: 1. Anatomy—outlines.   QS 18.2 L581h 1995]
QM31.L39   1995
611—dc20
DNLM/DLC
for Library of Congress   95-10041

9 8 7 6 5 4 3 2 1

Printed in the United States of America
on acid-free paper

For Bhasha,

Tanya and Satya

PREFACE

An in-depth understanding of human gross anatomy is fundamental to the practice of clinical medicine. Unfortunately, virtually all medical schools have severely curtailed the class hours allotted for anatomy instruction. As a result, anatomists have been challenged to develop more efficient educational methods in order to preserve high academic standard. This book was written as a response to this challenge.

The text presents gross anatomy in an expanded outline format. Its conciseness and logical organization permit easy previewing of the subject matter before a lecture or laboratory as well as allowing efficient learning and reviewing of the material before an examination. Notwithstanding its succinct style, the text's coverage of gross anatomy is comprehensive and contains a level of detail appropriate for the medical student.

The Introduction sets forth basic principles and terminology that will serve the student throughout the remainder of the text. Overviews of the nervous, muscular, skeletal, and vascular systems are also included in this Introduction. The main body of the text is organized on the basis of regional anatomy in the following sequence: the *back, thorax, abdomen, perineum* and *pelvis, head* and *neck, upper limb,* and *lower limb.* Clinical notes that highlight anatomy relevant to current medical practice appear throughout these chapters. Since each regional anatomy chapter is complete in itself, the order in which each is studied is optional.

During the writing of this text, some of the most difficult decisions involved the subject matter to be included in the chapters. A guidepost in this process was the question, "Will this information contribute significantly to a student's understanding of anatomy, especially as it relates to the practice of medicine?" When, for example, this question was posed for the study of the cranial nerves and autonomic nervous system, the details of this subject seemed highly relevant to clinical medicine. Thus, their anatomy was given extensive treatment. In contrast, when this criterion was applied to the relationship of the lumbricals, palmar interossei, and dorsal interossei to the deep transverse metacarpal ligaments, I thought this information was beyond the scope of applicable anatomy and excluded it from the text.

Other difficult deliberations involved the selection of and priority given to anatomical terms. Although the guidance offered by the sixth edition (1989) of *Nomina Anatomica* proved invaluable, common usage took precedence over strict adherence to *Nomina*

Anatomica. For example, dorsal and ventral roots of a spinal nerve were selected over posterior and anterior roots. When the commonly used terms were chosen, the *Nomina Anatomica* term was often noted in parentheses. Synonyms and eponyms were also parenthetically cited after *Nomina Anatomica* terms. Most terms were anglicized; for instance, foramen transversarium became transverse foramen.

Since this text was designed for use with an atlas, no illustrations were included. This decision was based on two considerations: (1) essentially all students of gross anatomy purchase an atlas, and (2) substantial classroom testing of the text indicated that additional illustrations were unnecessary.

Earlier versions of this text have been favorably received by my own students. Because it circumscribes the subject matter the student needs to master, anxiety that might have arisen from ambiguity about what the student would be examined upon was significantly reduced. Additionally, students showed more enthusiasm for self-instruction when the contours of the course were more clearly defined. This permitted a more Socratic method of teaching, whereby objectives for a formal lecture could be achieved through a more intellectually stimulating question-and-answer discussion. I hope other educators and students of anatomy will also find the book a valuable instructional and learning tool. I welcome their comments.

Riverside, Calif.   R.J.L.

ACKNOWLEDGMENTS

The impetus for this outline text was provided in large measure by my students and to all of them I extend much gratitude. I would especially like to acknowledge the sustained support and encouragement of Ramen Chmait, Jay Lee, Ravish Patwardhan, Richard Serrao, Chih-Wen Shi, and Kevin Taggart of the UCLA School of Medicine, Class of 1996. I would also like to extend special thanks to Nancy Price for typing the manuscript and to Kenneth Dorshkind, David M. Koester, Whitney R. Powers, Neal A. Cross, and Donald R. Cahill for their excellent suggestions for improving the manuscript.

Anatomy is that faculty which through inspection and dissection reveals the uses and actions of the parts.

WILLIAM HARVEY

CONTENTS

Human

Gross

Anatomy

Introduction

I. Anatomical Principles

   A. Anatomy

      1. The study of biological structure

      2. Structure and function are inextricably entwined; function is determined by structure and, in clinical medicine, the goal is often to restore structure so as to restore function

   B. Variation

      1. Human diversity is expressed in anatomical variation; variation in external human form reflects variation in internal form, consequently, one will not see the same face or the same liver twice

      2. Because of variation, anatomical descriptions and illustrations will often be unreliable; an appreciation for the anatomical uniqueness of an individual is part of the art of medicine

   C. Three-dimensional visualization

      1. One of the objectives of learning anatomy is to construct a three-dimensional mental image of the human body

      2. A three-dimensional appreciation of the human body is essential in many diagnostic procedures and may be facilitated by the study of cross-sectional anatomy, perhaps through the aid of magnetic resonance images (MRIs)

D. Living anatomy

    1. Since your knowledge of anatomy will be applied to the examination and treatment of a living individual, it is important to extrapolate your laboratory experience to the living individual

    2. Many of the structures you will study can be palpated through the skin, or their locations can be determined by palpable landmarks

E. Terminology

    1. The internationally recognized Latin terms for anatomical structures appear in the volume *Nomina Anatomica*; the meanings of their Latin names are usually noted in a medical dictionary and are often helpful in understanding their structure or function

    2. Other key words in the language of anatomical description are terms defining planes, locations, and muscle actions; they are utilized relative to the anatomical position, that is, an upright posture with the upper limbs by the sides and the palms of the hands facing forward, and are noted below

    3. Terms defining planes

       a. Sagittal plane: divides the body into right and left parts; a median (midsagittal) plane divides the body in the midline into right and left halves

       b. Coronal (frontal) plane: divides the body into front and back parts

       c. Transverse (horizontal, axial) plane: divides the body into upper and lower parts

    4. Terms defining locations

       a. Proximal—closer to the midline, point of origin, or entrance; distal—further from the midline, point of origin, or entrance

       b. Anterior (ventral)—toward the front of the body; posterior (dorsal)—toward the back of the body

       c. Superior (cranial)—toward the head; inferior (caudal)—toward the feet

       d. Medial—toward the midline; lateral—away from the midline

       e. Superficial (external)—toward the surface of the body; deep (internal)—away from the surface of the body

5. Terms defining muscle actions

    a. Flexion—a movement decreasing the angle between two bones or a movement in a ventral direction; extension—a movement increasing the angle between two bones or a movement in a dorsal direction

    b. Abduction—a movement away from the midline; adduction—a movement toward the midline

    c. Circumduction—a circular pivoting movement that describes a cone; involves a combination of flexion, extension, abduction, and adduction

    d. Medial rotation—a movement around a longitudinal axis in which the anterior surface turns medially; lateral rotation—a movement around a longitudinal axis in which the anterior surface turns laterally

    e. Lateral flexion—a movement of the vertebral column or head to the right or left within the coronal plane

II. Anatomical Systems

A. Nervous system

1. Composed of a central and peripheral nervous system

    a. The central nervous system consists of the brain and spinal cord; it receives and integrates sensory input and initiates motor output

    b. The peripheral nervous system consists of sensory (afferent) neurons that conduct impulses toward the central nervous system and motor (efferent) neurons that conduct impulses away from the central nervous system

2. Composed of a somatic and autonomic nervous system

    a. The somatic nervous system receives sensory information from the skin, muscles, and joints, and provides motor innervation to skeletal muscle

    b. The autonomic nervous system provides motor innervation to smooth muscle, cardiac muscle, and glands (the autonomic nervous system is generally regarded as a motor system, however, smooth muscle, cardiac muscle, and glands also have a sensory innervation)

B. Muscular system

  1. Muscles

    a. Span joints and contract; their actions can usually be deduced from their relationship to a joint

    b. Denervation of a muscle results in loss of its functions; the loss may be compensated for by other muscles with similar functions

  2. Deep fascia: represents the connective tissue sheaths of muscles (superficial fascia lies deep to the skin and usually contains fat)

C. Skeletal system

  1. Provides a protective casing for delicate structures, such as the brain and spinal cord, and provides a lever system of joints; joints are junctions between bones and are classified into the three major types noted below

  2. Synovial joint

    a. Characterized by a joint space between closely apposed hyaline-cartilage-covered, articular surfaces of bones; the joint space and articular surfaces are ensheathed in a collar of dense connective tissue called the fibrous capsule

    b. The fibrous capsule is lined by a synovial membrane which secretes synovial fluid into the joint space; synovial fluid is a viscous lubricating substance that reduces friction between the articular surfaces

  3. Cartilaginous joint: characterized by the imposition of hyaline cartilage or fibrocartilage between bones; in the former instance, the joint is called a synchondrosis and, in the latter instance, the joint is referred to as a symphysis

  4. Fibrous joint: bones are united by dense connective tissue

D. Vascular system

  1. A pumping, delivery, and drainage system

  2. Arteries: comprise a pulsatile, branching, tubular delivery system extending from the heart to the capillaries

  3. Veins: comprise a drainage system of expansile, tubular tributaries extending from the capillaries to the heart; when multiple veins accom-

pany a singular artery, they are sometimes referred to as venae comitantes (accompanying veins) of the named artery

4. Lymphatics: comprise a tubular drainage system for interstitial fluid or lymph; after passing through lymph nodes, lymph empties into the venous system

5. Valves: found within veins and lymphatics; prevent backflow of blood and lymph

part **I**

The

Back

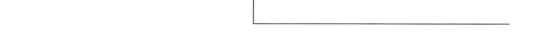

The Vertebral Column

I. General Features of Vertebrae

    A. Body: anterior, cylindrical, weight-bearing part; articular (hyaline) cartilage covers its superior and inferior surfaces

    B. Vertebral arch

        1. U-shaped element attached posteriorly to the body

            a. Consists of two laterally-placed, cylindrical pedicles united posteriorly by two platelike laminae

            b. The superior and inferior vertebral notches are indentations along the superior and inferior margins of each pedicle, respectively

        2. The vertebral arch and posterior surface of a body bound a vertebral foramen; collectively, the vertebral foramina form the vertebral canal which houses the spinal cord

    C. Processes

        1. Spinous process: projects posteriorly at the junction of the two laminae

        2. Transverse processes (two): project laterally at the junction of each pedicle and lamina

        3. Superior and inferior articular processes (two of each): project superiorly and inferiorly, respectively, at the junction of each pedicle and lamina

II. Regional Features of Vertebrae

    A. Cervical vertebrae (seven)

        1. Bodies: small

        2. Spinous processes: those of vertebrae C2 to C5 are short and bifid; vertebra C7 has a long, palpable spinous process, and is thus known as the vertebra prominens

        3. Transverse processes

            a. Perforated by transverse foramina; those of the upper six cervical vertebrae transmit the vertebral arteries

            b. Derived from two embryonic sources

                1. The posterior portion of a transverse process is the true transverse process; it ends in a posterior tubercle

                2. The anterior portion of a transverse process is the costal component and represents a rudimentary rib that has fused to the true transverse process; it ends in an anterior tubercle

                    a. The costal component of the transverse process of vertebra C7 occasionally fails to fuse with its posterior portion and forms a cervical rib

                    b. The large anterior tubercle of the transverse process of vertebra C6 is sometimes called the carotid tubercle because the common carotid artery crosses it and can be easily compressed against it

                    c. The sulcus for a spinal nerve lies between the anterior and posterior tubercles

        4. Articular processes: the articular surfaces of superior articular processes face posteriorly and superiorly; articular surfaces of inferior articular processes face anteriorly and inferiorly, thus, there is a tendency for lateral flexion to occur simultaneously with rotation (flexion and extension also occur at these joints)

        5. Atlas

            a. Consists of an anterior and posterior arch; it has no body

            b. The anterior arch has a facet for articulation with the dens on its posterior surface and the posterior arch has a posterior tubercle on its posterior surface (there is no spinous process); the sulcus for the vertebral artery grooves the superior surface of the posterior arch posterior to the superior articular surface

6. Axis: the dens or odontoid process is a toothlike extension of bone that projects superiorly from the body of the axis

B. Thoracic vertebrae (twelve)

1. Bodies: posterolaterally, they bear costal fovea (facets) for articulation with the heads of ribs, which usually articulate with the vertebral body of their segmental origin and the body of the adjacent superior vertebra (and the intervening intervertebral disc)

2. Spinous processes: usually point inferiorly

3. Transverse processes: usually bear costal fovea for articulation with the tubercles of ribs of the same segmental origin

4. Movements of the thoracic vertebrae are restricted by the articulation of the ribs to the sternum

C. Lumbar vertebrae (five)

1. Bodies: large

2. Articular processes: the articular surfaces approximate a sagittal plane, and thus permit a substantial amount of flexion and extension, however, little rotation is allowed; the articular surfaces of the inferior articular processes of vertebra L5 and the superior articular processes of vertebra S1 are more coronally placed, and thus prevent forward displacement of vertebra L5 (and the entire upper part of the human body) on the sloping superior surface of the sacrum

D. Sacrum

1. Triangular bone formed by the fusion of the five sacral vertebrae; its ventral surface faces inferiorly

2. Promontory: anteriorly projecting edge of the superior surface of the body of vertebra S1

3. Alae: lateral, winglike extensions on each side of the body of vertebra S1

4. Auricular surfaces: lateral, ear-shaped, articular regions that form synovial sacroiliac joints with the auricular surfaces of the ilia

5. Sacral canal: central canal transmitting the dorsal and ventral roots of spinal nerves S1 to S5 and the coccygeal spinal nerve

6. Ventral and dorsal sacral foramina (four pairs of each): apertures that transmit the ventral and dorsal rami of spinal nerves S1 to S4, respectively

E. Coccyx: small, triangular bone formed by three to five rudimentary coccygeal vertebrae; may occur in two or three separate parts

III. Articulations of the Vertebral Column

A. Synovial joints

1. Atlanto-occipital joints: oblong joints between the convex occipital condyles of the skull and the reciprocally concave superior articular surfaces of the atlas; allow flexion and extension of the head, but not rotation

2. Median atlantoaxial joints: an anterior joint lies between the dens of the axis and the articular facet on the posterior surface of the anterior arch of the atlas, and a posterior joint lies between the dens and the transverse ligament of the atlas; they permit rotation of the head and atlas on the axis

3. Facet (zygapophyseal) joints: between superior and inferior articular processes of adjacent vertebrae; provide for varying degrees of flexion, extension, lateral flexion, and rotation

B. Fibrous joints

1. Supraspinous (supraspinal) ligament: courses along the tips of the spinous processes; in the cervical region it is represented by the ligamentum nuchae, a median connective tissue septum separating the posterior neck muscles of each side

2. Interspinous (interspinal) ligaments: extend between adjacent spinous processes

3. Ligamenta flava: paired elastic ligaments between laminae of adjacent vertebrae; between the posterior arch of the atlas and the posterior margin of the foramen magnum of the skull, they are represented by the posterior atlanto-occipital membrane

4. Intertransverse ligaments: extend between adjacent transverse processes

5. Anterior longitudinal ligament: runs the length of the vertebral column along the anterior surfaces of vertebral bodies and intervertebral discs;

superiorly, it provides a narrow midline reinforcement for the anterior atlanto-occipital membrane, a fibrous band extending between the anterior arch of the atlas and the anterior margin of foramen magnum

6. Posterior longitudinal ligament: runs the length of the vertebral canal along the posterior surfaces of vertebral bodies and intervertebral discs

7. The ligamenta flava and the supraspinous, interspinous, intertransverse, and posterior longitudinal ligaments limit flexion of the vertebral column; the anterior longitudinal ligament limits extension of the vertebral column

C. Fibrocartilaginous joints (symphyses): intervertebral discs

1. Components

   a. Anulus fibrosus: outer, fibrocartilaginous portion; composed of concentric layers of fibers that insert superiorly and inferiorly into the articular cartilage plates covering the bodies of adjacent vertebrae

   b. Nucleus pulposus: central, mucoid portion encased by the anulus fibrosus as well as by the articular cartilage plates covering the bodies of adjacent vertebrae; serves as a shock absorber

   c. Clinical note: dehydration of an intervertebral disc, especially its nucleus pulposus, occurs after middle age; since the intervertebral discs account for about a quarter of the length of the vertebral column, a significant loss in height is often observed after middle age

2. Permit a slight tilting movement in any direction between two adjacent vertebrae (there is no intervertebral disc between the atlas and axis); the total movement provided by all of the intervertebral discs results in a substantial mobility of the vertebral column as a whole

3. Clinical notes: herniated intervertebral disc

   a. The posterior part of the anulus fibrosus may undergo degenerative changes and tear; the nucleus pulposus may herniate through the tear

   b. A herniated nucleus pulposus usually protrudes lateral to the posterior longitudinal ligament and may impinge on an exiting spinal nerve; intervertebral discs below vertebrae L4 and L5 are subjected to the greatest compressive forces and are particularly prone to herniation

    c. Occasionally, the nucleus pulposus will herniate into a vertebral body through a defect in the articular cartilage plate covering its superior or inferior surface; the herniated structure is known as a Schmorl body

IV. Curvatures of the Vertebral Column

    A. The vertebral column of the embryo forms an anteriorly-concave, C-shaped curve; it is called the primary curve and remains in the adult in the thoracic and sacral regions

    B. Following birth, the cervical and lumbar curves of the vertebral column begin to reverse themselves and form posteriorly-concave, secondary curves; the secondary curve of the cervical region develops when the infant begins to hold up its head, and the secondary curve of the lumbar region develops when the infant begins to walk

    C. Clinical note: abnormal curvatures of the vertebral column include kyphosis, an exaggeration of the thoracic curve, lordosis, an exaggeration of the lumbar curve, and scoliosis, a lateral deviation of the vertebral column; a lordosis commonly occurs during the latter part of a pregnancy as a means of compensating for the additional, anteriorly-placed weight of the fetus

The Muscles of the Back

I. Fasciae

    A. Superficial fascia: fibrous and tough

    B. Deep (thoracolumbar) fascia

        1. Thin in the thoracic region; in the lumbar region it is thick and consists of a posterior and an anterior layer as noted below

        2. Posterior layer: lies posterior to the deep back muscles; attaches medially to the spinous processes of lumbar vertebrae and gives origin to the latissimus dorsi

        3. Anterior layer: lies anterior to the deep back muscles, attaching medially to the transverse processes of lumbar vertebrae; fuses with the posterior layer lateral to the deep back muscles, forming a fascial sheet which provides origin for the transversus abdominis and internal abdominal oblique muscles

II. Superficial Back Muscles

    A. Involved in movements of the scapula, shoulder, head, and neck

    B. Trapezius

        1. Origin: medial part of the superior nuchal line, external occipital protuberance, ligamentum nuchae, and spinous processes of thoracic vertebrae

        2. Insertion: superior fibers—lateral clavicle; middle fibers—acromion and spine of the scapula; inferior fibers—base of the spine of the scapula

3. Action: superior fibers—extension of the head and neck and upward rotation, retraction, and elevation of the scapula; middle fibers—retraction of the scapula; inferior fibers—upward rotation, retraction, and depression of the scapula (movements of the scapula are described on p. 304)

4. Innervation: accessory nerve; descends on the deep surface of the trapezius with the superficial branches of the transverse cervical vessels

C. Latissimus dorsi

1. Origin: spinous processes of the inferior six thoracic vertebrae, spinous processes of the lumbar vertebrae (via the posterior layer of the thoracolumbar fascia), and the iliac crest

2. Insertion: intertubercular sulcus of the humerus

3. Action: adduction, medial rotation, and extension of the shoulder (movements of the shoulder are described on p. 315)

4. Innervation: thoracodorsal (middle subscapular) nerve

D. Levator scapulae

1. Origin: transverse processes of the atlas and axis and the posterior tubercles of the transverse processes of C3 and C4

2. Insertion: medial border of the scapula, superior to the base of the spine

3. Action: downward rotation, retraction, and elevation of the scapula

4. Innervation: ventral rami of spinal nerves C3 and C4, and a branch from the dorsal scapular nerve

E. Rhomboideus minor

1. Origin: inferior part of the ligamentum nuchae and the spinous process of T1

2. Insertion: medial border of the scapula, at the base of the spine

3. Action: downward rotation, retraction, and elevation of the scapula

4. Innervation: dorsal scapular nerve

5. May be fused with rhomboideus major

F. Rhomboideus major

   1. Origin: spinous processes of T2 to T5

   2. Insertion: medial border of the scapula, inferior to the base of the spine

   3. Action: downward rotation, retraction, and elevation of the scapula

   4. Innervation: dorsal scapular nerve; the thin dorsal scapular nerve descends on the deep surfaces of the levator scapulae, rhomboideus minor, and rhomboideus major near the medial border of the scapula, accompanied by the deep branches of the transverse cervical vessels

   5. Clinical note: the medial border of rhomboideus major, the superior border of latissimus dorsi, and the inferior border of trapezius form the triangle of auscultation; heart and lung sounds can be heard more clearly through this thinner region of the thoracic wall

III. Intermediate Back Muscles

   A. Assist in inspiration

   B. Serratus posterior superior

      1. Origin: inferior part of the ligamentum nuchae and the spinous processes of T1 and T2

      2. Insertion: ribs two to five

      3. Action: elevation of ribs two to five

      4. Innervation: ventral rami of spinal nerves T2 to T5

   C. Serratus posterior inferior

      1. Origin: spinous processes of T11 to L2

      2. Insertion: ribs nine to twelve

      3. Action: fixation of ribs nine to twelve during contraction of the diaphragm

      4. Innervation: ventral rami of spinal nerves T9 to T12

IV. Deep Back Muscles

   A. Involved in movements of the vertebral column, head, and neck

B. From superficial to deep, they are the splenius, erector spinae, and trans-versospinalis muscles; the distinctive orientation of their muscle fibers is noted below

  1. Splenius muscles: fibers originate along the posterior midline and as-cend laterally to their insertion

  2. Erector spinae muscles: fibers course vertically from their origin to insertion

  3. Transversospinalis muscles: fibers originate from transverse processes and ascend medially to spinous processes

C. Splenius muscles

  1. Splenius capitis

    a. Origin: inferior half of the ligamentum nuchae and the spinous pro-cesses of T1 to T3

    b. Insertion: lateral part of the superior nuchal line and mastoid process

  2. Splenius cervicis

    a. Origin: spinous processes of T4 to T6

    b. Insertion: transverse processes of C1 to C3

  3. Action: extension and lateral flexion of the head and neck; rotation of the head and neck to the same side

D. Erector spinae

  1. Origin: iliac crest, sacrum, spinous processes of lumbar vertebrae, and spinous processes of the inferior six thoracic vertebrae

  2. Insertion

    a. As the erector spinae ascends, it splits into three muscle columns; from lateral to medial, they are the iliocostalis, longissimus, and spinalis muscles, which insert as noted below

    b. Iliocostalis: angles of the ribs

    c. Longissimus: transverse processes of thoracic and cervical vertebrae; longissimus capitis inserts on the mastoid process

    d. Spinalis: spinous processes of T1 to T6

3. Action: extension and lateral flexion of the vertebral column; longissimus capitis extends the head and neck and rotates the head and neck to the same side

E. Transversospinalis

   1. Origin: transverse processes

   2. Insertion: spinous processes

   3. Three component muscles span the length of the vertebral column, each varying in fiber length, with the longest muscle lying most superficially; from superficial to deep, the component muscles are the semispinalis, multifidus, and rotatores

      a. Semispinalis

         1. Fibers span six vertebrae

         2. Exception: semispinalis capitis

            a. Origin: transverse processes of C7 to T7

            b. Insertion: between the superior and inferior nuchal lines

            c. Action: extension of the head and neck

      b. Multifidus: fibers span four vertebrae

      c. Rotatores: fibers span two or three vertebrae

   4. Action: extension of the vertebral column; rotation of the vertebral column to the opposite side

F. Innervation: dorsal rami of spinal nerves

G. Interspinales and intertransversarii: small muscles between adjacent spinous processes and adjacent transverse processes, respectively

V. Suboccipital Muscles

A. Involved in movements of the head; located deep to semispinalis capitis

B. Obliquus capitis inferior

   1. Origin: spinous process of the axis

2. Insertion: transverse process of the atlas

3. Action: rotation of the head to the same side

C. Obliquus capitis superior

1. Origin: transverse process of the atlas

2. Insertion: between the superior and inferior nuchal lines, deep to semi-spinalis capitis

3. Action: extension and lateral flexion of the head

D. Rectus capitis posterior major

1. Origin: spinous process of the axis

2. Insertion: lateral part of the inferior nuchal line

3. Action: extension of the head and rotation of the head to the same side

E. Rectus capitis posterior minor

1. Origin: posterior tubercle of the atlas

2. Insertion: medial part of the inferior nuchal line

3. Action: extension of the head

F. Innervation: suboccipital nerve (dorsal ramus of the first cervical spinal nerve)

G. Suboccipital triangle

1. Boundaries

a. Medial: rectus capitis posterior major

b. Lateral: obliquus capitis superior

c. Inferior: obliquus capitis inferior

2. Contents

a. Vertebral artery

   1. Ascends through the transverse foramina of the upper six cervical vertebrae; courses medially in the sulcus for the vertebral artery

(on the posterior arch of the atlas), deep within the suboccipital triangle

      2. Penetrates the posterior atlanto-occipital membrane and enters the skull through foramen magnum; gives rise to branches that supply the brain and spinal cord

   b. Suboccipital nerve: pierces the posterior atlanto-occipital membrane and emerges into the suboccipital triangle between the vertebral artery and posterior arch of the atlas; innervates the suboccipital muscles

3. Greater occipital nerve (dorsal ramus of the second cervical spinal nerve): emerges along the inferior border of obliquus capitis inferior, ascends superficial to the suboccipital triangle, and pierces the semispinalis capitis; emerges through the trapezius inferolateral to the external occipital protuberance and ascends on the back of the head with the occipital artery to provide sensory innervation to the scalp

The Meninges and Spinal Cord

I. Meninges

   A. The spinal cord is enclosed within three meningeal sheaths; from superficial to deep, they are the dura mater, arachnoid, and pia mater

   B. Dura mater

      1. Tube of dense connective tissue; superiorly, it is continuous with the cranial dura mater at the foramen magnum and, inferiorly, it is closed, ending blindly at vertebra S2

      2. Epidural space

         a. Located between the dura mater and the wall of the vertebral canal; contains loose fatty connective tissue and the internal vertebral venous plexus

         b. Clinical note: the internal vertebral venous plexus drains the vertebral column and spinal cord, and anastomoses with intracranial dural venous sinuses through foramen magnum and with the external vertebral venous plexus through intervertebral foramina; the external vertebral venous plexus, in turn, anastomoses with veins of the thorax, abdomen, and pelvis—this system of interconnecting venous channels commonly serves as a conduit for the widespread dispersion of metastatic cancer

   C. Arachnoid

      1. Translucent connective tissue membrane deep to the dura mater; from its deep surface, delicate connective tissue strands traverse the subarachnoid space and merge with the pia mater covering the spinal cord

2. Subarachnoid space

    a. Space between the arachnoid and pia mater; filled with cerebrospinal fluid (CSF)

    b. Since the spinal cord ends at vertebra L1, and the arachnoid extends with the dura mater to vertebra S2, the subarachnoid space is expansive between vertebrae L1 and S2, and called the lumbar cistern

        1. The lumbar cistern contains the dorsal and ventral roots of spinal nerves which exit the vertebral canal below the end of the spinal cord; the appearance of these roots is likened to a horse's tail, and thus they are collectively known as the cauda equina

        2. Clinical note: a needle can be inserted between laminae of adjacent lower lumbar vertebrae and into the lumbar cistern without risk of injury to the spinal cord; this procedure is known as a lumbar puncture

D. Pia mater

    1. Microscopic, connective tissue layer intimately bound to the surface of the spinal cord

    2. Denticulate ligaments

        a. Two flattened bands of pia-derived connective tissue that extend laterally from each side of the spinal cord

        b. Along their lateral margins, 21 pointed projections extend laterally, penetrate the arachnoid between exiting spinal nerves, and secure the spinal cord to the dura mater

    3. From the inferior tip of the spinal cord, a tough, silvery-white, pia-derived thread, the filum terminale, descends through the lumbar cistern; it emerges from the tip of the dural sac and attaches to the coccyx

E. The dura mater and arachnoid extend laterally around exiting dorsal and ventral roots, forming a sleeve that becomes continuous with the connective tissue covering of the spinal nerve

II. Spinal Cord

A. Spinal nerves

    1. Thirty-one pairs: eight cervical, twelve thoracic, five lumbar, five sacral, and one coccygeal

2. Tiny dorsal and ventral rootlets arise along the length of a spinal cord segment and unite to form a dorsal and a ventral root of a spinal nerve; the dorsal root exhibits a swelling, the spinal (dorsal root) ganglion, which contains cell bodies of sensory neurons

3. A dorsal and a ventral root fuse within an intervertebral foramen to form a spinal nerve, which divides almost immediately into a dorsal and a ventral ramus (do not confuse a root with a ramus); dorsal rami supply the deep muscles of the back and the overlying skin, whereas ventral rami supply the muscles and skin of the neck, limbs, and trunk

4. Except for spinal nerve C8, which exits the intervertebral foramen below vertebra C7, cervical spinal nerves exit the vertebral canal above their respective vertebrae; in contrast, thoracic, lumbar, sacral, and coccygeal spinal nerves exit below their respective vertebrae

5. Intervertebral foramen

   a. The superior and inferior vertebral notches of pedicles of adjacent vertebrae form the inferior and superior borders of an intervertebral foramen, respectively

   b. An intervertebral foramen is bordered anteriorly by a vertebral body superiorly, and an intervertebral disc inferiorly; posteriorly, it is bounded by the inferior and superior articular processes of adjacent vertebrae and their associated facet joint

   c. Clinical notes

      1. Narrowing of an intervertebral foramen, perhaps as the result of a bony outgrowth or exostosis, may compress the exiting spinal nerve and produce pain

      2. A spinal nerve traverses the superior portion of an intervertebral foramen, in relation to the vertebral body and superior to the intervertebral disc; consequently, the spinal nerve exiting the intervertebral foramen at the level of the herniated disc is usually not compressed, however, the spinal nerve roots exiting the intervertebral foramen immediately below the herniated disc may be compressed

B. Regions

   1. Cervical enlargement: occurs at spinal cord levels C5 to T1 where there are massive numbers of neurons responsible for the innervation of the upper limbs

   2. Lumbar enlargement: occurs at spinal cord levels L2 to S4 where there are massive numbers of neurons responsible for the innervation of the lower limbs

3. Conus medullaris

    a. Tapered end of the spinal cord; lies at the level of vertebra L1 in the adult and at the level of vertebra L3 in the newborn

    b. The discrepancy between the position of a spinal cord segment and its corresponding vertebra results because a spinal cord segment is not as long as a vertebral segment; thus, the further the spinal cord is traced caudally, the greater the discrepancy

    c. Clinical note: a lesion of a particular vertebra may affect a different segment (or segments) of the spinal cord; for example, lumbar spinal cord segments are on a level with the bodies of vertebrae T11 and T12 and sacral spinal cord segments are on a level with the body of vertebra L1

C. Internal organization

    1. Neuron cell bodies are concentrated in a central, butterfly-shaped mass called the gray matter; the ventral and dorsal parts of the "wings" of the gray matter are called the ventral and dorsal horns, respectively

        a. Neuron cell bodies within a dorsal horn receive sensory impulses brought in by a dorsal root; a ventral horn contains motor neuron cell bodies whose axons exit the spinal cord in a ventral root and innervate skeletal muscle

        b. A lateral horn extends laterally between the dorsal and ventral horns at spinal cord levels T1 to L2 and S2 to S4; it contains cell bodies of preganglionic autonomic neurons whose axons exit the spinal cord in a ventral root and innervate smooth muscle, cardiac muscle, and glands

    2. Myelinated axons located peripheral to the gray matter form the white matter

D. Vessels

    1. The spinal cord is supplied by an anterior spinal artery and two posterior spinal arteries derived from the vertebral arteries within the skull; as they descend on the spinal cord, they are augmented by arteries that pass through the intervertebral foramina

    2. Corresponding veins drain into the internal vertebral venous plexus

part **II**

The

Thorax

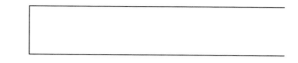

The Thoracic Wall

I. Bones and Bony Landmarks

    A. Thoracic vertebrae (twelve)

        1. Bodies: posterolaterally, they bear costal fovea for articulation with the heads of ribs

        2. Transverse processes: usually bear costal fovea for articulation with the tubercles of ribs

    B. Ribs

        1. Twelve pairs

            a. The costal cartilages of the upper seven rib pairs articulate with the sternum at synovial sternocostal joints

            b. The lower five rib pairs do not articulate with the sternum

                1. The eighth, ninth, and tenth rib pairs articulate anteriorly with the costal cartilages of the adjacent superior rib pair at synovial interchondral joints

                2. The short eleventh and twelfth rib pairs are called "floating" ribs because they do not articulate anteriorly

            c. Eleven intercostal spaces separate the ribs; they are numbered according to the bordering superior rib

2. Typical rib

    a. Head: posterior, expanded end; typically articulates at a synovial costovertebral joint with the body of the correspondingly numbered thoracic vertebra, the body of the adjacent superior vertebra, and their intervening intervertebral disc

    b. Neck: located between the head and tubercle

    c. Tubercle: posterior enlargement at the junction of the neck and body; forms a synovial costotransverse joint with the transverse process of the correspondingly numbered thoracic vertebra

    d. Body

        1. Extends from the tubercle to the anterior end of the rib; rounded along its superior border and thin along its inferior border, where it exhibits a recess, the costal groove, on its inner surface

        2. A short distance lateral to the tubercle, the body bends sharply anteriorly; this point is termed the angle of the rib

3. Atypical ribs

    a. First rib

        1. Broad, short, flat, and highly curved

        2. At about midshaft, its superior surface is marked by a slight projection, the tubercle for the scalenus anterior muscle; anterior and posterior to the tubercle are the grooves for the subclavian vein and subclavian artery, respectively

    b. Eleventh and twelfth rib pairs: they lack tubercles and, consequently, do not participate in costotransverse articulations

4. Costal arch: anteroinferior concavity of the thorax formed by the costal margins of each side; bordered by the costal cartilages of rib pairs seven through ten

C. Sternum

    1. A tripartite, sword-shaped bone in the midline of the anterior thoracic wall; its three parts are noted below

    2. Manubrium

        a. Wide, superior, handlelike part; the jugular (suprasternal) notch is its superior concave margin

b. On each side of the jugular notch, clavicular notches receive the sternal ends of the clavicles to form synovial sternoclavicular joints; inferior to the clavicular notches are costal notches that receive the costal cartilages of the first rib pair

c. The symphysial manubriosternal joint between the manubrium and body forms a forward-projecting, palpable ridge, the sternal angle; it is on a level with the sternocostal joints of the second rib pair (and the fourth thoracic vertebra posteriorly)

3. Body

a. Middle part of the sternum composed of four fused segments called sternebrae; lateral margins have costal notches for sternocostal joints

b. Clinical note: the body of the sternum is a common site for obtaining bone marrow by needle biopsy

4. Xiphoid process: inferior, pointed process of the sternum; the symphysial xiphisternal joint between the body and xiphoid process is on a level with the sternocostal joints of the seventh rib pair (and the tenth thoracic vertebra posteriorly)

D. Thoracic apertures

1. Superior thoracic aperture: opening bounded by the manubrium, the first rib pair, and the first thoracic vertebra

2. Inferior thoracic aperture: opening bounded by the costal arch, rib pairs eleven and twelve, and the twelfth thoracic vertebra

II. Pectoral Region

A. Superficial fascia

1. Superiorly, it contains the inferior part of a thin, sheetlike muscle in the neck, the platysma

2. Cutaneous nerves

a. Intercostal nerves: lateral and anterior cutaneous branches of the upper six intercostal nerves (ventral rami of spinal nerves T1 to T6) supply the pectoral region; the lateral cutaneous branch of the second intercostal nerve may also supply the skin of the upper medial arm and is then called the intercostobrachial nerve

b. Supraclavicular nerves: derived from ventral rami of spinal nerves C3 and C4; descend deep to the platysma to supplement the innervation to the superior part of the pectoral region

3. Cephalic vein: ascends along the anterolateral aspect of the arm; passes through the deltopectoral triangle between the deltoid, pectoralis major, and clavicle, and then courses deep to pectoralis major to drain into the axillary vein

4. Breast

  a. Glandular tissue

    1. Embedded in the fat and connective tissue of the superficial fascia of the pectoral region

    2. Extends from the second to the sixth rib and from the sternum to the midaxillary line; a portion of the glandular tissue extends toward the armpit or axilla and is called the axillary tail

    3. Composed of about 15 lobes; each lobe drains into an expanded lactiferous sinus whose associated lactiferous duct opens on the nipple

    4. Clinical note: after menopause, the glandular tissue decreases or disappears and is replaced by fat and connective tissue

  b. The superficial fascia of the breast has a deep membranous layer

    1. Between the deep membranous layer of the superficial fascia and the deep fascia covering the pectoralis major lies a retromammary space filled with loose connective tissue; this loose connective tissue provides for significant mobility of the breast on the anterior thoracic wall

    2. Clinical note: loss of mobility or fixation of the breast may result following extension of carcinoma of the breast into the retromammary space and underlying muscles

  c. Suspensory ligaments (of Cooper)

    1. Supportive connective tissue bands within the superficial fascia; they extend from the membranous layer of the superficial fascia to the skin of the breast

    2. Clinical note: carcinoma of the breast may produce fibrosis and shortening of the suspensory ligaments; this, in turn, may pro-

duce a characteristic orange-peel dimpling of the skin of the breast

   d. Nipple: cylindrical projection at the level of the fourth intercostal space in the male and more inferiorly in the female; the areola is the pigmented skin surrounding the nipple

   e. Vessels

      1. Perforating branches of the internal thoracic artery, anterior and posterior intercostal arteries, and the lateral thoracic artery supply the breast; veins accompany their corresponding arteries

      2. Most lymphatic drainage is to lymph nodes within the axilla; some lymphatics follow the perforating branches of the internal thoracic artery and drain to parasternal nodes along the internal thoracic artery (some lymphatics may cross the midline)

      3. Clinical note: anastomoses between the posterior intercostal veins and vertebral venous plexuses provide a route for metastasis of carcinoma of the breast to the vertebrae, spinal cord, and brain; carcinoma of the breast also metastasizes by way of lymphatics

B. Deep fascia

  1. Envelops the muscles of the pectoral region, covering their superficial and deep surfaces

  2. Clavipectoral fascia

    a. Deep fascia ensheathing pectoralis minor

    b. Extends from the medial border of pectoralis minor to the clavicle, enclosing the subclavius muscle; pierced superiorly by the cephalic vein, lateral pectoral nerve, and thoracoacromial vessels

    c. Extends from the lateral border of pectoralis minor to the deep fascia forming the floor of the axilla; this portion of the clavipectoral fascia produces the hollow of the armpit when the arm is abducted and is sometimes called the suspensory ligament of the axilla

C. Muscles

  1. Pectoralis major

    a. Origin: medial clavicle, sternum, and the upper six costal cartilages

b. Insertion: crest of the greater tubercle of the humerus

c. Action: medial rotation, adduction, flexion (clavicular part), and extension (sternocostal part) of the shoulder (movements of the shoulder are described on p. 315)

d. Innervation: medial and lateral pectoral nerves

2. Pectoralis minor

a. Origin: third to fifth ribs, near their costochondral junctions

b. Insertion: coracoid process

c. Action: downward rotation, protraction, and depression of the scapula (movements of the scapula are described on p. 304)

d. Innervation: medial and lateral pectoral nerves

3. Subclavius

a. Origin: first rib, near its costochondral junction

b. Insertion: groove for the subclavius muscle on the inferior surface of the clavicle near midshaft

c. Action: helps prevent upward dislocation of the sternoclavicular joint

d. Innervation: nerve to the subclavius

e. Clinical note: the subclavius may protect the subjacent subclavian vessels and brachial plexus from the sharp, splintered ends of a fractured clavicle

4. Serratus anterior

a. Origin: upper nine ribs

b. Insertion: costal surface of the scapula, along the medial border

c. Action: upward rotation, protraction, and depression (lower fibers only) of the scapula

d. Innervation: long thoracic nerve

e. Clinical note: paralysis of serratus anterior, perhaps following injury to the long thoracic nerve while excising axillary lymph nodes during a mastectomy, is characterized by winging of the scapula, where the medial border stands away from the thoracic wall; also, in the absence of the upward rotation of the scapula provided by serratus anterior, the affected individual is unable to abduct the arm above the horizontal

D. Nerves

1. Lateral pectoral nerve: branches from the lateral cord of the brachial plexus, hence its name, notwithstanding its medial position on the thoracic wall relative to the medial pectoral nerve; sends a branch to pectoralis minor, pierces the clavipectoral fascia medial to pectoralis minor, and ends in pectoralis major

2. Medial pectoral nerve: branches from the medial cord of the brachial plexus, hence its name; supplies pectoralis minor as it pierces it and then ends in pectoralis major

3. Nerve to the subclavius: branches from the superior trunk of the brachial plexus; innervates subclavius

4. Long thoracic nerve: formed by contributions from ventral rami of spinal nerves C5, 6, and 7; descends on serratus anterior, innervating it

E. Vessels

1. Superior (supreme) thoracic artery: small branch from the proximal part of the axillary artery; supplies the superior part of the pectoral region

2. Thoracoacromial artery

   a. Arises from the axillary artery posterior to pectoralis minor; emerges through the clavipectoral fascia medial to pectoralis minor and, deep to pectoralis major, gives rise to the four branches noted below

   b. Clavicular branch—courses medially, inferior to the clavicle; pectoral branch—descends on the deep surface of pectoralis major; deltoid branch—courses laterally and emerges from the deltopectoral triangle; acromial branch—courses toward the acromion, deep to the deltoid

3. Lateral thoracic artery: arises from the axillary artery posterior to pectoralis minor, distal to the origin of the thoracoacromial artery; descends on the lateral thoracic wall near the lateral border of pectoralis minor

4. Veins: course with their respective arteries and drain into the axillary vein

III. Intercostal Spaces

    A. Muscles

        1. Each intercostal space contains, from superficial to deep, an external intercostal, internal intercostal, and innermost intercostal muscle

        2. External intercostal muscle

            a. Extends from the tubercles of adjacent ribs to their costochondral junctions; an external intercostal membrane continues from the anterior end of the muscle to the sternum

            b. On the posterior thoracic wall their fibers run inferiorly and laterally; on the anterior thoracic wall their fibers run inferiorly and medially

        3. Internal intercostal muscle

            a. Extends from the angles of adjacent ribs to the sternum; anteriorly, lateral to the sternum, it is visible through the external intercostal membrane and, posteriorly, an internal intercostal membrane extends from the angles of adjacent ribs to the vertebral column

            b. Fibers run perpendicular to those of the external intercostal muscle

        4. Innermost intercostal muscle

            a. Occupies about the middle third of an intercostal space

            b. Its fibers run in the same direction as those of the internal intercostal muscle and are distinguished from them by an intervening neurovascular plane containing the intercostal nerve and vessels

            c. The innermost intercostal, subcostal, and transversus thoracis muscles comprise the deepest muscle layer of the thoracic wall

                1. The subcostal muscles span two intercostal spaces, attaching near the angles of the ribs; their fibers run in the same direction as the innermost and internal intercostals

                2. Transversus thoracis muscle fibers extend from the posteroinferior surface of the sternum to the costal cartilages of the second to sixth ribs

        5. Innervation: intercostal nerves

        6. Action: assist in respiration

B. Intercostal nerves (ventral rami of spinal nerves T1 to T11)

1. Course

    a. An intercostal nerve courses laterally from an intervertebral foramen and, near the angle of its respective rib, enters the neurovascular plane between the innermost and internal intercostal muscles; as it courses anteriorly within the costal groove, it gives off a lateral cutaneous branch about midway along the intercostal space

    b. The upper six intercostal nerves are confined to the thorax and terminate as anterior cutaneous branches that emerge from the upper six intercostal spaces lateral to the sternum

    c. Intercostal nerves seven to eleven leave their intercostal spaces and enter the anterior abdominal wall by descending deep to the costal arch; they are sometimes called thoracoabdominal nerves

2. Function: innervate external intercostal, internal intercostal, innermost intercostal, subcostal, and the transversus thoracis muscles; supply the skin of the thorax, except for the skin of the medial part of the posterior thorax, which is supplied by dorsal rami of spinal nerves

C. Vessels

1. Posterior intercostal arteries

    a. Those for the first two intercostal spaces arise from the supreme intercostal artery, a branch of the costocervical trunk, which is, in turn, a branch of the subclavian artery; the remaining nine posterior intercostal arteries arise from the thoracic aorta

    b. Course in the costal grooves with a posterior intercostal vein above and an intercostal nerve below; they anastomose anteriorly with anterior intercostal arteries

2. Anterior intercostal arteries

    a. Those for the upper six intercostal spaces course laterally from the internal thoracic artery; the internal thoracic artery is a branch of the subclavian artery which descends posterior to the costal cartilages and anterior to the transversus thoracis muscle, about one centimeter lateral to the sternum

    b. Near the sixth sternocostal joint the internal thoracic artery divides into the musculophrenic and superior epigastric arteries

1. The musculophrenic artery passes inferiorly and laterally, deep to the costal margin and superficial to the costal attachment of the diaphragm; it gives rise to the lower five anterior intercostal arteries

2. The superior epigastric artery descends vertically into the anterior abdominal wall, posterior to the rectus abdominis muscle

3. Perforating branches of the internal thoracic artery: emerge lateral to the sternum accompanied by perforating veins of the internal thoracic vein and anterior cutaneous branches of the upper six intercostal nerves

4. Posterior intercostal veins: right posterior intercostal veins drain mainly into the azygos vein, which empties into the superior vena cava; left posterior intercostal veins drain mainly into the hemiazygos and accessory hemiazygos veins, which drain into the azygos vein

5. Anterior intercostal veins: drain into the musculophrenic and internal thoracic veins; the musculophrenic vein drains into the internal thoracic vein and the internal thoracic vein drains into the brachiocephalic vein

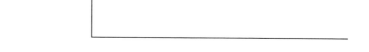

The Lungs

I. Pleural Cavity

   A. A slitlike, closed space surrounding each lung and lined by a serous membrane called the pleura; contains a small amount of serous fluid that lubricates the apposed moving surfaces of the visceral and parietal pleurae

   B. Visceral pleura: lines the inner wall of the pleural cavity; covers the lobes and root of the lung (a bilayered sheet of pleura called the pulmonary ligament drapes from the root of the lung)

   C. Parietal pleura

      1. Lines the outer wall of the pleural cavity; it is divided into the four parts noted below

      2. Diaphragmatic pleura: covers the superior surface of the diaphragm

      3. Mediastinal pleura: covers structures within the mediastinum, the region between the two pleural cavities; it is continuous with the visceral pleura that covers the root of the lung

      4. Costal pleura: covers the inner surface of the thoracic wall; it is attached to the thoracic wall by endothoracic fascia, the deep fascia covering the inner surfaces of the deepest muscle layer of the thoracic wall

      5. Cervical pleura (cupola): rounded, apical portion that projects into the neck, superior to the first rib; the endothoracic fascia associated with the cervical pleura is called the suprapleural membrane (Sibson's fascia), a thickened, tentlike structure which extends from the transverse process of the seventh cervical vertebra to the inner border of the first rib

D. Pleural recesses

    1. Regions within the pleural cavities where parietal pleura doubles back and contacts itself; the lungs expand into the pleural recesses only during maximal inspiration

    2. Costodiaphragmatic recess: deep gutter where the costal pleura reflects onto the superior surface of the diaphragm to become diaphragmatic pleura

    3. Sternocostal (costomediastinal) recess: located behind the sternum where costal pleura doubles back to become mediastinal pleura; sometimes it is described only on the left side

E. Innervation and blood supply: the cervical and costal pleurae and the outer portion of the diaphragmatic pleura are supplied by intercostal nerves and vessels; the inner portion of the diaphragmatic pleura and the mediastinal pleura are supplied by the phrenic nerve and its accompanying pericardiacophrenic vessels, which are branches of the internal thoracic vessels (the visceral pleura is supplied by the pulmonary and bronchial vessels; it has no nerve supply)

F. Respiration

    1. Inspiration

        a. An increase in thoracic wall dimensions during inspiration generates a negative pressure within the pleural cavity, which brings about expansion of the elastic lung

        b. Approximately two-thirds of the increase in thoracic wall dimensions is due to contraction and descent of the diaphragm; the remaining increase is produced by movements of the ribs

    2. Expiration: brought about by relaxation of the diaphragm and passive contraction of the thoracic wall and lung; in forced expiration, such as in sneezing, the muscles of the abdominal wall contract forcibly and push the abdominal viscera and diaphragm superiorly

G. Clinical notes

    1. Pneumothorax: condition in which a negative pressure cannot be generated within the pleural cavity because outside air enters the pleural cavity through a defect in the parietal or visceral pleurae; may result from a penetrating wound of the thoracic wall or rupture of an emphysematous bulla

2. Pleural tap: procedure involving the withdrawal of fluid from the pleural cavity; the needle should be inserted through an intercostal space along the superior border of a rib, where there is minimal risk of injury to the intercostal nerve and vessels

3. Pleurisy: inflammation of the pleura; since the parietal pleura is innervated by somatic nerves, that is, the intercostal and phrenic nerves, it is very sensitive to painful stimuli (the visceral pleura is insensitive to pain)

II. External Anatomy of the Lungs

   A. Surfaces

      1. Costal surface: convex surface contacting the inner surface of the thoracic wall

      2. Diaphragmatic surface: concave, inferior surface which contacts the diaphragm in deep inspiration

      3. Mediastinal surface

         a. Concave, medial surface contacting the mediastinum

         b. Hilum

            1. Central region on the mediastinal surface where structures within the root of the lung enter and exit the lung

            2. Within the hilum of both lungs, the pulmonary artery lies anteriorly and superiorly, and the pulmonary veins lie anteriorly and inferiorly

            3. Within the hilum of the left lung, the principal bronchus lies posteriorly; within the hilum of the right lung there are two bronchi, a superior lobar or eparterial bronchus which lies superior and posterior to the pulmonary artery, and an intermediate bronchus, which is located posteriorly in the hilum (the intermediate bronchus subsequently divides into the middle and inferior lobar bronchi)

            4. Bronchial vessels, autonomic nerves, and lymphatics also pass through the hilum

         c. Impressions

            1. The heart produces deep cardiac impressions anterior to the hilum of each lung, being especially pronounced on the left; posterior to the hilum, the right and left lungs are grooved by the esophagus and thoracic aorta, respectively

    2. Superior to the hilum, the right and left lungs are grooved by the azygos vein and aortic arch, respectively

B. Borders

    1. Inferior border: thin margin at the junction of the costal and diaphragmatic surfaces

    2. Anterior border

        a. Thin margin at the junction of the costal and mediastinal surfaces

        b. The anterior border of the superior lobe of the left lung has a deep indentation, the cardiac notch; the tonguelike portion of the superior lobe located between the cardiac notch and oblique fissure is called the lingula

C. Fissures

    1. Oblique fissures: commence posteriorly near the base of the spine of the scapula and intersect the inferior border of the lung near the costochondral junction of the sixth rib (posteriorly, the oblique fissures approximate the medial borders of the scapulae when the upper limbs are raised vertically above the head); in the left lung, the oblique fissure divides the superior from the inferior lobe and, in the right lung, the oblique fissure divides the superior and middle lobes from the inferior lobe

    2. Horizontal fissure: diverges from the oblique fissure of the right lung about halfway along the fourth intercostal space and intersects the anterior border of the lung at the level of the fourth rib; divides the superior lobe from the middle lobe

III. Trachea and Bronchi

A. Trachea

    1. Descends into the thorax anterior to the esophagus

    2. It is a patent tube supported anteriorly and laterally by a series of horseshoe-shaped, cartilaginous bars united by ligaments; posteriorly, the tracheal wall is completed by a musculofibrous membrane

3. Bifurcates into the right and left principal bronchi posterior to the ascending aorta, at about the level of the fifth thoracic vertebra; at its bifurcation, an internal ridge, the carina, deviates to the left

B. Principal (main, primary) bronchi

1. Right principal bronchus

   a. Wider than the left principal bronchus; diverges from the trachea at an angle of about 25 degrees

   b. The azygos vein arches from posterior to anterior above the right principal bronchus to enter the superior vena cava

2. Left principal bronchus: diverges from the trachea at an angle of about 45 degrees and passes through the aortic arch

3. Clinical note: because the right principal bronchus is wider and more vertical than the left principal bronchus, and because the carina deviates toward the left, inhaled foreign objects are more likely to lodge in the right versus the left lung

C. Lobar (secondary) bronchi

1. Aerate the lobes of the lungs

2. In the right lung, there is a superior, a middle, and an inferior lobar bronchus (the middle and inferior lobar bronchi arise from the intermediate bronchus); in the left lung, there is a superior and an inferior lobar bronchus

D. Segmental (tertiary) bronchi

1. Aerate portions of the lobes called bronchopulmonary segments; the names of the segmental bronchi of each lobar bronchus are listed below (bronchopulmonary segments are similarly named)

   a. Right superior lobar bronchus: apical, posterior, and anterior segmental bronchi

   b. Left superior lobar bronchus: apicoposterior (aerates the apical and posterior bronchopulmonary segments), anterior, superior lingular, and inferior lingular segmental bronchi

   c. Right middle lobar bronchus: medial and lateral segmental bronchi

   d. Right and left inferior lobar bronchi: superior, medial basal, lateral basal, anterior basal, and posterior basal segmental bronchi (there is often a shared anterior-medial basal segmental bronchus in the inferior lobe of the left lung that aerates the anterior basal and medial basal bronchopulmonary segments)

2. Clinical note: after a segmental bronchus and its associated vessels are secured and severed, a bronchopulmonary segment may be teased away from the surrounding lung tissue with minimal blood loss; this surgical procedure is called a segmental resection

IV. Vessels

A. Pulmonary arteries

1. Arise at the bifurcation of the pulmonary trunk within the concavity of the aortic arch

2. Right pulmonary artery: courses laterally through the aortic arch; passes posterior to the superior vena cava and anterior to the intermediate bronchus before entering the hilum

3. Left pulmonary artery: attached at its origin to the underside of the aortic arch by a fibrous cord, the ligamentum arteriosum; courses anterior to the left principal bronchus before entering the hilum

4. Pulmonary artery branches accompany the bronchi and are termed intrasegmental

B. Pulmonary veins

1. The right superior pulmonary vein drains the right superior and middle lobes, and the left superior pulmonary vein drains the left superior lobe; the right and left inferior pulmonary veins drain their respective inferior lobes

2. Within the lungs, the tributaries of pulmonary veins are described as intersegmental because they course between the bronchi and at the periphery of a bronchopulmonary segment; however, as they approach the hilum, they course more closely with their respective bronchi

C. Bronchial vessels: one or more bronchial arteries from the thoracic aorta enter the hilum of each lung to supply the bronchi and bronchioles; bronchial veins from the left and right lungs drain into the accessory hemiazygos and azygos veins, respectively

D. Lymphatics

    1. Pulmonary lymph nodes are located within the substance of the lung, bronchopulmonary nodes lie near the hilum, tracheobronchial nodes occur inferior to the tracheal bifurcation, and paratracheal nodes ascend along the sides of the trachea

    2. Paratracheal lymphatics join parasternal lymphatics to form a bronchomediastinal trunk, which joins the thoracic duct on the left side and the right lymphatic duct on the right side; lymphatic drainage of the lung is to the same side, except for the inferior lobe of the left lung, which drains to right paratracheal nodes

    3. Clinical notes

        a. Carbon particles inhaled by urban dwellers and smokers are taken up by the lymphatics and lymph nodes of the lung, thus, their lungs appear black instead of pink

        b. Carcinoma of the lung metastasizes by way of the lymphatics

V. Pulmonary Plexus

    A. Network of autonomic nerve fibers within the root of the lung, near the hilum; from the pulmonary plexus, nerve fibers course within the lung on bronchi, bronchioles, and blood vessels (see also The Autonomic Nervous System, p. 65)

    B. Fibers contributing to the pulmonary plexus

        1. Parasympathetic efferents: preganglionic vagal fibers pass through the pulmonary plexus to synapse on postganglionic parasympathetic cell bodies in the bronchial and bronchiolar walls; postganglionic parasympathetic fibers function in bronchoconstriction

        2. Sympathetic efferents: postganglionic sympathetic fibers derived from medial branches of the upper four thoracic sympathetic ganglia pass through the pulmonary plexus to supply bronchi, bronchioles, and blood vessels; they function in bronchodilation and vasodilation

        3. Parasympathetic afferents: leave the pulmonary plexus in the vagus nerves; fibers detect stretch and mediate pain, and are involved in the stretch reflex, which inhibits inspiration, and the cough reflex, respectively

        4. Sympathetic afferents: absent

The Middle Mediastinum

I. Mediastinum

   A. Median region between the mediastinal pleurae of the two pleural sacs; extends from the superior thoracic aperture to the diaphragm and from the sternum to the thoracic vertebral bodies

   B. Divisions

      1. Superior mediastinum: extends from the superior thoracic aperture to an imaginary transverse plane passing through the sternal angle anteriorly, and the lower border of the fourth thoracic vertebra posteriorly

      2. Inferior mediastinum

         a. Lies between the superior mediastinum and diaphragm; it is subdivided into the middle, anterior, and posterior mediastinum

         b. Middle mediastinum: occupied by the pericardial sac, heart, and roots of the great vessels, that is, the aorta, pulmonary trunk, superior vena cava, inferior vena cava, and the four pulmonary veins

         c. Anterior mediastinum: lies between the pericardial sac and sternum; contains the thymus, sternopericardial ligaments, parasternal lymph nodes, internal thoracic vessels, and the transversus thoracis muscle

         d. Posterior mediastinum: lies between the lower eight thoracic vertebral bodies and the pericardial sac superiorly, and the sloping, posterior portion of the diaphragm inferiorly; its contents include the esophagus, thoracic aorta, and thoracic duct

II. Pericardial Sac

   A. Encloses the pericardial cavity and surrounds the heart and roots of the great vessels; it is composed of a fibrous and serous pericardium

   B. Fibrous pericardium

      1. Tough, outer layer of the pericardial sac; limits distention of the pericardial cavity

      2. Inferiorly, it is fused to the diaphragm; anteriorly, it is attached to the sternum by connective tissue condensations termed the sternopericardial ligaments

   C. Serous pericardium

      1. Parietal layer: completely lines the inner aspect of the fibrous pericardium, except for a narrow strip between the entrances of the inferior vena cava, superior vena cava, and pulmonary veins; here, the parietal layer reflects onto the roots of the great vessels and becomes the visceral layer of the serous pericardium

      2. Visceral layer (epicardium, visceral pericardium)

         a. Serous membrane covering the roots of the great vessels, the myocardium, and the blood vessels on the surface of the heart; the loose connective tissue between the epicardium and myocardium may contain large amounts of fat

         b. Completely invests the surface of the heart, except for a narrow strip between the entrances of the inferior vena cava, superior vena cava, and pulmonary veins; here, the myocardium may contact the fibrous pericardium

   D. Pericardial cavity

      1. Potential space between the visceral and parietal layers of the serous pericardium; contains a small amount of serous fluid that lubricates the apposed moving surfaces of the serous pericardium

      2. Transverse pericardial sinus: passageway within the pericardial cavity between the ascending aorta and pulmonary trunk anteriorly, and the superior vena cava posteriorly; it is separated from the upper, blind end of the oblique pericardial sinus by two layers of serous pericardium between the superior vena cava and left superior pulmonary vein

      3. Oblique pericardial sinus: cul-de-sac posterior to the left atrium; bounded by the inverted L-shaped reflection of the parietal layer of the serous

pericardium to the visceral layer of the serous pericardium, where the inferior vena cava, superior vena cava, and pulmonary veins enter the heart

E. Innervation and blood supply: the fibrous pericardium and parietal layer of the serous pericardium are supplied by the phrenic nerves and pericardiacophrenic vessels; the visceral layer of the serous pericardium is supplied by sympathetic and vagal afferents, and the coronary arteries and cardiac veins

F. Clinical note: accumulation of blood or serous fluid within the pericardial sac results in a condition known as cardiac tamponade; since the fibrous pericardium is relatively rigid, this condition can compress the atria and prevent adequate filling

III. External Anatomy of the Heart

A. Hollow, muscular organ resembling a flattened cone whose rounded apex points anteriorly and to the left and whose base faces posteriorly

B. Surfaces

1. Posterior surface (base): formed by the left atrium and part of the right atrium

2. Diaphragmatic surface

a. Faces inferiorly, toward the diaphragm

b. Formed by the left ventricle and a narrow strip of the right ventricle with the posterior interventricular sulcus intervening; the inferior part of the coronary (atrioventricular) sulcus separates the posterior and diaphragmatic surfaces (except for its interruption by the ascending aorta, the coronary sulcus completely encircles the heart between the atria and ventricles)

3. Sternocostal surface

a. Faces anteriorly, superiorly, and to the left; formed centrally by the right ventricle with the right atrium and left ventricle on their respective sides

b. The right ventricle is separated from the right atrium by the coronary sulcus and from the left ventricle by the anterior interventricular sulcus (the anterior and posterior interventricular sulci indicate the position of the interventricular septum)

4. Clinical note: the clinical base of the heart is the region where the pulmonary trunk, aorta, and superior vena cava emerge from the heart; it lies deep to the part of the sternum immediately below the sternal angle and includes the adjacent portions of the second intercostal spaces—it is a frequent site for inspection and auscultation

C. Borders

1. The right border of the heart is formed by the right atrium; the left border is formed mainly by the left ventricle with the left auricle most superiorly

2. The inferior border of the heart is formed by the right ventricle and a narrow portion of the left ventricle near the apex

3. Clinical note: in radiology, mediastinal, rather than cardiac borders, are described; from superior to inferior, the right mediastinal border consists of the superior vena cava, right atrium, and inferior vena cava, and the left mediastinal border consists of the aortic arch (aortic knob, aortic knuckle), pulmonary trunk, left auricle, and left ventricle

IV. Coronary Arteries and Cardiac Veins

A. Coronary arteries

1. Right coronary artery

a. Arises from the ascending aorta within the sinus of the right aortic cusp, descends in the coronary sulcus between the right atrium and right ventricle, curves around the right border of the heart, and courses to the left in the coronary sulcus, between the posterior and diaphragmatic surfaces of the heart; its branches are noted below

b. Sinuatrial nodal artery: arises near the origin of the right coronary artery and encircles the superior vena cava posteriorly before emerging anteriorly to supply the sinuatrial node at the junction of the superior vena cava and right atrium; often arises from the circumflex artery

c. Marginal artery: arises from the right coronary artery before it curves around the right border of the heart; courses toward the apex, superior to the inferior border of the heart

d. Posterior interventricular artery (posterior descending artery, PDA): continuation of the right coronary artery after it leaves the coronary sulcus and descends toward the apex in the posterior interventricular sulcus; since the right coronary artery gives rise to the posterior interventricular artery in about 85 percent of individuals, it is often referred to as the "dominant" coronary artery (even though it supplies less myocardium than the left coronary artery)

   e. Clinical note: the sinuatrial node sets the heart rate and is thus called the pacemaker of the heart; stenosis of the sinuatrial nodal artery may result in ischemic injury to the sinuatrial node and cardiac arrythmia

2. Left coronary artery

   a. Arises from the ascending aorta within the sinus of the left aortic cusp; courses anteriorly between the pulmonary trunk and left auricle, and bifurcates into the anterior interventricular (left anterior descending, LAD) and circumflex arteries

   b. Anterior interventricular artery: descends toward the apex in the anterior interventricular sulcus

   c. Circumflex artery: curves around the left border of the heart in the coronary sulcus; it may be the source of the posterior interventricular artery, in which case the left coronary artery would be the "dominant" coronary artery

3. Clinical notes: coronary bypass surgery

   a. The coronary arteries are common sites of occlusive atherosclerosis

   b. Coronary bypass surgery involves the placement of a vascular graft (usually harvested from a great saphenous vein or internal thoracic artery) between the ascending aorta and a coronary artery, distal to the site of potentially life-threatening occlusive atherosclerosis

B. Cardiac veins

1. Great cardiac vein

   a. Ascends in the anterior interventricular sulcus adjacent to the anterior interventricular artery; when it reaches the coronary sulcus, it curves around the left border of the heart with the circumflex artery

   b. After being joined by the oblique vein of the left atrium inferior to the left pulmonary veins, it becomes the coronary sinus

2. Coronary sinus

   a. Courses to the right in the coronary sulcus and empties into the right atrium; its tributaries are noted below

     b. Middle cardiac vein: ascends in the posterior interventricular sulcus adjacent to the posterior interventricular artery; drains into the coronary sinus near its entry into the right atrium

     c. Small cardiac vein: courses with the marginal artery, and then curves around the right border of the heart with the right coronary artery; drains into the coronary sinus at its point of entry into the right atrium

   3. Anterior cardiac veins (two or three): ascend on the anterior wall of the right ventricle, span the coronary sulcus, and drain directly into the right atrium

   4. Thebesian or smallest cardiac veins: tiny veins within the myocardium that drain directly into the four chambers of the heart

V. Internal Anatomy of the Heart

  A. Right atrium

    1. Crista terminalis

      a. Lateral, vertical, muscular ridge; partially divides the right atrium into an anterior part, the atrium proper, and a posterior part, the sinus venarum

      b. Atrium proper: lined by pectinate muscles which extend transversely, like the teeth of a comb, from the crista terminalis; includes the auricle, an ear-shaped appendage projecting toward the left

      c. Sinus venarum: smooth-walled, posterior part; receives the superior vena cava superiorly, the inferior vena cava and coronary sinus inferiorly, and includes the interatrial septum

    2. Fossa ovalis: oval depression in the interatrial septum; its prominent superior and lateral borders form the limbus

    3. Ostium of the coronary sinus: situated between the orifice of the inferior vena cava and the right atrioventricular orifice

  B. Right ventricle

    1. Its lumen is crescentic in transverse section, since the higher pressure in the left ventricle pushes the interventricular septum to the right

    2. Trabeculae carneae

a. Consist of elevated myocardial ridges, bridges, and nipplelike papillary muscles

b. Papillary muscles: the anterior papillary muscle is large, the posterior papillary muscle is often bipartite, and the septal papillary muscles are small and multiple

c. Septomarginal trabecula (moderator band): bridge of myocardium between the interventricular septum and the base of the anterior papillary muscle

3. Chordae tendineae

a. Thin, dense connective tissue strands; arise from papillary muscles and attach to the free margins and ventricular surfaces of the cusps of the right atrioventricular valve

b. Contraction of the papillary muscles and the resultant tautness developed in the chordae tendineae prevents the cusps of the atrioventricular valve from being driven into the atrium when the ventricle contracts

4. Right atrioventricular orifice: guarded by the right atrioventricular or tricuspid valve

5. Right atrioventricular (tricuspid) valve: cusps are designated anterior, posterior, and septal; often the septal cusp is not well defined

6. Infundibulum or conus arteriosus: smooth-walled, outflow tract proximal to the pulmonary orifice

7. Pulmonary orifice

a. The most anterior of the four valvular orifices; contains the pulmonary semilunar valve whose three pouchlike cusps are designated anterior, left, and right

b. The pouchlike cavities of the cusps are called sinuses; near the middle of the lunulae, or free inner borders of the cusps, there is a fibrous thickening called the nodule

C. Left atrium: its anterior portion has pectinate muscles and includes the auricle; its posterior portion is smooth-walled and receives the four pulmonary veins (the left pulmonary veins often fuse before entering the left atrium)

D. Left ventricle

   1. The lumen of the left ventricle is circular in transverse section and roughened by trabeculae carneae; its wall is about three times as thick as that of the right ventricle

   2. Aortic vestibule: smooth-walled, outflow tract proximal to the aortic orifice

   3. Aortic orifice: contains the aortic semilunar valve, which is similar in structure to the pulmonary semilunar valve and has three cusps designated right, left, and posterior (noncoronary); it lies posterior and to the right of the pulmonary orifice

   4. Left atrioventricular orifice: located posterior and to the left of the aortic orifice, and to the left of the right atrioventricular orifice; it is guarded by the left atrioventricular (bicuspid, mitral) valve

   5. Left atrioventricular (bicuspid, mitral) valve: cusps are designated anterior and posterior; chordae tendineae arise from an anterior and a posterior papillary muscle and attach to the free margins and ventricular surfaces of the cusps

   6. Interventricular septum

     a. Muscular part: extensive, thick, inferior part

     b. Membranous part: thin, superior part; located just inferior to the attached margins of the right and noncoronary cusps of the aortic valve (it is about the size of the tip of the thumb)

     c. Clinical note: patency of the membranous part of the interventricular septum is a common congenital cardiac defect

E. Skeleton of the heart

   1. Components

     a. Anuli fibrosi: four thick, fibrous rings of dense connective tissue that encircle each valvular orifice and provide attachment and support for the valvular cusps

     b. Fibrous trigones: two triangular, connective tissue thickenings; the left fibrous trigone lies toward the left between the anuli fibrosi of the aortic and left atrioventricular orifices, and the right fibrous trigone lies between the anuli fibrosi of the aortic, right atrioventricular, and left atrioventricular orifices

2. Atrial cardiac muscle fibers take origin from the superior surface of the fibrous skeleton; ventricular cardiac muscle fibers take origin from its inferior surface

VI. Innervation and Conducting System of the Heart

A. Innervation

1. The superficial and deep cardiac plexuses are composed of networks of nerves and intermingled postganglionic parasympathetic cell bodies near the ligamentum arteriosum and tracheal bifurcation, respectively; from the cardiac plexuses, fibers are distributed to the vessels of the heart and elements of the conducting system (see also The Autonomic Nervous System, p. 65)

2. Fibers contributing to the cardiac plexuses

a. Parasympathetic efferents: preganglionic parasympathetic fibers from the vagus nerves synapse on postganglionic parasympathetic cell bodies within the cardiac plexuses or, after passing through the cardiac plexuses, on postganglionic parasympathetic cell bodies within the walls of the atria; postganglionic parasympathetic fibers function in vasoconstriction, slowing the heart rate, and reducing the force of contraction

b. Sympathetic efferents: postganglionic sympathetic fibers to the cardiac plexuses travel within superior, middle, and inferior cervical cardiac nerves (derived from medial branches of the superior, middle, and inferior cervical sympathetic ganglia, respectively) and within thoracic cardiac nerves (derived from medial branches of the upper four thoracic sympathetic ganglia); function in vasodilation and in increasing the heart rate and force of contraction

c. Parasympathetic afferents: pass through the cardiac plexuses to travel with the vagus nerves; function in the reflex control of the heart rate

d. Sympathetic afferents

1. Pass through the cardiac plexuses and travel within the cervical and thoracic cardiac nerves; they mediate pain

2. Clinical note: sympathetic afferent fibers concerned with cardiac pain caused by myocardial ischemia terminate in spinal cord segments T1 to T4; by a phenomenon known as referred pain, visceral pain from the heart is referred to the skin along the inner

border of the left upper limb and the upper part of the left pectoral region as angina pectoris, presumably because these areas of skin also send their afferent fibers into spinal cord segments T1 to T4 to synapse on the same neurons as incoming sympathetic afferent fibers (the brain preferentially interprets incoming pain as coming from the skin regardless of whether it originates from the viscera or skin)

B. Conducting system

    1. Sinuatrial (SA) node: a crescentic collection of specialized cardiac muscle fibers within the superior end of the crista terminalis, at the junction of the superior vena cava and right atrium

    2. Atrioventricular (AV) node: an oval collection of specialized cardiac muscle fibers in the inferior part of the interatrial septum, above the septal cusp of the tricuspid valve

    3. Atrioventricular (AV) bundle (bundle of His)

        a. Threadlike extension of the AV node that descends through the right fibrous trigone; upon entering the muscular part of the interventricular septum, it divides into a right and a left bundle branch

            1. Right bundle branch: passes from the interventricular septum to the base of the anterior papillary muscle of the right ventricle within the septomarginal trabecula; from here, branches are distributed to the right ventricular wall

            2. Left bundle branch: gives rise to multiple branches that pass to the left ventricular wall within a number of trabeculae carneae

        b. Initiates ventricular contraction near the apex of the heart, thus producing an efficient expulsion of blood toward the pulmonary and aortic outflow tracts

The Posterior and
Superior Mediastinum

I. Contents of the Posterior Mediastinum

   A. Esophagus

      1. Superiorly, it descends on the anterior surfaces of thoracic vertebral bodies to the right of the thoracic aorta, and posterior to the left atrium; inferiorly, it crosses in front of the thoracic aorta and enters the abdomen through the esophageal hiatus of the diaphragm, anterior and to the left of the thoracic aorta

      2. Esophageal plexus

         a. Nerve network formed by the vagus nerves; supplies the muscle and glands of the esophagus, and functions to increase peristaltic and secretory activity

         b. Just above the diaphragm the fibers of the esophageal plexus coalesce to form the anterior and posterior vagal trunks which lie on the corresponding surfaces of the esophagus; the anterior and posterior vagal trunks are derived from fibers of the left and right vagus nerves, respectively

      3. Vessels

         a. Supplied by the inferior thyroid arteries, esophageal branches of the thoracic aorta, and branches of the left gastric artery that ascend through the esophageal hiatus of the diaphragm; venous drainage is into the inferior thyroid, azygos, hemiazygos, accessory hemiazygos, and left gastric veins

b. Lymphatic drainage is to posterior mediastinal and celiac nodes, which, in turn, drain into paratracheal nodes and the cisterna chyli, respectively (the cisterna chyli is the inferior, dilated, abdominal portion of the thoracic duct)

4. Clinical note: enlargement of the left atrium may produce an indentation in the esophagus that may be visible on X-ray following a barium swallow

B. Thoracic (descending) aorta

1. Inferior continuation of the aortic arch at the lower border of the fourth thoracic vertebra; descends on thoracic vertebral bodies and, anterior to the twelfth thoracic vertebra, penetrates the aortic hiatus of the diaphragm to become the abdominal aorta

2. Branches

a. Gives rise to nine pairs of posterior intercostal arteries for the third to eleventh intercostal spaces and one pair of subcostal arteries, which course along the inferior borders of the twelfth ribs (the posterior intercostal arteries for the first and second intercostal spaces are derived from the supreme intercostal artery, a branch of the costo-cervical trunk)

b. A variable number of bronchial, esophageal, and tracheal arteries supply their respective structures; a pair of superior phrenic arteries supply the diaphragm just before the thoracic aorta passes through the aortic hiatus

C. Azygos venous system

1. Consists of two parallel, highly variable, longitudinal venous drainage systems on the anterior surfaces of the thoracic vertebral bodies; on the right is the azygos vein and on the left are the hemiazygos and accessory hemiazygos veins

2. Azygos vein

a. Formed inferiorly by the union of the right subcostal and right ascending lumbar veins; ascends posterior to the esophagus and, superiorly, arches forward over the right principal bronchus to empty into the superior vena cava

b. Receives the right posterior intercostal veins from the fifth to eleventh intercostal spaces; right posterior intercostal veins from the second to fourth intercostal spaces unite to form the right superior intercostal vein, which drains inferiorly into the azygos vein (the supreme intercostal vein drains the right first intercostal space and empties into the right brachiocephalic vein)

3. Hemiazygos and accessory hemiazygos veins

   a. Hemiazygos vein

      1. Formed inferiorly by the union of the left subcostal and left ascending lumbar veins; ascends posterior to the thoracic aorta and receives the left posterior intercostal veins from the eighth to eleventh intercostal spaces

      2. It crosses to the right, anterior to the body of the eighth thoracic vertebra, to empty into the azygos vein

   b. Accessory hemiazygos vein: descends posterior to the thoracic aorta and receives the left posterior intercostal veins of the fourth to seventh intercostal spaces; drains into the hemiazygos vein or crosses the vertebral column to drain into the azygos vein (the left superior intercostal vein receives the left posterior intercostal veins of the first to third intercostal spaces and ascends anterior to the aortic arch to drain into the left brachiocephalic vein)

D. Thoracic duct

   1. Thin-walled, pale channel; ascends between the thoracic aorta and azygos vein, anterior to the right posterior intercostal arteries and posterior to the esophagus

   2. In the superior mediastinum it lies to the left of the esophagus, and in the base of the neck it deviates to the left, anterior to the left vertebral artery and vein

   3. Empties into the angle of junction of the left subclavian and left internal jugular veins; near its termination, it receives the left jugular, left subclavian, and left bronchomediastinal trunks

E. Sympathetic trunks

   1. Superiorly, they lie posterior to the costal pleura against the necks of the ribs; inferiorly, they are located on the sides of the thoracic vertebral bodies (since the sympathetic trunks do not lie anterior to the thoracic vertebral bodies, they are not actually in the posterior mediastinum)

   2. Each sympathetic trunk has twelve thoracic ganglia (the first thoracic ganglion is frequently fused to the inferior cervical ganglion to form the

stellate or cervicothoracic ganglion); each ganglion lies inferior to its respective ventral ramus and is connected to it by a white and a gray ramus communicans

    a. White ramus communicans: the more lateral ramus; carries preganglionic sympathetic fibers from a ventral ramus into a sympathetic ganglion and sympathetic afferents from a sympathetic ganglion into a ventral ramus

    b. Gray ramus communicans: carries postganglionic sympathetic fibers from postganglionic cell bodies in a sympathetic ganglion into a ventral ramus

    c. The white and gray rami communicantes may be fused into a single ramus

3. Greater, lesser, and least splanchnic nerves

    a. The greater splanchnic nerve is formed by medial branches of the fifth to ninth thoracic sympathetic ganglia, the lesser splanchnic nerve is formed by medial branches of the tenth and eleventh thoracic sympathetic ganglia, and the least splanchnic nerve is derived from the medial branch of the twelfth thoracic sympathetic ganglion; they descend on the thoracic vertebral bodies medial to the sympathetic trunks

    b. The greater, lesser, and least splanchnic nerves are composed of preganglionic sympathetic fibers that have passed through their respective sympathetic ganglia without synapsing; they penetrate the diaphragm and synapse on postganglionic sympathetic cell bodies in the celiac, superior mesenteric, and aorticorenal ganglia within the abdomen

    c. They have no function in the thorax

II. Contents of the Superior Mediastinum

  A. Thymus

    1. Lies between the manubrium of the sternum and the aortic arch; usually extends superiorly into the neck and inferiorly into the anterior mediastinum

    2. Appears pink and bilobular in the infant; begins to involute around age 15 and is largely replaced by fat and connective tissue in the adult

3. Supplied by the internal thoracic arteries; a single thymic vein drains into the left brachiocephalic vein

B. Trachea and esophagus: descend through the superior thoracic aperture between the lungs; contacted on the right by the azygos vein and on the left by the aortic arch

C. Aortic arch

1. Commences near the second right sternocostal articulation and arches backward and to the left, reaching its summit about midway up the manubrium (the ascending aorta is the short segment that precedes the aortic arch and gives rise to the coronary arteries); its branches are noted below

2. The brachiocephalic trunk arises from the aortic arch just proximal to its summit; ascends on the right side of the trachea and, near the superior thoracic aperture, bifurcates into the right subclavian and right common carotid arteries

3. The left common carotid artery and then the left subclavian artery arise from the summit of the aortic arch; they ascend on the left side of the trachea with the common carotid artery lying anterior to the subclavian artery

D. Brachiocephalic veins

1. Formed on the sides of the superior thoracic aperture by the union of the internal jugular and subclavian veins; the left brachiocephalic vein crosses to the right along the summit of the aortic arch and unites with the right brachiocephalic vein near the right border of the manubrium to form the superior vena cava

2. The right brachiocephalic vein receives the right internal thoracic and supreme intercostal veins; the left brachiocephalic vein receives the left internal thoracic, left superior intercostal, and thymic veins

E. Superior vena cava: descends along the right border of the sternum; receives the azygos vein posteriorly and enters the right atrium at about the level of the third right sternocostal articulation

F. Vagus nerves

1. Superiorly, they descend anterior to their respective subclavian arteries; in their course, each vagus nerve gives rise to a recurrent laryngeal nerve

2. Right vagus nerve

    a. The right recurrent laryngeal nerve loops posteriorly under the right subclavian artery and ascends in the groove between the trachea and esophagus on the right side

    b. The right vagus nerve then descends on the right side of the trachea and then posterior to the root of the right lung where it breaks up into numerous branches that contribute to the esophageal plexus

3. Left vagus nerve

    a. As the left vagus nerve descends anterior to the aortic arch, the left recurrent laryngeal nerve loops posteriorly through the concavity of the aortic arch, on the left side of the ligamentum arteriosum; the left recurrent laryngeal nerve ascends in the groove between the trachea and esophagus on the left side

    b. The left vagus nerve then descends posterior to the root of the left lung where it breaks up into numerous branches that contribute to the esophageal plexus

G. Phrenic nerves

  1. Derived from ventral rami of spinal nerves C3, 4, and 5, especially C4

  2. The right phrenic nerve descends on the lateral surface of the superior vena cava; the left phrenic nerve descends anterior to the aortic arch

  3. Both phrenic nerves descend anterior to the roots of their respective lungs, between the fibrous pericardium and mediastinal pleurae; they are accompanied by the pericardiacophrenic vessels

  4. The right and left phrenic nerves enter the diaphragm near the inferior vena cava and apex of the heart, respectively; they innervate the skeletal muscle of the diaphragm and provide sensory innervation to the fibrous pericardium, parietal layer of the serous pericardium, mediastinal pleurae, and the inner portions of the diaphragmatic pleurae

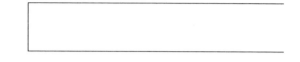

The Autonomic Nervous System

I. General Remarks

    A. Involuntary (visceral) motor system

        1. Innervates smooth muscle, cardiac muscle, and glands via two neurons designated preganglionic and postganglionic (in contrast, the voluntary or somatic motor system innervates skeletal muscle via one neuron)

        2. Preganglionic neuron cell bodies are located in nuclei, collections of neuron cell bodies within the central nervous system; postganglionic neuron cell bodies are located in ganglia, collections of neuron cell bodies outside the central nervous sytem

    B. Composed of a parasympathetic and sympathetic nervous system

        1. The parasympathetic nervous system regulates vegetative functions, such as digestion, and the sympathetic nervous system produces effects appropriate for a "fight or flight" response, such as an increase in heart rate

        2. Generally, the effects of the parasympathetic and sympathetic nervous systems are reciprocal; for example, the parasympathetic and sympathetic innervation to the eye produces pupillary constriction and pupillary dilation, respectively

II. Parasympathetic Nervous System

    A. Preganglionic neurons

        1. Cell bodies are located in nuclei within the brainstem and lateral horns

of spinal cord segments S2 to S4, thus, the parasympathetic nervous system is sometimes referred to as the craniosacral system

2. Preganglionic parasympathetic fibers from nuclei within the brainstem travel with the oculomotor, facial, glossopharyngeal, and vagus nerves; preganglionic fibers from nuclei within the lateral horns of spinal cord segments S2 to S4 form the pelvic splanchnic nerves

3. Preganglionic parasympathetic fibers associated with the oculomotor, facial, and glossopharyngeal nerves are described in Chapter V; preganglionic fibers that travel with the vagus and pelvic splanchnic nerves are described subsequently

B. Postganglionic neurons: cell bodies are located in ganglia near or within the wall of the organ to be innervated; postganglionic parasympathetic fibers terminate on smooth muscle, cardiac muscle, or gland cells to produce their effects

C. Vagus nerve

1. Preganglionic parasympathetic fibers that travel with the vagus nerve originate from the dorsal motor nucleus of the vagus in the brainstem; they branch from the vagus nerve as noted below

2. Cardiac branches leave the vagus nerve in the neck and thorax to synapse on postganglionic parasympathetic cell bodies within the cardiac plexuses or walls of the atria; postganglionic parasympathetic fibers terminate on the blood vessels and conducting system of the heart and function in vasoconstriction, slowing the heart rate, and reducing the force of contraction

3. Bronchial branches arise in the thorax, pass through the pulmonary plexus, and synapse on postganglionic parasympathetic cell bodies in the bronchial and bronchiolar walls; postganglionic parasympathetic fibers function in bronchoconstriction

4. Esophageal branches arise in the thorax and form a nerve network, the esophageal plexus, whose fibers synapse on postganglionic parasympathetic neurons within the wall of the esophagus; postganglionic parasympathetic fibers increase peristaltic and secretory activity

5. Above the diaphragm, fibers of the esophageal plexus coalesce into the anterior and posterior vagal trunks, which pass into the abdomen on the esophagus, through the celiac and superior mesenteric plexuses, and along branches of the celiac trunk and superior mesenteric artery to postganglionic parasympathetic cell bodies within the abdominal portion of the esophagus, stomach, duodenum, pancreas, liver, gall bladder, bile

ducts, jejunum, ileum, appendix, cecum, ascending colon, and the proximal half of the transverse colon; postganglionic parasympathetic fibers increase peristaltic and secretory activity

D. Pelvic splanchnic nerves

1. Formed by fibers of preganglionic parasympathetic cell bodies located in nuclei within the lateral horns of spinal cord segments S2 to S4; they exit the spinal cord in their respective ventral roots and spinal nerves, emerge from corresponding ventral rami, and are distributed to viscera within the abdomen and pelvis

2. Pelvic splanchnic nerve fibers which ascend out of the pelvis and into the abdomen pass through the inferior mesenteric plexus and are distributed along branches of the inferior mesenteric artery to postganglionic parasympathetic cell bodies within the walls of the distal half of the transverse colon, descending colon, sigmoid colon, rectum, and proximal half of the anal canal; postganglionic parasympathetic fibers increase peristaltic and secretory activity

3. Pelvic splanchnic nerve fibers which remain in the pelvis, pass forward through the inferior hypogastric plexus and are distributed along branches of the internal iliac artery to postganglionic parasympathetic cell bodies within perineal and pelvic organs; postganglionic parasympathetic fibers are responsible for the engorgement of erectile tissue with blood

III. Sympathetic Nervous System

A. Preganglionic neurons

1. Cell bodies are located in nuclei within the lateral horns of spinal cord segments T1 to L2, thus, the sympathetic nervous system is sometimes referred to as the thoracolumbar system

2. Preganglionic sympathetic fibers leave the spinal cord in their respective ventral root, spinal nerve, and ventral ramus and enter the associated sympathetic ganglion through a white ramus communicans; since preganglionic sympathetic fibers are only within ventral rami of spinal nerves T1 to L2, white rami communicantes are present only at these levels

3. Once in a sympathetic ganglion, a preganglionic sympathetic fiber may remain within that ganglion or ascend or descend in the sympathetic trunk to a ganglion at a higher or lower level; preganglionic sympathetic fibers that emerge from sympathetic ganglia without synapsing are noted below

a. Preganglionic sympathetic fibers that emerge as medial branches of sympathetic ganglia T5 to T9 unite to form the greater splanchnic nerve

b. Preganglionic sympathetic fibers that emerge as medial branches of sympathetic ganglia T10 and T11 unite to form the lesser splanchnic nerve

c. Preganglionic sympathetic fibers that emerge as the medial branch of sympathetic ganglion T12 constitute the least splanchnic nerve; although the greater, lesser, and least splanchnic nerves originate in the thorax, they descend into the abdomen to produce their effects

d. Preganglionic sympathetic fibers that emerge as medial branches of sympathetic ganglia L1 to L5 constitute the lumbar splanchnic nerves

e. Preganglionic sympathetic fibers that emerge as medial branches of sympathetic ganglia S1 to S5 constitute the sacral splanchnic nerves

B. Postganglionic neurons

1. Cell bodies are located in sympathetic ganglia along the sympathetic trunk as well as in collateral ganglia; the latter include the celiac, superior mesenteric, aorticorenal, and inferior mesenteric ganglia within the abdomen, and the inferior hypogastric plexus within the pelvis

2. Sympathetic ganglia

a. Postganglionic sympathetic cell bodies within a sympathetic ganglion give rise to postganglionic sympathetic fibers that leave the sympathetic ganglion and join a ventral ramus via a gray ramus communicans; these fibers may remain within the ventral ramus or join its associated dorsal ramus and are distributed to blood vessels as well as to sweat glands and arrector pili muscles to produce sweating and goose flesh, respectively

b. Postganglionic sympathetic cell bodies within the superior, middle, and inferior cervical ganglia and sympathetic ganglia T1 to T4 also give rise to postganglionic sympathetic fibers that emerge as medial branches (although there are eight cervical spinal nerves, their respective sympathetic ganglia fuse to form only three cervical sympathetic ganglia)

   1. Postganglionic sympathetic fibers that leave the cervical sympathetic ganglia as medial branches form cervical cardiac nerves; they descend into the thorax and terminate on the blood vessels and conducting system of the heart and function in vasodilation and in increasing the heart rate and force of contraction

2. Some postganglionic sympathetic fibers that leave sympathetic ganglia T1 to T4 as medial branches form thoracic cardiac nerves which terminate on the blood vessels and conducting system of the heart and function in vasodilation and in increasing the heart rate and force of contraction; other postganglionic sympathetic fibers that leave sympathetic ganglia T1 to T4 as medial branches pass through the pulmonary plexus to supply bronchi, bronchioles, and blood vessels and function in bronchodilation and vasodilation

3. Collateral ganglia

   a. Celiac ganglia (two)

      1. Located within the celiac plexus, a network of nerves surrounding the origin of the celiac trunk from the abdominal aorta; they receive preganglionic sympathetic fibers from the greater splanchnic nerves, which are formed by medial branches of sympathetic ganglia T5 to T9 (recall that the medial branches of cervical sympathetic ganglia and sympathetic ganglia T1 to T4 are composed of postganglionic sympathetic fibers)

      2. Postganglionic sympathetic fibers from the celiac ganglia are distributed to the abdominal portion of the esophagus, stomach, spleen, the proximal half of the duodenum, the neck, body, tail, and superior part of the head of the pancreas, liver, gall bladder, and bile ducts along branches of the celiac trunk and function to inhibit peristaltic and secretory activity

   b. Superior mesenteric ganglion

      1. Located within the superior mesenteric plexus, a network of nerves surrounding the origin of the superior mesenteric artery from the abdominal aorta; it receives preganglionic sympathetic fibers from the greater and lesser splanchnic nerves, which are formed by medial branches of sympathetic ganglia T5 to T9 and medial branches of sympathetic ganglia T10 and T11, respectively

      2. Postganglionic sympathetic fibers from the superior mesenteric ganglion are distributed to the distal half of the duodenum, the inferior part of the head of the pancreas, the jejunum, ileum, appendix, cecum, ascending colon, and the proximal half of the transverse colon along branches of the superior mesenteric artery and function to inhibit peristaltic and secretory activity

c. Aorticorenal ganglion

   1. Located within the renal plexus, a network of nerves surrounding the origin of a renal artery from the abdominal aorta; it receives preganglionic sympathetic fibers from the lesser and least splanchnic nerves, which are formed by medial branches of sympathetic ganglia T10 and T11 and the medial branch of sympathetic ganglion T12, respectively

   2. Postganglionic sympathetic fibers from the aorticorenal ganglion are distributed to the renal artery and its branches and function in vasoconstriction

d. Inferior mesenteric ganglion

   1. Located within the inferior mesenteric plexus, a network of nerves surrounding the origin of the inferior mesenteric artery from the abdominal aorta; it receives some preganglionic sympathetic fibers from the greater, lesser, and least splanchnic nerves via the intermesenteric plexus, but most are from the lumbar splanchnic nerves, which represent the medial branches of sympathetic ganglia L1 to L5

   2. Postganglionic sympathetic fibers from the inferior mesenteric ganglion are distributed to the distal half of the transverse colon, descending colon, sigmoid colon, rectum, and the proximal half of the anal canal along branches of the inferior mesenteric artery and function to inhibit peristaltic and secretory activity

e. Inferior hypogastric plexuses

   1. Nerve networks containing clusters of postganglionic sympathetic cell bodies; located in the pelvis within the extraperitoneal connective tissue on either side of the rectum

   2. They receive some preganglionic sympathetic fibers from the greater, lesser, and least splanchnic nerves via the superior hypogastric plexus and hypogastric nerves, but most are from the sacral splanchnic nerves, which represent the medial branches of sympathetic ganglia S1 to S5; postganglionic sympathetic fibers from the inferior hypogastric plexuses are distributed to perineal and pelvic organs along branches of the internal iliac arteries and, in the male, are responsible for the smooth muscle contractions that expel semen during ejaculation

4. Blood vessels are supplied by postganglionic sympathetic fibers derived from all sympathetic and collateral ganglia; they function in both vaso-

constriction and vasodilation, for example, in a "fight or flight" response, blood vessels to the gut will be constricted, whereas blood vessels to skeletal muscle will be dilated (blood vessels, like sweat glands and arrector pili muscles, do not receive a parasympathetic innervation)

IV. Autonomic Afferents

A. Although the autonomic nervous system is generally regarded as a motor system, smooth muscle, cardiac muscle, and glands also have an afferent or sensory supply; afferent fibers travel with their respective parasympathetic and sympathetic efferents and, like their somatic afferent counterparts, have their cell bodies in spinal and cranial ganglia

B. Parasympathetic afferents

1. Vagal afferents from the lung detect stretch and mediate pain, and are involved in the stretch reflex, which inhibits inspiration, and the cough reflex, respectively; vagal afferents from the heart function in the reflex control of the heart rate and vagal afferents from the abdomen mediate the feeling of nausea and function in gastrointestinal reflexes

2. Pelvic splanchnic afferents associated with the gut mediate the feeling of nausea and function in gastrointestinal reflexes

C. Sympathetic afferents

1. Although sympathetic afferents enter sympathetic ganglia at all levels via cervical and thoracic cardiac nerves, and the greater, lesser, least, lumbar, and sacral splanchnic nerves, they only enter ventral rami of spinal nerves T1 to L2 via white rami communicantes (after descending or ascending in the sympathetic trunk, if needed); they function in the mediation of pain

2. Sympathetic afferents are absent in the lungs; sympathetic afferents from the heart travel with the cervical and thoracic cardiac nerves, sympathetic afferents from the abdomen travel with the greater, lesser, least, and lumbar splanchnic nerves, and sympathetic afferents from the pelvis travel with the sacral splanchnic nerves

part III

The
Abdomen

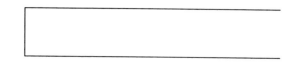

The Anterior Abdominal Wall

I. Fasciae

    A. Superficial fascia

        1. Camper's fascia: superficial, fatty layer

        2. Scarpa's fascia

            a. Deep, membranous layer; usually well developed in the lower part of the anterior abdominal wall

            b. Attaches to the deep fascia of the thigh a few centimeters inferior to the inguinal ligament

    B. Deep fascia

        1. Envelops the anterior abdominal wall muscles, covering their superficial and deep surfaces; a cleavage plane usually exists between Scarpa's fascia and the deep fascia

        2. Transversalis (endoabdominal) fascia: deep fascia covering the inner surface of the deepest muscle layer of the abdominal wall; it is the abdominal equivalent of the endothoracic fascia

II. Muscles

    A. External abdominal oblique

        1. Origin: external surfaces of the lower eight ribs; interdigitates superiorly with serratus anterior

2. Insertion: fibers run inferiorly and medially to insert on the iliac crest, anterior superior iliac spine and, through the aponeurosis of the external abdominal oblique, on the pubic tubercle, pubic crest, and into the linea alba, a midline connective tissue seam; it has a free posterior border

    a. The thick, posteriorly upturned, lower free border of the aponeurosis of the external abdominal oblique constitutes the inguinal ligament; it extends from the anterior superior iliac spine to the pubic tubercle

    b. A portion of the medial end of the inguinal ligament diverges posteriorly and attaches to the pecten pubis; it is termed the lacunar ligament

    c. The pectineal ligament is a strong fibrous band that continues posteriorly from the lacunar ligament along the pecten pubis

3. Clinical note: since no major nerves or vessels cross the midline of the anterior abdominal wall, the linea alba is frequently used as a site for surgical incisions

B. Internal abdominal oblique

1. Origin: thoracolumbar fascia, iliac crest, and the lateral two-thirds of the inguinal ligament

2. Insertion: most fibers run superiorly and medially to insert along the inferior borders of the last three ribs and, through the aponeurosis of the internal abdominal oblique, into the linea alba; inferior fibers course inferiorly and medially above and parallel to the inguinal ligament and, through the aponeurosis of the internal abdominal oblique, insert on the pecten pubis and pubic crest

C. Transversus abdominis

1. Origin: inner aspect of the costal margin, thoracolumbar fascia, and iliac crest

2. Insertion: fibers run transversely and, through the aponeurosis of the transversus abdominis, insert into the linea alba; inferiorly, its aponeurosis inserts on the pecten pubis and pubic crest, fusing with the insertion of the aponeurosis of the internal abdominal oblique to form the conjoint tendon or falx inguinalis

D. Rectus abdominis

1. Origin: pubic crest

2. Insertion: from its narrow origin it widens as it ascends to insert on the costal cartilages of the fifth, sixth, and seventh ribs, and the xiphoid process; tendinous intersections divide the muscle transversely

3. Rectus sheath

   a. Dense connective tissue envelope enclosing the rectus abdominis; composed of an anterior and posterior layer formed by the aponeuroses of the external abdominal oblique, internal abdominal oblique, and transversus abdominis muscles

   b. The aponeurosis of the external abdominal oblique contributes to the anterior layer of the rectus sheath, the aponeurosis of the internal abdominal oblique contributes to the anterior and posterior layers of the rectus sheath, and the aponeurosis of the transversus abdominis contributes to the posterior layer of the rectus sheath

   c. Inferior to the midpoint between the umbilicus and pubic symphysis, the aponeuroses of the internal abdominal oblique and transversus abdominis pass only to the anterior layer of the rectus sheath, thus, the posterior layer of the rectus sheath is absent inferiorly and the rectus abdominis is in direct contact with transversalis fascia; the inferior limit of the posterior layer of the rectus sheath is indicated by a curved border called the arcuate line

E. Action: support the abdominal contents and compress the abdominal contents as for maximal expiration and coughing; flexion and rotation of the vertebral column and stabilization of the thorax, vertebral column, and pelvis relative to one another, especially when performing forceful actions such as lifting heavy objects

F. Innervation: thoracoabdominal, subcostal, iliohypogastric, and ilioinguinal nerves

III. Nerves

A. Ventral rami of spinal nerves T7 to T11 continue from the thorax into the anterior abdominal wall and, thus, are sometimes referred to as thoracoabdominal nerves; other nerves of the anterior abdominal wall are the ventral ramus of spinal nerve T12 or the subcostal nerve and the iliohypogastric and ilioinguinal nerves which are derived from the ventral ramus of spinal nerve L1

   1. Nerves of the anterior abdominal wall course inferiorly and medially within the neurovascular plane between the internal abdominal oblique and transversus abdominis, providing motor innervation to the exter-

nal abdominal oblique, internal abdominal oblique, and transversus abdominis

2. Lateral cutaneous branches emerge near the origin of the external abdominal oblique; anteriorly, the nerves of the anterior abdominal wall pierce the rectus sheath, innervate the rectus abdominis, and emerge as anterior cutaneous branches (the ilioinguinal nerve traverses the inguinal canal and supplies the anterior scrotum/labium majus and upper medial thigh with cutaneous innervation)

B. Dermatomes

1. A dermatome is a circumscribed region of skin which receives most of its sensory innervation from one spinal cord segment; it is designated according to the spinal cord segment which provides most of its innervation (transsection of one spinal nerve will not produce complete anesthesia within a dermatome because of overlapping innervation by adjacent spinal nerves)

2. Some landmarks indicating dermatome levels on the anterior abdominal wall are: xiphoid process—dermatome T7; umbilicus—dermatome T10; dermatome L1 lies above the pubis

3. Clinical note: a knowledge of dermatomes is useful in cases of referred pain, for example, in appendicitis, pain may be felt over dermatome T10 near the umbilicus because sympathetic afferents that mediate pain from the appendix travel with the lesser splanchnic nerve, enter spinal cord segment T10, and are "referred" to the dermatome supplied by the same spinal cord segment

IV. Vessels

A. Arteries

1. Superior epigastric artery: branches from the internal thoracic artery and descends within the rectus sheath posterior to the rectus abdominis; here, it anastomoses with the inferior epigastric artery

2. Inferior epigastric artery: branches from the external iliac artery proximal to the inguinal ligament and courses superiorly and medially in the extraperitoneal connective tissue on the deep aspect of the lower anterior abdominal wall; penetrates the transversalis fascia to ascend anterior to the arcuate line and then within the rectus sheath posterior to the rectus abdominis

3. Deep circumflex iliac artery: branches from the external iliac artery adjacent to the origin of the inferior epigastric artery; courses laterally

in the extraperitoneal connective tissue posterior to the inguinal ligament, supplying the lower part of the anterior abdominal wall

4. Posterior intercostal arteries 7 to 11 and the subcostal artery: arise from the thoracic aorta and course inferiorly and medially within the neurovascular plane between the internal abdominal oblique and transversus abdominis; anteriorly, they pierce the rectus sheath to anastomose with the superior and inferior epigastric arteries

5. Clinical note: when the aortic arch is narrowed just beyond the origin of the left subclavian artery (coarctation of the aorta), sufficient arterial blood may still reach the lower part of the body through anastomoses between the ventrally placed internal thoracic, superior epigastric, and inferior epigastric arteries and the dorsally placed aorta, provided by the anterior intercostal, posterior intercostal, and subcostal arteries; the internal thoracic and epigastric arteries themselves constitute an anastomosis between the subclavian and external iliac arteries

B. Veins

1. Course with their corresponding arteries, except that posterior intercostal veins 7 to 11 and the subcostal vein drain into the azygos, hemiazygos, and accessory hemiazygos veins; within the rectus sheath the tributaries of the posterior intercostal and subcostal veins anastomose with those of the superior and inferior epigastric veins

2. Clinical notes

   a. As with the arteries, anastomoses of corresponding veins provide for a collateral circulation in cases of obstruction of the superior or inferior vena cava

   b. In obstruction of the superior vena cava, perhaps as the result of compression by a tumor, blood from the head, neck, and upper limbs can reach the right atrium via the inferior vena cava through anastomoses provided by the brachiocephalic, internal thoracic, superior epigastric, inferior epigastric, external iliac, and common iliac veins; blood would flow in the reverse direction in the same venous channels in an obstruction of the inferior vena cava (blood within valved veins can reverse direction if the veins become distended to such a degree that the valves are rendered incompetent)

3. Thoracoepigastric (superficial epigastric) vein

   a. Longitudinal vein in the superficial fascia of the lateral part of the thorax and abdomen; drains into the superior vena cava via the lateral thoracic, axillary, subclavian, and brachiocephalic veins and into the inferior vena cava via the great saphenous, femoral, external iliac, and common iliac veins

    b. Clinical notes

        1. The thoracoepigastric vein provides another important anastomotic link between the superior vena cava and the inferior vena cava in cases of obstruction of the superior or inferior vena cava

        2. Tributaries of the thoracoepigastric vein near the umbilicus anastomose with tributaries of the paraumbilical veins which course along the ligamentum teres hepatis (round ligament of the liver) and drain into the portal vein; in portal hypertension, blood flow through the portal vein may be impeded to the degree that there is a significant retrograde flow through the paraumbilical veins, which may result in visibly enlarged and tortuous paraumbilical and thoracoepigastric tributaries radiating from the umbilicus, a condition known as caput medusae

  C. Superficial lymphatics of the superior and inferior parts of the anterior abdominal wall drain into axillary and superficial inguinal nodes, respectively; lymphatics from abdominal wall muscles drain along the posterior intercostal, superior epigastric, and inferior epigastric arteries to posterior mediastinal, parasternal, and external iliac nodes, respectively

V. Inguinal Canal

  A. General remarks

    1. A 4-centimeter oblique passage through the fascial and muscular layers of the inferomedial anterior abdominal wall; connects the scrotum/labium majus to the retroperitoneal region and transmits the spermatic cord/round ligament of the uterus

    2. Lies above and parallel to the medial end of the inguinal ligament, extending from the superficial inguinal ring to the deep inguinal ring

  B. Superficial inguinal ring

    1. Triangular opening in the aponeurosis of the external abdominal oblique; its base is the pubic crest, the lateral crus (margin) is formed by the medial end of the inguinal ligament, and the medial crus (margin) is formed by the aponeurosis of the external abdominal oblique attaching on the pubic crest (intercrural fibers bind the two crura superiorly)

    2. A tube of deep fascia, the external spermatic fascia, extends from the borders of the superficial inguinal ring to ensheath the spermatic cord and testis

C. "Intermediate inguinal ring"

  1. The inferior fibers of the internal abdominal oblique arise from the lateral two-thirds of the inguinal ligament; as these fibers run medially and inferiorly, they lie in front of the deep inguinal ring

  2. About halfway along the inguinal canal, the internal abdominal oblique splits to allow the spermatic cord to pass through an "intermediate inguinal ring"; deep fascia, the cremasteric fascia, and muscle fibers, the cremaster muscle, extend from the margins of the "intermediate inguinal ring" to ensheath the spermatic cord and testis

D. Deep inguinal ring

  1. Represents the mouth of a tubular evagination of transversalis fascia that extends into the inguinal canal and scrotum; the evagination of transversalis fascia ensheaths the spermatic cord and testis, and is termed the internal spermatic fascia

  2. The deep inguinal ring is located about midway between the anterior superior iliac spine and pubic symphysis, about one centimeter superior to the inguinal ligament; lies just lateral to the inferior epigastric vessels and superficial to the parietal peritoneum and extraperitoneal connective tissue (the lower free border of the transversus abdominis arches above it)

E. Walls

  1. Floor: laterally, it is formed by the inguinal ligament, which is upturned posteriorly to form a gutter; medially, it is formed by the lacunar ligament

  2. Roof: formed by the external abdominal oblique at the superficial inguinal ring, the internal abdominal oblique at the "intermediate inguinal ring", and the transversus abdominis above the deep inguinal ring; superiorly, it opens into two cleavage planes, one between the external and internal abdominal obliques, and the other between the internal abdominal oblique and transversus abdominis

  3. Anterior wall: laterally, it is formed by the aponeurosis of the external abdominal oblique and the inferior muscle fibers of the internal abdominal oblique; medially, it is formed by the aponeurosis of the external abdominal oblique (when the transversus abdominis contracts, it descends and forms part of the anterior wall overlying the deep inguinal ring)

  4. Posterior wall: laterally, it is formed by the transversalis fascia between the inferior border of the transversus abdominis and the inguinal ligament; medially, it is formed by the conjoint tendon and transversalis fascia

F. Inguinal (Hesselbach's) triangle: bounded medially by the lower lateral border of the rectus abdominis, inferiorly by the medial part of the inguinal ligament, and laterally by the lower portion of the inferior epigastric vessels; its posterior wall is formed laterally by transversalis fascia, and medially by the conjoint tendon and transversalis fascia

G. Clinical notes: inguinal hernias

1. An inguinal hernia is a protrusion of a loop of intestine through a defect in the musculofascial walls of the inguinal canal; they are much more frequent in males, perhaps because the inguinal canal is wider

2. Direct inguinal hernia: a hernia in which a loop of intestine protrudes through the inguinal triangle (medial to the inferior epigastric vessels) and emerges through the superficial inguinal ring into the scrotum/labium majus

3. Indirect inguinal hernia

   a. Acquired: a hernia in which a loop of intestine protrudes through the deep inguinal ring (lateral to the inferior epigastric vessels), traverses the inguinal canal, and emerges through the superficial inguinal ring into the scrotum/labium majus

   b. Congenital: a hernia in which a loop of intestine protrudes through the deep inguinal ring, traverses the inguinal canal, and emerges through the superficial inguinal ring into the scrotum/labium majus within a persisting processus vaginalis that, in the male, is still continuous with the cavity of the tunica vaginalis surrounding the testis

VI. Peritoneal Folds on the Inner Surface of the Lower Anterior Abdominal Wall

A. Retroperitoneal structures extending superiorly from the region of the bladder produce folds in the parietal peritoneum

B. The median umbilical ligament, the remains of the embryonic urachus, extends from the apex of the bladder to the umbilicus and produces the median umbilical fold

C. The medial umbilical folds, one on each side of the median umbilical fold, are produced by the medial umbilical ligaments, fibrous remnants of the distal portions of the umbilical arteries; they extend from just lateral to the bladder to the umbilicus

D. The lateral umbilical folds, located lateral to the medial umbilical folds, are produced by the inferior epigastric vessels as they course superiorly and medially to enter the rectus sheath

The Scrotum, Spermatic Cord, and Testis

I. Scrotum

    A. Pouch derived from the skin and fascia of the inferomedial anterior abdominal wall and perineum; divided by a median septum with each half containing a spermatic cord and testis

    B. Superficial fascia

        1. Superficial layer: continuous with Camper's fascia, but it is devoid of fat; contains smooth muscle, the dartos muscle, that wrinkles the scrotal skin to reduce heat loss from the testis

        2. Deep layer (dartos fascia): membranous layer continuous with Scarpa's fascia; lies superficial to the external spermatic fascia and is separated from it by a cleavage plane

    C. Deep fascia: represented by the external spermatic, cremasteric, and internal spermatic fasciae, derivatives of the deep fascia associated with anterior abdominal wall musculature

II. Spermatic Cord

    A. Thick bundle that passes through the inguinal canal and connects the testis with the extraperitoneal region of the lower anterior abdominal wall; its component structures are noted below

    B. Fasciae

        1. External spermatic fascia: outermost fascial covering of the spermatic

cord and testis; it is continuous at the superficial inguinal ring with the deep fascia enveloping the external abdominal oblique

2. Cremasteric fascia

   a. Intermediate fascial covering of the spermatic cord and testis; it is continuous at the "intermediate inguinal ring" with the deep fascia enveloping the internal abdominal oblique

   b. Ensheaths the cremaster muscle which is derived from the internal abdominal oblique muscle

      1. The cremasteric muscle is composed of observable muscle bundles that loop down into the spermatic cord and are innervated by the genital branch of the genitofemoral nerve; the genital branch of the genitofemoral nerve passes into the deep inguinal ring and descends within the spermatic cord deep to the internal spermatic fascia (distal to the superficial inguinal ring, sensory branches of the genital branch of the genitofemoral nerve leave the spermatic cord to supply skin of the anterior scrotum and upper medial thigh)

      2. The cremaster muscle draws the testis toward the abdominal wall to reduce heat loss

      3. Clinical note: in the male, stroking of the upper medial thigh normally elicits the cremaster reflex evidenced by contraction of the cremaster muscle and elevation of the testis; the presence of this reflex confirms the integrity of spinal cord segments L1 and L2 since both the skin of the upper medial thigh and cremaster muscle are supplied by the genitofemoral nerve, which is derived from spinal cord segments L1 and L2

3. Internal spermatic fascia: innermost fascial covering of the spermatic cord and testis; it is continuous with the transversalis fascia at the deep inguinal ring

4. The transversus abdominis does not contribute to the fascial coverings of the spermatic cord because it lies above the deep inguinal ring and does not serve as a barrier to the descending testis

C. Ductus (vas) deferens

   1. Continuous with the epididymis; commences at the inferior pole of the testis and ascends in the posterior aspect of the spermatic cord, forming a hard palpable cord

2. Traverses the inguinal canal and, at the deep inguinal ring, bends sharply medially behind the inferior epigastric vessels to descend on the bladder

D. Vessels

1. Testicular artery: arises from the abdominal aorta and passes inferiorly in the extraperitoneal connective tissue to the deep inguinal ring; lies anteriorly in the spermatic cord and is surrounded by the pampiniform plexus of veins that drain the testis

2. Pampiniform plexus: consists of about a dozen veins which emerge from the back of the testis, anastomose with one another as they ascend around the testicular artery, and then coalesce to form the testicular vein after emerging into the abdomen through the deep inguinal ring; the close association of the testicular artery and pampiniform plexus allows for the transfer of heat from the blood in the testicular artery to the cooler blood within the pampiniform plexus, thus promoting spermatogenesis by keeping the testis below body temperature

3. Cremasteric artery: branch of the inferior epigastric artery; enters the deep inguinal ring and supplies the cremaster muscle

4. Artery of the ductus deferens: branch of a superior vesical artery; enters the deep inguinal ring on the ductus deferens and anastomoses with the cremasteric and testicular arteries within the spermatic cord

5. Lymphatics from the testis pass through the inguinal canal and along the testicular vessels to drain to lumbar nodes (lymphatics from the scrotum drain to superficial inguinal nodes)

6. Clinical note: the anastomoses between the cremasteric artery, artery of the ductus deferens, and testicular artery usually safeguard against avascular necrosis of the testis if the testicular artery is occluded

E. Ilioinguinal nerve

1. Enters the spermatic cord in the distal part of the inguinal canal, in the plane between the aponeurosis of the external abdominal oblique and cremasteric fascia

2. Just inferior to the superficial inguinal ring the ilioinguinal nerve lies laterally within the spermatic cord; here, it penetrates the external spermatic fascia and provides sensory innervation to the skin of the anterior scrotum and upper medial thigh

F. Round ligament of the uterus

1. Not part of the spermatic cord, but represents the comparable female structure occupying the inguinal canal; it is a band of fibrous tissue that courses retroperitoneally from the uterus to the deep inguinal ring and then through the inguinal canal

2. At the superficial inguinal ring, the ilioinguinal nerve lies lateral to the round ligament of the uterus; it provides cutaneous innervation to the anterior labium majus and upper medial thigh (the genital branch of the genitofemoral nerve also traverses the inguinal canal and also provides cutaneous innervation to the anterior labium majus and upper medial thigh)

3. After emerging from the superficial inguinal ring, the round ligament of the uterus spreads out and merges with the superficial fascia of the labium majus; since the round ligament of the uterus develops *in situ*, it does not descend through the anterior abdominal wall, and is thus devoid of fascial sheaths

III. Testis

A. Oval organ covered by a dense connective tissue capsule, the tunica albuginea; divided into pyramidal lobules by fine connective tissue septa that extend inward from the tunica albuginea (each lobule contains about three seminiferous tubules)

B. Associated structures

1. Epididymis

    a. C-shaped structure consisting of a single convoluted tube divided into three regions; the head or caput lies on the superior pole of the testis, the body or corpus descends along the posterior aspect of the testis, and the tail or cauda is located at the inferior pole of the testis (the tail is continuous with the ductus deferens)

    b. About 15 efferent ductules transport spermatozoa from the superior pole of the testis into the head of the epididymis

2. Processus and tunica vaginalis

    a. In the embryo, the processus vaginalis is a diverticulum of the parietal peritoneum that evaginates into the inguinal canal and scrotum; it nearly surrounds the testis and epididymis as the tunica vaginalis and normally closes off from the peritoneal cavity

    b. The visceral layer of the tunica vaginalis covers the epididymis and the tunica albuginea of the testis, except at the mediastinum testis, the posterior region of the testis where blood vessels, nerves, and exit lymphatics enter and exit the testis; it also lines a deep groove, the sinus of the epididymis, that intervenes between the testis and body of the epididymis

c. The parietal layer of the tunica vaginalis is fused to the internal spermatic fascia

d. The closed cavity of the tunica vaginalis contains a small amount of serous fluid that moistens the apposed parietal and visceral layers of the tunica vaginalis and allows the testis to move freely in the scrotum

e. Clinical note: an abnormal accumulation of serous fluid within the cavity of the tunica vaginalis is known as a hydrocele

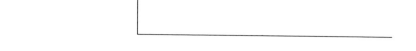

The Abdominopelvic or Peritoneal Cavity

I. General Structure

   A. Peritoneum

      1. Serous membrane lining the peritoneal cavity; it is composed of a parietal and visceral peritoneum

         a. Parietal peritoneum lines the outer wall of the peritoneal cavity, that is, the inner surface of the abdominal and pelvic walls; it receives its sensory innervation from the same somatic nerves that supply the abdominal and pelvic walls

         b. Visceral peritoneum covers the abdominal and pelvic viscera; it receives its sensory innervation from the autonomic nerves that supply the viscera

      2. At particular locations, the parietal peritoneum is reflected off the outer wall of the peritoneal cavity to form bilayered peritoneal sheets called mesenteries; the peritoneal sheets forming the mesenteries suspend viscera, transmit the nerves and vessels that subserve the viscera, and are continuous with the visceral peritoneum enclosing the viscera

         a. Viscera suspended by mesenteries are often said to lie within the peritoneal cavity or to be intraperitoneal; viscera not suspended within the peritoneal cavity by mesenteries are said to lie outside the peritoneal cavity or to be retroperitoneal

         b. Some mesenteries are called omenta or "ligaments"

B. Greater sac

1. Main region of the peritoneal cavity extending from the diaphragm to the floor of the pelvis; its associated mesenteries, recesses, and gutters are noted below

2. Subphrenic recesses

   a. The right and left subphrenic recesses are narrow spaces of the greater sac between the liver and diaphragm on the right and left sides of the falciform ligament

      1. The falciform ligament is a bilayered peritoneal sheet connecting the liver to the anterior abdominal wall and diaphragm; its peritoneal layers are continuous with the parietal peritoneum covering the inner surface of the anterior abdominal wall, the parietal peritoneum covering the inferior surface of the diaphragm, and the visceral peritoneum covering the diaphragmatic surface of the liver

      2. The ligamentum teres hepatis (round ligament of the liver) lies within the inferior free border of the falciform ligament; it is a fibrous remnant of the left umbilical vein and extends from the umbilicus to the portal vein

   b. The right subphrenic recess is limited posteriorly by the coronary ligament

      1. The coronary ligament is a single peritoneal sheet that attaches the superior surface of the liver to the inferior surface of the diaphragm; it is continuous anteriorly with the right layer of the falciform ligament

      2. Laterally, on the right, the coronary ligament reflects back on itself to form the bilayered right triangular ligament

      3. The posterior layer of the right triangular ligament becomes the hepatorenal ligament, as it diverges from the anterior layer to enclose the bare area of the liver; the hepatorenal ligament attaches the posterior surface of the liver to the posterior abdominal wall and right kidney

   c. The left subphrenic recess is limited posteriorly by the anterior layer of the left triangular ligament, which is continuous anteriorly with the left layer of the falciform ligament; laterally, on the left, the anterior layer of the left triangular ligament reflects back on itself, however, in contrast to the right triangular ligament, the posterior layer of the left triangular ligament does not separate from the anterior layer to enclose a bare area of the liver

   d. The posterior layer of the left triangular ligament and the hepatorenal ligament unite posteriorly at the junction of the caudate and left lobes of the liver to form a bilayered peritoneal sheet called the lesser omentum; the attachment of the lesser omentum to the liver extends inferiorly on the visceral surface of the liver in the groove for the ligamentum venosum between the caudate and left lobes of the liver and, most inferiorly, encloses the porta hepatis

3. Hepatorenal recess (pouch): region of the greater sac located between the right lobe of the liver and the right kidney; it is bounded superiorly by the hepatorenal ligament and, in the supine position, is the lowest point in the peritoneal cavity

4. The gutter to the right of the mesentery of the small intestine is limited superiorly by the transverse mesocolon and inferiorly by the ileocolic junction; the gutter to the left of the mesentery of the small intestine is limited superiorly by the transverse mesocolon and opens inferiorly into the pelvis

5. The right and left paracolic gutters lie lateral to the ascending and descending colons, respectively

   a. The right paracolic gutter communicates superiorly with the hepatorenal recess, and the left paracolic gutter is limited superiorly by the phrenicocolic ligament, a fold of peritoneum between the left colic flexure and diaphragm; inferiorly, both paracolic gutters extend into the pelvis

   b. Clinical note: gutters provide pathways for the spread of infectious material within the peritoneal cavity; for example, the right paracolic gutter may serve as a conduit for the spread of infectious material from the appendix to the hepatorenal recess

C. Lesser sac (omental bursa)

   1. Small region of the peritoneal cavity posterior to the stomach and lesser omentum; its omenta and recesses are noted below

   2. Lesser omentum

   a. Bilayered peritoneal sheet extending from the groove for the ligamentum venosum and porta hepatis on the visceral surface of the liver to the abdominal portion of the esophagus, the lesser curvature of the stomach, and the superior part of the duodenum; it is composed of the hepatogastric and hepatoduodenal ligaments

b. Hepatogastric ligament: the part of the lesser omentum extending from the groove for the ligamentum venosum to the abdominal portion of the esophagus and lesser curvature of the stomach

c. Hepatoduodenal ligament: the part of the lesser omentum extending from the porta hepatis to the superior part of the duodenum; it terminates inferiorly in a free border which contains the common bile duct, proper hepatic artery, portal vein, autonomic nerve fibers, and lymphatics

3. Greater omentum

   a. Extends from the greater curvature of the stomach to the posterior abdominal wall; composed of the gastrocolic, gastrosplenic (gastro-lienal), and splenorenal (lienorenal) ligaments

   b. Gastrocolic ligament (often referred to as the greater omentum)

      1. A large and often fat-laden apron composed of two bilayered peritoneal sheets that enclose the inferior recess of the lesser sac; the two bilayered peritoneal sheets of the gastrocolic ligament (greater omentum) are often fused and the inferior recess of the lesser sac obliterated

      2. Its anterior bilayer drapes from the distal two-thirds of the greater curvature of the stomach anterior to the transverse colon and small intestine before reflecting superiorly as the posterior bilayer; the posterior bilayer ascends posterior to the anterior bilayer on the small intestine and transverse colon, adhering to the latter and to the superior surface of the transverse mesocolon before attaching to the posterior abdominal wall just above the attachment of the transverse mesocolon

      3. Clinical note: the greater omentum can prevent the spread of infection by adhering to and walling off an inflamed area

   c. Gastrosplenic and splenorenal ligaments

      1. Superior to the transverse colon and to the left, the gastrocolic ligament becomes continuous with the gastrosplenic ligament, which extends from the proximal one-third of the greater curvature of the stomach to the spleen; the splenorenal ligament extends from the spleen to the posterior abdominal wall and left kidney

      2. The outer layer of the gastrosplenic ligament extends from the stomach to the hilum of the spleen, covers the surface of the spleen,

and then becomes continuous with the outer layer of the spleno-renal ligament; the outer layer of the gastrosplenic ligament, the visceral peritoneum covering the spleen, and the outer layer of the splenorenal ligament face into the greater sac

3. The inner layer of the gastrosplenic ligament passes from the stomach to the splenic hilum, and then, without covering the spleen, passes posteriorly as the inner layer of the splenorenal ligament; the inner layers of the gastrosplenic and splenorenal ligaments line the splenic recess of the lesser sac

4. Superior recess of the lesser sac: its anterior wall is formed by the caudate lobe of the liver, the posterior wall is the part of the diaphragm covering the thoracic aorta, and the left and right walls are formed by the abdominal portion of the esophagus and inferior vena cava, respectively

5. The lesser sac communicates with the greater sac through the epiploic or omental foramen (of Winslow); the epiploic foramen is bounded superiorly by the caudate lobe of the liver, inferiorly by the superior part of the duodenum, posteriorly by the inferior vena cava, and anteriorly by the hepatoduodenal ligament

II. The Foregut

A. In the abdomen, the foregut extends from the abdominal portion of the esophagus to midway along the duodenum

B. Abdominal portion of the esophagus

1. Short, distal segment of the esophagus between the esophageal hiatus of the diaphragm and cardia of the stomach; it indents the liver posteriorly between its caudate and left lobes

2. Its right border continues inferiorly as the lesser curvature of the stomach and its left border forms an acute angle, the cardiac incisure, with the fundus of the stomach

C. Stomach

1. Highly distensible portion of the gastrointestinal tract between the abdominal portion of the esophagus and duodenum; although usually located primarily above the left costal margin, its position varies considerably

2. Curvatures: the lesser curvature comprises the short, right, concave border; the greater curvature is the long, left, convex border

3. Regions

    a. Cardia: small region distal to the cardioesophageal junction

    b. Fundus and body: divided from each other by an imaginary transverse plane through the cardioesophageal junction; the fundus lies superior to the imaginary plane and the body lies inferior to the plane

    c. Pyloric antrum: the angular notch, an indentation along the lesser curvature, indicates the junction between the body and pyloric antrum

    d. Pyloric canal: narrow, distal region of the stomach between the pyloric antrum and pylorus; the boundary between the pyloric antrum and pyloric canal is indistinct

    e. Pylorus: orifice between the pyloric canal and duodenum; it is encircled by the pyloric sphincter

4. Sphincters

    a. Cardiac sphincter: not an anatomical sphincter; however, radiological evidence demonstrating constriction at the cardioesophageal junction suggests the existence of a physiologic sphincter that prevents the reflux of chyme into the esophagus

    b. Pyloric sphincter: anatomical sphincter formed by a thickening of the inner circular layer of the muscularis externa at the pylorus; regulates the flow of chyme from the stomach into the duodenum

5. Internally, there may be longitudinal ridges called rugae

6. Relations

    a. Anterior surface: on the left, the anterior surface of the stomach contacts the diaphragm; on the right, the anterior surface contacts the left lobe of the liver superiorly, and the anterior abdominal wall inferiorly

    b. Posterior surface: on the left, the posterior surface contacts the spleen; on the right, the posterior surface faces the lesser sac and through it contacts most of the pancreas, the superior pole of the left kidney, and the left suprarenal gland

D. Spleen

1. Not an embryologic derivative of the foregut, but included here for simplicity

2. Suspended between the proximal one-third of the greater curvature of the stomach and the posterior abdominal wall (in the region of the left kidney) by the gastrosplenic and splenorenal ligaments, respectively; inferiorly, it is supported by the phrenicocolic ligament, a fold of peritoneum between the left colic flexure and diaphragm

3. The longitudinal axis of the spleen follows the tenth rib, with the center of the spleen lying near the posterior axillary line; its convex diaphragmatic surface is related, through the diaphragm, to the costodiaphragmatic recess of the left pleural cavity

4. Concave indentations on the visceral surface of the spleen are made by the left colic flexure (anteriorly), the stomach (superiorly), and the left kidney (inferiorly); the tail of the pancreas contacts the hilum, the central region on the visceral surface where vessels and nerves enter and exit the spleen

5. Its superior border is sharp and often notched; its inferior border is rounded

6. Clinical notes

   a. Because of its thin capsule and friable consistency, the spleen is easily ruptured by traumatic injury

   b. Enlargement of the spleen is called splenomegaly; an enlarged spleen may be palpable below the left costal margin or may produce an indentation in the stomach or left colic flexure that is visible on barium X-ray

   c. Small accessory spleens along the splenic vessels are common

E. Duodenum

   1. General remarks

      a. Extends from the pylorus to the jejunum, forming almost a complete circle which encloses the head of the pancreas; except for its very proximal and very distal ends, the duodenum lies retroperitoneally

      b. Its proximal half, including the major duodenal papilla, is a foregut derivative; its distal half, although derived from the midgut, is included with the foregut for simplicity

   2. Parts

      a. Superior part

         1. Lies anterior to the body of vertebra L1

2. Its proximal part is called the duodenal ampulla, duodenal bulb, or duodenal cap; in barium X-ray its wall appears smooth due to the absence of internal folds called plicae circulares (plicae circulares are present in the remainder of the duodenum and present a feathery appearance in barium X-ray)

3. The hepatoduodenal ligament attaches to its upper margin; its posterior surface contacts the inferior vena cava, portal vein, common bile duct, and gastroduodenal artery

4. Clinical note: about 95 percent of duodenal ulcers occur in the superior part

b. Descending part

1. Descends to the right of vertebral bodies L1, 2, and 3

2. About halfway along its length, the hepatopancreatic ampulla (of Vater) opens into its lumen medially (the hepatopancreatic ampulla is formed by the union of the main pancreatic duct and common bile duct); its site of penetration is marked internally by the major duodenal papilla

3. A minor duodenal papilla, if present, is located about 2 centimeters superior to the major duodenal papilla; it marks the site of penetration of the accessory pancreatic duct

4. Its posterior surface contacts the hilum of the right kidney and right renal vein; medially, it is related to the head of the pancreas and, laterally, to the right colic flexure

c. Horizontal part: courses to the left, anterior to the body of vertebra L3, and contacts, in close succession, the right ureter, right testicular/ovarian vessels, inferior vena cava, abdominal aorta, and inferior mesenteric artery; the superior mesenteric vessels descend on its anterior surface

d. Ascending part

1. Ascends on the left side of vertebral body L2 and, at its junction with the jejunum, turns abruptly anteriorly and inferiorly, forming the duodenojejunal flexure; the duodenojejunal flexure is suspended from the right crus of the diaphragm by a fibromuscular band called the suspensory ligament of the duodenum or the ligament of Treitz

2. The superior attachment of the root of the mesentery of the small intestine to the posterior abdominal wall crosses the anterior surfaces of the horizontal and ascending parts of the duodenum

F. Pancreas

1. Lobulated, retroperitoneal, exocrine and endocrine gland; extends transversely from the duodenum to the spleen

2. Parts

a. Head

   1. Almost completely encircled by the duodenum

   2. From the inferior and left part of the head, the hooklike uncinate process of the pancreas projects behind the superior mesenteric vessels; the superior part of the head is continuous to the left with the neck

b. Neck: narrow part between the head and body; lies anterior to the superior mesenteric vessels

c. Body: part above and to the left of the duodenojejunal flexure

d. Tail: tapering end within the splenorenal ligament

3. The transverse mesocolon attaches transversely across the anterior surface of the head, neck, and body of the pancreas; the parts of the pancreas superior and inferior to the attachment of the transverse mesocolon face into the lesser and greater sacs, respectively

4. Pancreatic ducts

a. Main pancreatic duct: traverses the pancreas from left to right, draining pancreatic enzymes from the tail, body, neck, and head; within the wall of the duodenum, about halfway along the medial side of its descending part, the main pancreatic duct joins the common bile duct to form the hepatopancreatic ampulla, which opens onto the major duodenal papilla

b. Accessory pancreatic duct: drains part of the head of the pancreas; opens into the descending part of the duodenum at the minor duodenal papilla, about 2 centimeters superior to the major duodenal papilla

G. Liver

1. Wedge-shaped; lies superior to the right costal margin and extends across the midline to the left midclavicular line

2. Surfaces

    a. Diaphragmatic surface

        1. Includes the anterior, superior, posterior, and right surfaces; part of the diaphragmatic surface lacks a peritoneal covering and is called the bare area of the liver

        2. Peritoneal ligaments associated with the diaphragmatic surface are the falciform, left triangular, coronary, right triangular, and hepatorenal ligaments

    b. Visceral surface

        1. Faces inferiorly, posteriorly, and to the left; inferiorly, it is separated from the diaphragmatic surface by the sharp, inferior border of the liver

        2. Fossa for the gall bladder: extends posteriorly from the inferior border of the liver to the groove for the inferior vena cava; the fossa for the gall bladder and the groove for the inferior vena cava comprise the right sagittal fossa

        3. Fissure for the ligamentum teres hepatis: lies to the left of the fossa for the gall bladder, extending posteriorly from the inferior border of the liver to the fissure for the ligamentum venosum; the fissure for the ligamentum teres hepatis and the fissure for the ligamentum venosum comprise the left sagittal fissure

        4. Porta hepatis: transverse fissure between the right sagittal fossa and left sagittal fissure, about midway along their lengths; at the porta hepatis, the right and left hepatic ducts, the right and left branches of the portal vein, the right and left hepatic arteries, autonomic nerves, and lymphatics enter and exit the liver

3. Lobes

    a. Right lobe: located to the right of the right sagittal fossa; drained by the right hepatic duct and supplied by the right branch of the portal vein and right hepatic artery

    b. Left lobe: lies to the left of the left sagittal fissure; drained by the left hepatic duct and supplied by the left branch of the portal vein and left hepatic artery

    c. Quadrate lobe: lies between the fossa for the gall bladder and the fissure for the ligamentum teres hepatis, anterior to the porta hepatis;

drained by the left hepatic duct and supplied by the left branch of the portal vein and left hepatic artery

    d. Caudate lobe: lies between the groove for the inferior vena cava and the fissure for the ligamentum venosum, posterior to the porta hepatis; drained by the right and left hepatic ducts and supplied by right and left branches of the portal vein, and the right and left hepatic arteries

    e. Clinical note: surgeons often divide the liver into right and left surgical lobes, based on arterial supply; in this case, the right surgical lobe would consist of the right lobe and part of the caudate lobe, and the left surgical lobe would consist of the left, quadrate, and part of the caudate lobe

  4. Relations

    a. Diaphragmatic surface (peritoneal area): through the subphrenic recesses and diaphragm, the diaphragmatic surface of the liver is related to the right pleural cavity, pericardial cavity, and part of the left pleural cavity

    b. Diaphragmatic surface (bare area): related to the diaphragm, superior pole of the right kidney, right suprarenal gland, and inferior vena cava

    c. Visceral surface

       1. To the right of the right sagittal fossa, the visceral surface of the liver is related to the right colic flexure anteriorly and the inferior pole of the right kidney posteriorly

       2. To the left of the right sagittal fossa, the left and quadrate lobes are related anteriorly to the transverse colon and posteriorly to the proximal and distal portions of the stomach, respectively; through the superior recess of the lesser sac, the caudate lobe is related to the diaphragm

H. Gall bladder and bile ducts

  1. Gall bladder

    a. Pear-shaped reservoir for bile

    b. Regions: the fundus of the gall bladder is the expanded, inferior part that protrudes below the inferior border of the liver; the body lies between the fundus and a narrow neck, which angles downward near the porta hepatis to become the cystic duct

c. Relations

1. The anterior surface of the fundus of the gall bladder is covered by visceral peritoneum and contacts the posterior surface of the anterior abdominal wall at the junction of the lateral margin of the right rectus abdominis and right costal margin; the anterior surfaces of the body and neck are devoid of peritoneum and are in direct contact with the substance of the liver within the fossa for the gall bladder

2. The peritoneum-covered, posterior surfaces of the fundus, body, and neck contact the transverse colon, descending part of the duodenum, and superior part of the duodenum, respectively

2. Bile ducts

a. Common hepatic duct: formed within the porta hepatis by the union of the right and left hepatic ducts

b. Cystic duct

1. Joins the common hepatic duct inferior to the porta hepatis to form the common bile duct

2. The cystohepatic triangle (of Calot) is formed by the common hepatic duct, cystic duct, and visceral surface of the liver; the right hepatic artery, cystic artery (which supplies the gall bladder), and most accessory hepatic ducts traverse the cystohepatic triangle

c. Common bile duct

1. Descends in the hepatoduodenal ligament to the right of the proper hepatic artery and anterior to the portal vein; passes behind the superior part of the duodenum to the right of the gastroduodenal artery

2. Penetrates the head of the pancreas and unites with the main pancreatic duct within the wall of the duodenum to form the hepatopancreatic ampulla; flow of bile and pancreatic enzymes through the hepatopancreatic ampulla is regulated by the encircling hepatopancreatic sphincter (of Oddi)

3. Clinical note: gallstones are concretions of cholesterol and bile pigments that form in the gall bladder; they may exit the gall bladder and lodge in the cystic or common bile ducts

I. Celiac trunk

  1. The celiac trunk ("the artery of the foregut") arises from the abdominal aorta anterior to the body of vertebra L1; its three branches, the common hepatic, splenic, and left gastric arteries, course retroperitoneally behind the lesser sac

  2. Common hepatic artery

    a. Courses to the right, above the superior part of the duodenum; here, it divides into its terminal branches, the proper hepatic and gastroduodenal arteries

    b. Proper hepatic artery

      1. Ascends in the hepatoduodenal ligament to the left of the common bile duct and anterior to the portal vein; gives rise to the right gastric artery which courses to the left within the lesser omentum along the lesser curvature of the stomach

      2. Inferior to the porta hepatis, it divides into the right and left hepatic arteries; the right hepatic artery gives rise to the cystic artery

    c. Gastroduodenal artery: descends posterior to the superior part of the duodenum and divides into the right gastroepiploic (gastro-omental) and superior pancreaticoduodenal arteries; the right gastroepiploic artery courses to the left within the greater omentum along the greater curvature of the stomach and the superior pancreaticoduodenal artery divides into anterior and posterior branches that descend through the head of the pancreas and supply the superior part of the head of the pancreas and the proximal half of the duodenum (the gastroduodenal artery may also give rise to small supraduodenal and retroduodenal arteries that supply the superior and posterior surfaces of the superior part of the duodenum, respectively)

  3. Splenic artery

    a. Takes a tortuous course to the left, superior to the body of the pancreas, and then passes forward within the splenorenal ligament to enter the hilum of the spleen; its branches are noted below

    b. Numerous branches supply the neck, body, and tail of the pancreas

    c. Left gastroepiploic (gastro-omental) artery: arises near the hilum of the spleen and traverses the gastrosplenic ligament; courses to the right within the greater omentum along the greater curvature of the stomach and anastomoses with the right gastroepiploic artery

    d. Short gastric arteries (five to seven): arise from the splenic artery distal to the origin of the left gastroepiploic artery; they reach the fundus of the stomach within the gastrosplenic ligament

  4. Left gastric artery: small branch which ascends to the cardioesophageal junction; some branches ascend on the abdominal portion of the esophagus and others descend within the lesser omentum along the lesser curvature of the stomach and anastomose with branches of the right gastric artery

J. Veins

  1. Veins corresponding to branches of the celiac trunk ultimately drain into the portal vein (there is no celiac vein); the portal vein is formed behind the neck of the pancreas by the union of the superior mesenteric and splenic veins

  2. Splenic vein

    a. Receives the short gastric and left gastroepiploic veins near the hilum of the spleen

    b. After leaving the splenorenal ligament the splenic vein courses to the right, posterior to the pancreas, and receives tributaries from the pancreas as well as the inferior mesenteric vein, which ascends to the left of the duodenojejunal flexure; alternatively, the inferior mesenteric vein may drain into the superior mesenteric vein or the angle of junction between the superior mesenteric and splenic veins

  3. Superior mesenteric vein: ascends anterior to the horizontal part of the duodenum to the right of the superior mesenteric artery; receives the right gastroepiploic vein (there is no gastroduodenal vein) which, in turn, receives the inferior pancreaticoduodenal vein

  4. Portal vein: receives the right and left gastric veins, the superior pancreaticoduodenal vein, and the paraumbilical veins (paraumbilical veins course from the umbilicus to the portal vein along the round ligament of the liver; there are no paraumbilical arteries)

  5. Hepatic veins: drain the sinusoids of the liver; three large hepatic veins empty into the inferior vena cava where it lies in its groove on the bare area of the liver, just before it pierces the diaphragm to enter the right atrium

6. Clinical notes

    a. There are three primary sites where anastomoses of the portal and systemic venous systems may become distended and hemorrhage due to portal hypertension, a condition in which portal venous blood that would normally flow through the liver flows in a retrograde fashion through valveless tributaries of the portal vein to sites of portal-systemic anastomoses; from these sites, blood returns to the heart through the systemic venous system

        1. Esophageal varices are varicose veins that may occur within the wall of the esophagus where tributaries of the left gastric vein (portal) anastomose with tributaries of the azygos and hemiazygos veins (systemic)

        2. A caput medusae may occur around the umbilicus where tributaries of the paraumbilical veins (portal) anastomose with tributaries of the thoracoepigastric veins (systemic)

        3. Hemorrhoids or submucosal varicosities may occur in the anal canal where tributaries of the superior rectal vein (portal) anastomose with tributaries of the inferior rectal veins (systemic)

    b. Secondary sites of portal-systemic anastomoses exist wherever "bare" areas of portal drained structures, such as the duodenum, ascending colon, descending colon, liver, and pancreas, are in contact with the body wall, which is drained by the systemic venous system

    c. Cancers of the gastrointestinal tract often metastasize to the liver via the portal venous system

K. Lymphatics

    1. Lymph from the abdominal portion of the esophagus, stomach, spleen, duodenum, pancreas, liver, gall bladder, and bile ducts drains to celiac nodes near the celiac trunk; celiac nodes drain into the cisterna chyli via the intestinal lymphatic trunk

    2. Some of the lymph from the bare area of the liver drains into posterior mediastinal nodes, which drain superiorly to tracheobronchial nodes

L. Celiac plexus

    1. Network of nerves surrounding the celiac trunk and containing two large celiac ganglia, one on each side of the celiac trunk; its efferent contributions are noted below

a. Preganglionic parasympathetic efferent fibers which pass through the celiac plexus are derived from the anterior and posterior vagal trunks and are distributed to the abdominal portion of the esophagus, stomach, the proximal half of the duodenum, the neck, body, tail, and superior part of the head of the pancreas, liver, gall bladder, and bile ducts along branches of the celiac trunk; they synapse on postganglionic parasympathetic cell bodies in ganglia within the wall of the organ to be innervated and postganglionic fibers increase peristaltic and secretory activity

b. Preganglionic sympathetic efferent fibers to the celiac plexus are derived from the greater splanchnic nerves which are formed by medial branches of sympathetic ganglia T5 to T9; they synapse in the celiac ganglia on postganglionic sympathetic cell bodies, which give rise to postganglionic sympathetic fibers that are distributed to the abdominal portion of the esophagus, stomach, spleen, the proximal half of the duodenum, the neck, body, tail, and superior part of the head of the pancreas, liver, gall bladder, and bile ducts along branches of the celiac trunk and function to inhibit peristaltic and secretory activity

c. Clinical note: vagotomy or surgical sectioning of the vagal trunks may be performed to reduce the secretion of acid by the stomach

2. Afferent contributions to the celiac plexus

a. Parasympathetic afferent fibers that pass through the celiac plexus travel with the vagal trunks; they mediate the feeling of nausea and function in gastrointestinal reflexes

b. Sympathetic afferent fibers that pass through the celiac plexus travel with the greater splanchnic nerves to sympathetic ganglia T5 to T9; from the ganglia they enter their respective ventral rami through white rami communicantes and terminate in the dorsal gray horns of spinal cord segments T5 to T9 to mediate pain

c. Clinical note: because sympathetic afferent fibers from the gall bladder travel with the right greater splanchnic nerve, pain from the gall bladder may be referred to dermatomes T5 to T9 on the right side of the trunk; since the inner portion of the parietal peritoneum on the inferior surface of the right dome of the diaphragm is innervated by the right phrenic nerve (C3, 4, and 5), an inflamed gall bladder irritating this portion of the parietal peritoneum may present as referred pain to the right shoulder region, the location of dermatomes for spinal nerves C3, 4, and 5

III. The Midgut and Hindgut

    A. The midgut extends from midway along the duodenum to midway along the transverse colon; the hindgut extends from midway along the transverse colon to midway along the anal canal

    B. Small intestine

        1. Composed of the duodenum (see pp. 95-96), jejunum, and ileum, and measures about 7 meters in length; the jejunal and ileal loops are almost completely framed by the large intestine

        2. Jejunum: commences at the duodenojejunal flexure on the left side of vertebral body L2 and generally occupies the region above the umbilicus; internal folds called plicae circulares are abundant

        3. Ileum

            a. Comprises about the distal three-fifths of the small intestine, generally occupies the region below the umbilicus, and usually extends into the pelvis; joins the large intestine between the cecum and ascending colon

            b. Within its wall there are lymphoid follicle aggregations called Peyer's patches; plicae circulares are few or absent

            c. Clinical note: a Meckel's diverticulum is a fingerlike pouch that projects from the ileum about 1 meter proximal to the ileocecal junction; it represents a persistent vitelline duct, is present in about 2 percent of individuals, and may contain gastric or pancreatic tissue

        4. Mesentery of the small intestine (the mesentery)

            a. Fan-shaped; its intestinal border is about 40 times longer than its root, which is attached diagonally across the posterior abdominal wall from the duodenojejunal to the ileocecal junction

            b. Between the two peritoneal sheets of the mesentery are blood vessels, lymphatics, lymph nodes, and nerve plexuses that serve the jejunum and ileum

    C. Large intestine

        1. Consists of the appendix, cecum, ascending colon, transverse colon, descending colon, sigmoid colon, rectum, and anal canal; measures about 1.5 meters in length

2. Appendix

    a. Vermiform diverticulum of the cecum; arises about 3 centimeters inferior to the ileocecal orifice

    b. Connected to the terminal end of the ileum by a mesentery, the mesoappendix; most commonly, the appendix lies in a retrocecal position

3. Cecum and colon

    a. General features

        1. The longitudinal musculature of the muscularis externa is concentrated into three bands called taeniae coli; because the taeniae coli are shorter than the wall of the cecum and colon, they produce characteristic sacculations called haustra (plicae semilunares are the internal crescentic folds between the haustra)

        2. Appendices epiploicae are small, peritoneum-covered bodies of fat associated with the cecum and colon

    b. Cecum

        1. Blind-ending portion of the large intestine located in the right iliac fossa; its extent of fusion to the posterior abdominal wall and, thus, its degree of mobility, varies considerably

        2. The junction of the cecum with the ascending colon is marked internally along its medial wall by the ileocecal orifice

    c. Colon

        1. Ascending colon: ascends retroperitoneally from the ileocecal junction to the liver; anterior to the inferior pole of the right kidney, it bends to the left at the hepatic or right colic flexure

        2. Transverse colon: extends from the right colic flexure to the more superior and posterior splenic or left colic flexure; suspended from the posterior abdominal wall by the transverse mesocolon

        3. Descending colon: extends from the left colic flexure, which lies anterior to the inferior pole of the left kidney, to the left iliac fossa

        4. Sigmoid colon: extends from the left iliac fossa to the third sacral vertebra; suspended by the sigmoid mesocolon

5. Clinical notes: diverticulosis

   a. Characterized by mucosal-lined diverticula that protrude through the muscularis externa of the colon; in a barium X-ray the diverticula appear as radiopaque-filled blebs

   b. Feces tends to stagnate in the diverticula; this predisposes to inflammation (diverticulitis), rupture, and peritonitis

4. Rectum (see pp. 152–154)

5. Anal canal (see pp. 125–129)

D. Superior mesenteric artery ("the artery of the midgut")

   1. Arises from the abdominal aorta anterior to the body of vertebra L1, inferior to the origin of the celiac trunk; descends anterior to the left renal vein and horizontal part of the duodenum, and then courses retroperitoneally adjacent to the root of the mesentery

   2. Supplies the inferior part of the head of the pancreas, the distal half of the duodenum, the jejunum, ileum, appendix, cecum, ascending colon, and the proximal half of the transverse colon; its branches are noted below

   3. Inferior pancreaticoduodenal artery: arises posterior to the pancreas and divides into anterior and posterior branches that ascend within the head of the pancreas; they supply the inferior part of the head of the pancreas and the distal half of the duodenum and anastomose with the anterior and posterior branches of the superior pancreaticoduodenal artery, a branch of the gastroduodenal artery

   4. Middle colic artery: arises anterior to the uncinate process of the pancreas; passes into the transverse mesocolon and, as it nears the transverse colon, divides into right and left branches which supply the proximal half of the transverse colon

   5. Right colic artery: courses retroperitoneally to the right and divides into ascending and descending branches which supply the ascending colon; often arises from the ileocolic artery

   6. Ileocolic artery

      a. Courses retroperitoneally to the right iliac fossa and gives rise to the branches noted below

      b. Colic branches supply the proximal end of the ascending colon; an ileal branch supplies the distal end of the ileum and anastomoses with the last ileal artery off the superior mesenteric artery

c. Anterior and posterior cecal arteries supply the cecum; the appendicular artery descends posterior to the ileum, and then within the mesoappendix to supply the appendix

7. Intestinal (jejunal and ileal) arteries

a. Number about 15; arise from the left side of the superior mesenteric artery and course within the mesentery of the small intestine

b. Each artery branches and unites with similar branches of adjacent arteries to form a series of arches or arcades; branches from the arcades may again divide and unite to form another series of arcades, a pattern which may continue for up to five series of arcades

c. Straight vessels or vasa recta arise from the distal series of arcades to supply the jejunum and ileum (vasa recta are also present in the colon)

E. Inferior mesenteric artery ("the artery of the hindgut")

1. Arises from the abdominal aorta anterior to the body of vertebra L3 and posterior to the horizontal part of the duodenum; descends retroperitoneally along the left side of the abdominal aorta and gives rise to the branches noted below

2. Left colic artery: courses retroperitoneally to the left; divides into ascending and descending branches which supply the distal half of the transverse colon and descending colon

3. Sigmoid arteries (two to four): form anastomosing arcades in the sigmoid mesocolon; supply the sigmoid colon

4. Superior rectal artery: represents the continuation of the inferior mesenteric artery after the sigmoid arteries are given off; enters the pelvis to supply the rectum and proximal half of the anal canal

F. Marginal artery (of Drummond)

1. Composite artery that courses along the inner border of the colon from the ileocecal to the rectosigmoid junction

2. Component arteries include the colic branches of the ileocolic artery, the ascending and descending branches of the right colic artery, the right and left branches of the middle colic artery, the ascending and descending branches of the left colic artery, and the anastomosing arcades of the sigmoid arteries

3. Clinical note: the marginal artery may provide an adequate collateral circulation to the colon if one of its major contributing arteries is ligated

G. Veins: tributaries of the superior and inferior mesenteric veins travel with their respective arteries; the superior and inferior mesenteric veins drain into the portal and splenic veins, respectively

H. Lymphatics

1. Course with branches of the superior and inferior mesenteric arteries to superior and inferior mesenteric nodes located near the origins of their respective arteries

2. Superior mesenteric nodes drain into the intestinal trunk which empties into the cisterna chyli

3. Inferior mesenteric nodes drain to lumbar nodes along the inferior vena cava and abdominal aorta; lumbar nodes drain into the lumbar trunks which empty into the cisterna chyli

I. Nerve supply

1. Superior mesenteric plexus

   a. Network of nerves surrounding the origin of the superior mesenteric artery and containing the superior mesenteric ganglion; its efferent contributions are noted below

   b. Preganglionic parasympathetic efferent fibers which pass through the superior mesenteric plexus are derived from the anterior and posterior vagal trunks and are distributed to the inferior part of the head of the pancreas, distal half of the duodenum, the jejunum, ileum, appendix, cecum, ascending colon, and the proximal half of the transverse colon along branches of the superior mesenteric artery; they synapse on postganglionic parasympathetic cell bodies in ganglia within the wall of the organ to be innervated and postganglionic fibers increase peristaltic and secretory activity

   c. Preganglionic sympathetic efferent fibers to the superior mesenteric plexus are derived from the greater and lesser splanchnic nerves which are formed by medial branches of sympathetic ganglia T5 to T9 and medial branches of sympathetic ganglia T10 and T11, respectively; they synapse in the superior mesenteric ganglion on postganglionic sympathetic cell bodies which give rise to postganglionic sympathetic fibers that are distributed to the inferior part of the head of the pancreas, the distal half of the duodenum, the jejunum, ileum, appendix, cecum, ascending colon, and the proximal half of the transverse colon along branches of the superior mesenteric artery and function to inhibit peristaltic and secretory activity

2. Inferior mesenteric plexus

   a. Network of nerves surrounding the origin of the inferior mesenteric artery and containing the inferior mesenteric ganglion; its efferent contributions are noted below

   b. Preganglionic parasympathetic efferent fibers which pass through the inferior mesenteric plexus are derived from the pelvic splanchnic nerves and are distributed to the distal half of the transverse colon, descending colon, sigmoid colon, rectum, and the proximal half of the anal canal along branches of the inferior mesenteric artery; they synapse on postganglionic parasympathetic cell bodies in ganglia within the wall of the organ to be innervated and postganglionic fibers increase peristaltic and secretory activity (preganglionic parasympathetic cell bodies for the pelvic splanchnic nerves reside in the lateral horns of spinal cord segments S2 to S4; their axons leave the spinal cord in the ventral roots of spinal nerves S2 to S4, emerge from their respective ventral rami, and ascend out of the pelvis to join the inferior mesenteric plexus)

   c. Preganglionic sympathetic efferent fibers to the inferior mesenteric plexus are derived from lumbar splanchnic nerves which represent medial branches of the lumbar sympathetic ganglia; they synapse in the inferior mesenteric ganglion on postganglionic sympathetic cell bodies which give rise to postganglionic sympathetic fibers that are distributed to the distal half of the transverse colon, descending colon, sigmoid colon, rectum, and the proximal half of the anal canal along branches of the inferior mesenteric artery and function to inhibit peristaltic and secretory activity

3. Afferent contributions to the superior and inferior mesenteric plexuses

   a. Parasympathetic afferent fibers that pass through the superior and inferior mesenteric plexuses travel with the vagal trunks and pelvic splanchnic nerves, respectively; they mediate the feeling of nausea and function in gastrointestinal reflexes

   b. Sympathetic afferents

      1. Pass through the superior and inferior mesenteric plexuses and travel with their corresponding efferents (greater, lesser, and lumbar splanchnic nerves) to sympathetic ganglia T5 to T11 and L1 to L5, respectively; from the sympathetic ganglia they enter ventral rami T5 to L2 via white rami communicantes and termi-

nate in the dorsal gray horns of spinal cord segments T5 to L2 to mediate pain (sympathetic afferents that travel with lumbar splanchnic nerves associated with sympathetic ganglia L3 to L5 ascend in the sympathetic trunk to sympathetic ganglion L2 to gain access to a white ramus communicans)

2. Clinical note: pain from viscera within the fields of distribution of the superior and inferior mesenteric arteries is referred to dermatomes T5 to T11 and L1 to L2, respectively

4. Intermesenteric plexus: network of nerves located on the abdominal aorta between the origins of the superior and inferior mesenteric arteries; comprised of greater, lesser, least, and lumbar splanchnic nerve fibers

The Posterior Abdominal Wall

I. Muscles

    A. Quadratus lumborum

        1. Origin: iliac crest

        2. Insertion: transverse processes of lumbar vertebrae and the twelfth rib

        3. Action: lateral flexion of the lumbar vertebrae; assists in inspiration by anchoring the twelfth rib during contraction and descent of the diaphragm

        4. Innervation: subcostal nerve and ventral rami L1, 2, 3, and 4

        5. Along its lateral border the transversus abdominis takes origin from the thoracolumbar fascia; medially, its anterior surface is covered by the psoas major

    B. Psoas major

        1. Origin: bodies and transverse processes of lumbar vertebrae

        2. Insertion: descends lateral to the pelvic brim, fuses with the iliacus to form the iliopsoas, and inserts on the lesser trochanter of the femur

        3. Action: flexion of the hip; flexion of the lumbar vertebrae

        4. Innervation: ventral rami L1, 2, and 3

5. Lumbar plexus

   a. Derived from ventral rami of spinal nerves L1 to L5 and formed within the substance of the psoas major; its component nerves, as well as the spinal cord level(s) contributing to their formation, are noted below

   b. Iliohypogastric and ilioinguinal nerves (L1)

      1. Emerge along the lateral border of the upper part of the psoas major, inferior to the subcostal nerve (they may arise as a single nerve which then divides); the iliohypogastric nerve courses superior to the ilioinguinal nerve

      2. Course laterally across the quadratus lumborum and then penetrate the transversus abdominis above the iliac crest

      3. The iliohypogastric nerve courses anteriorly in the neurovascular plane between the transversus abdominis and internal abdominal oblique, enters the rectus sheath, and then emerges from it as the lowest anterior cutaneous branch of the anterior abdominal wall

      4. The ilioinguinal nerve also courses anteriorly in the neurovascular plane between the transversus abdominis and internal abdominal oblique, but then enters the cleavage plane between the internal and external abdominal obliques; from this plane it enters the inguinal canal and, after emerging from the superficial inguinal ring, supplies the skin of the upper medial thigh and anterior scrotum/labium majus

   c. Genitofemoral nerve (L1, 2)

      1. Emerges from the anterior surface of the psoas major and descends on it

      2. Its genital branch enters the deep inguinal ring and, in the male, descends in the spermatic cord, supplying the cremaster muscle; distal to the superficial inguinal ring, it gives rise to cutaneous branches that supply the skin of the upper medial thigh and anterior scrotum/labium majus

      3. The femoral branch of the genitofemoral nerve accompanies the femoral artery and supplies the skin of the thigh

   d. Lateral femoral cutaneous nerve (L2, 3): emerges about midway along the lateral border of the psoas major and takes an oblique course across the iliacus muscle; enters the thigh through or deep to the lateral attachment of the inguinal ligament to supply the skin of the lateral thigh

    e. Femoral nerve (L2, 3, 4): descends in the gutter between the psoas major and iliacus; enters the thigh deep to the inguinal ligament to supply muscles and skin of the lower limb

    f. Obturator nerve (L2, 3, 4): descends along the medial border of the psoas major; courses forward in the obturator groove and then leaves the pelvis through the obturator canal to supply muscles and skin of the lower limb

    g. Accessory obturator nerve (L3, 4): present in about 10 percent of individuals; descends along the medial border of psoas major and then passes above the superior ramus of the pubis to supplement the innervation to the pectineus muscle in the thigh

    h. Lumbosacral trunk (L4, 5): descends on the ala of the sacrum, medial to the psoas major; contributes to the sacral plexus in the pelvis

C. Psoas minor

    1. Origin: bodies and transverse processes of vertebrae L1 and L2

    2. Insertion: descends on the anterior surface of the psoas major and inserts on the iliopubic eminence

    3. Action: flexion of the lumbar vertebrae

    4. Innervation: ventral rami L1 and L2

    5. Absent in about 40 percent of individuals

D. Iliacus

    1. Origin: iliac fossa

    2. Insertion: fuses with the psoas major to form the iliopsoas and inserts on the lesser trochanter of the femur

    3. Action: flexion of the hip

    4. Innervation: femoral nerve

E. Diaphragm

    1. Musculoaponeurotic sheet with right and left domes; separates the thoracic and abdominopelvic cavities

2. Parts

    a. Central tendon: aponeurotic portion; serves as an insertion site for the muscular parts noted below

    b. Sternal part: muscle fibers originate from the posterior surface of the xiphoid process

    c. Costal part: muscle fibers originate from the inner surfaces of the lower six rib pairs, near the perimeter of the inferior thoracic aperture

    d. Lumbar parts

        1. The left and right crura of the diaphragm originate from the bodies of vertebrae L1, 2, and 3

        2. Some lumbar muscle fibers originate from fascial bands termed the medial and lateral arcuate ligaments

            a. Medial arcuate ligament: spans the upper part of psoas major, extending from the body to the transverse process of vertebra L1

            b. Lateral arcuate ligament: spans the upper part of quadratus lumborum, extending from the transverse process of vertebra L1 to the twelfth rib

3. Apertures

    a. Aortic hiatus

        1. Median aperture bordered posteriorly by the body of the twelfth thoracic vertebra and anteriorly by the median arcuate ligament, a U-shaped, fibrous thickening of the medial margins of the left and right crura of the diaphragm; the thoracic aorta descends through the aortic hiatus and becomes the abdominal aorta

        2. Posteriorly, the aortic hiatus transmits the thoracic duct

    b. Esophageal hiatus

        1. Located anterior and to the left of the aortic hiatus, on a level with the tenth thoracic vertebra, and bounded by muscle fibers of the right crus of the diaphragm

        2. Transmits the esophagus, the anterior and posterior vagal trunks, and the esophageal branches/tributaries of the left gastric artery/vein

c. Foramen for the inferior vena cava

   1. Located to the right of the midline, further anterior than the esophageal hiatus, and within the central tendon at the level of the eighth thoracic vertebra

   2. Transmits the inferior vena cava

d. Other structures traversing the diaphragm

   1. The superior epigastric vessels penetrate the diaphragm between its sternal and costal parts

   2. The greater, lesser, and least splanchnic nerves enter the abdomen through the crura of the diaphragm; the azygos and hemiazygos veins are formed posterior to the crura (by the union of ascending lumbar and subcostal veins) and then ascend on lumbar and thoracic vertebral bodies

   3. The sympathetic trunks and subcostal nerves descend into the abdomen posterior to the medial arcuate and lateral arcuate ligaments, respectively

4. Blood supply: superior phrenic, inferior phrenic, musculophrenic, and pericardiacophrenic vessels

5. Innervation: phrenic nerves; derived from ventral rami C3, 4, and 5, especially C4 (the parietal peritoneum covering the inferior surface of the diaphragm receives its sensory innervation from the phrenic and intercostal nerves)

II. Vessels

A. Abdominal aorta

   1. Descends on the upper four lumbar vertebral bodies, to the left of the inferior vena cava; its branches are noted below

   2. Three unpaired branches, the celiac trunk, superior mesenteric artery, and inferior mesenteric artery, were described earlier (see pp. 101–102 and 107–108)

   3. Inferior phrenic arteries: arise immediately below the aortic hiatus; give rise to the superior suprarenal arteries for the suprarenal glands and supply the diaphragm

   4. Middle suprarenal arteries: arise at vertebral level L1 on either side of the superior mesenteric artery; supply the suprarenal glands

5. Renal arteries: arise at vertebral level L2, inferior to the origin of the superior mesenteric artery; supply the kidneys

6. Testicular/ovarian arteries: arise at vertebral level L2, inferior to the renal arteries, and descend on the psoas major muscles; supply the testes/ovaries

7. Lumbar arteries (four pairs): arise below the renal arteries; the upper and lower two pairs course laterally deep to the crura of the diaphragm and psoas major muscles, respectively, and supply the muscles of the posterior abdominal wall and the deep back muscles

8. Median sacral artery: small artery arising from the dorsal side of the abdominal aorta above its bifurcation; descends into the pelvis on the sacrum and supplies the rectum

9. Common iliac arteries: terminal branches of the aortic bifurcation at vertebral level L4; the umbilicus usually lies just above the level of the aortic bifurcation

B. External and internal iliac arteries: terminal branches of the common iliac artery near the sacroiliac joint; the internal iliac artery descends into the pelvis and the external iliac artery becomes the femoral artery as it passes deep to the inguinal ligament to enter the thigh

C. Inferior vena cava

1. Commences at the junction of the common iliac veins on the body of vertebra L5; the inferior vena cava is crossed anteriorly, from superior to inferior, by the superior part of the duodenum, the head of the pancreas, the horizontal part of the duodenum, the root of the mesentery, and the right testicular/ovarian artery

2. Tributaries: from inferior to superior, the inferior vena cava receives the lumbar veins, right testicular/ovarian vein, renal veins, right suprarenal vein, right inferior phrenic vein, and hepatic veins (the left suprarenal vein and left testicular/ovarian vein drain into the left renal vein; the left inferior phrenic vein drains into the left suprarenal vein)

D. Ascending lumbar vein: ascends anterior to the transverse processes of the lumbar vertebrae where it anastomoses with the lumbar veins; inferiorly, it anastomoses with the common iliac vein and, superiorly, it unites with the subcostal vein to form the hemiazygos vein on the left and the azygos vein on the right

E. Cisterna chyli

1. Inferior dilatation of the thoracic duct; receives lymphatic drainage from

structures inferior to the diaphragm via two lumbar trunks and a single intestinal trunk

2. Located to the right of the abdominal aorta on the bodies of vertebrae L1 and L2; absent in about 75 percent of individuals

III. Nerves

A. Lumbar plexus: derived from ventral rami of spinal nerves L1 to L5; its component nerves and their relation to the psoas major muscle were described earlier (see pp. 114–115)

B. Lumbar sympathetic trunks

1. Descend along the medial borders of the psoas major muscles; the left sympathetic trunk lies to the left of the abdominal aorta and the right sympathetic trunk lies posterior to the inferior vena cava

2. The first two lumbar sympathetic ganglia are connected to their respective ventral rami by white and gray rami communicantes; the inferior three lumbar sympathetic ganglia are connected to their respective ventral rami by gray rami communicantes only, since preganglionic sympathetic fibers do not exit the spinal cord below level L2

3. Medial branches of the lumbar sympathetic ganglia form the lumbar splanchnic nerves

IV. Kidney

A. Morphology

1. Bean-shaped, retroperitoneal organ surmounted by a suprarenal (adrenal) gland; its posterior surface contacts the diaphragm superiorly and the psoas major, quadratus lumborum, and transversus abdominis inferiorly

2. The superior poles of the right and left kidneys are on a level with the twelfth and eleventh ribs, respectively; both kidneys extend inferiorly to vertebral level L3

3. The hilum is the vertical, medial fissure through which vessels, nerves, and the renal pelvis enter or exit the kidney; lateral to the hilum, these structures pass through a fat-filled cavity called the renal sinus

4. Renal parenchyma

a. Renal cortex: granular appearing tissue located beneath the fibrous capsule; another part of the renal cortex, the renal columns, extends inward between the renal pyramids of the renal medulla

    b. Renal medulla: composed of five to eighteen cone-shaped renal pyramids whose bases are outwardly directed; the apex of a renal pyramid is called a renal papilla and extends into the renal sinus

    c. Lobe: consists of a renal pyramid and its overlying renal cortex

B. Renal pelvis and ureter

    1. Within the renal sinus the funnel-shaped renal pelvis lies posteriorly; it gives rise to two or three major calyces, each of which gives rise to several minor calyces which cap the renal papillae

    2. The renal pelvis narrows near the inferior pole of the kidney and becomes the ureter; it descends retroperitoneally on the anterior surface of the psoas major, passes posterior to the testicular/ovarian vessels, courses anterior to the bifurcation of the common iliac artery, and enters the pelvis

    3. Clinical note: since sympathetic afferents from the ureter travel with the lesser, least, lumbar, and sacral splanchnic nerves, visceral pain from the ureter, perhaps as the result of an impacted kidney stone, is referred to dermatomes T10 to L2 (lumbar and sacral splanchnic sympathetic afferents entering sympathetic ganglia L3 to S5 ascend in the sympathetic trunk to sympathetic ganglion L2 to gain access to a white ramus communicans)

C. Fat and fascia

    1. Perirenal fat: adipose tissue between the fibrous capsule and renal fascia; continuous with the fat within the renal sinus

    2. Renal fascia: membranous connective tissue layer surrounding the perirenal fat; merges medially with the adventitia of the renal vessels

    3. Pararenal fat: adipose tissue superficial to the renal fascia; covered by parietal peritoneum anteriorly, and transversalis fascia posteriorly

D. Vessels

    1. Renal arteries

        a. Course laterally, posterior to the renal veins; before entering the hilum, each renal artery divides into anterior and posterior rami that pass anterior and posterior to the renal pelvis, respectively, and which, in turn, divide into segmental branches

b. The right renal artery is longer than the left; it courses posterior to the inferior vena cava

c. Clinical notes

    1. Segmental branches of a renal artery do not anastomose, therefore, obstruction of a segmental artery or one of its branches leads to avascular necrosis of the part of the kidney supplied by the segmental artery or its branch

    2. Accessory renal arteries from the abdominal aorta are present in about 20 percent of individuals; usually, they do not pass through the hilum, but enter the kidney on its extrahilar surface

2. Renal veins

a. Drain into the inferior vena cava; at the hilum, tributaries emerge anterior and posterior to the renal pelvis

b. The left renal vein courses posterior to the pancreas and anterior to the abdominal aorta, just below the origin of the superior mesenteric artery; tributaries include the left suprarenal vein and left testicular/ovarian vein

c. The short right renal vein courses posterior to the descending part of the duodenum and head of the pancreas; it has no tributaries

3. Suprarenal arteries: a number of superior suprarenal arteries branch from the inferior phrenic artery; usually a single middle suprarenal artery arises from the abdominal aorta above the renal artery and one or more inferior suprarenal arteries arise from the renal artery

4. Suprarenal vein: emerges from an anterior hilum; on the left it drains into the left renal vein and on the right it drains into the inferior vena cava

5. Lymphatics from the kidneys and suprarenal glands drain into lumbar nodes which drain via the lumbar trunks into the cisterna chyli

E. Nerves

1. Innervation of the kidney: an aorticorenal ganglion on the renal artery receives preganglionic sympathetic fibers from the lesser and least splanchnic nerves which are formed by medial branches of sympathetic ganglia T10 and T11 and the medial branch of sympathetic ganglion T12, respectively; postganglionic sympathetic fibers from the aorticorenal ganglion are distributed to the renal artery and its branches and function in vasoconstriction (sympathetic afferents travel with the lesser

and least splanchnic nerves to spinal cord levels T10, 11, and 12, and mediate pain)

2. Innervation of the suprarenal medulla: receives preganglionic sympathetic fibers from the greater splanchnic nerve; cells of the suprarenal medulla are themselves modified postganglionic sympathetic neurons and, upon stimulation by fibers of the greater splanchnic nerve, release epinephrine and norepinephrine into the blood to produce a generalized sympathetic response (afferents are absent)

3. The kidney and suprarenal gland do not receive a parasympathetic innervation; the suprarenal cortex does not receive a sympathetic innervation

F. Clinical notes

1. The embryologic development of the kidney begins in the pelvis, however, due to differential growth, it assumes a position on the posterior abdominal wall; if this fails to occur, a pelvic or ectopic kidney results

2. Occasionally, as the kidneys ascend out of the pelvis, they fuse below the origin of the inferior mesenteric artery, forming a single "horseshoe" kidney

part **IV**

The Perineum and Pelvis

The Anal Triangle

I. Perineum

    A. Diamond-shaped area between the thighs and buttocks

    B. Boundaries

        1. Anterolateral: pubic arch; formed by the pubic symphysis, bodies and inferior rami of the pubic bones, and the rami of the ischia

        2. Posterolateral: sacrotuberous ligaments

        3. Roof: pelvic diaphragm (a muscular hammock within the bony pelvic ring)

        4. Floor: skin

    C. Divided by an imaginary line between the ischial tuberosities into a urogenital triangle anteriorly, and an anal triangle posteriorly

II. Structures of the Anal Triangle

    A. Anal canal

        1. Terminal portion of the large intestine between the rectum and anus; its length is about 2.5 centimeters

        2. Internal anatomy

            a. Anal columns

                1. Five to ten longitudinal mucosal ridges in the superior half of the anal canal; the inferior ends of the anal columns are joined by small, crescentic folds of mucosa called anal valves

2. A sinuous border, the pectinate line, lies immediately below the anal valves; the pocketlike recess above each anal valve is termed an anal sinus

3. Clinical note: fecal material may be retained by the anal sinuses or tear the anal valves; this may result in an infection or anal fissure (linear ulcer)

b. Transitional zone (pecten): extends inferiorly from the pectinate line to the white line (of Hilton); the white line is situated at the bottom of the palpable intersphincteric groove between the subcutaneous part of the external anal sphincter and the inferior border of the internal anal sphincter (it appears white due to its relative avascularity)

c. Anal verge: the distal portion of the anal canal from the white line to the perianal skin

3. The pectinate line represents the point of junction between the embryonic hindgut and an invagination of embryonic skin, the proctodeum, and thus, indicates a dividing line between two types of epithelia and two sources of nerve and arterial supply; it also represents a lymphatic and venous drainage "divide"

a. Anal canal above the pectinate line

1. Lined by simple columnar epithelium

2. Sensory innervation to the mucosa is provided by sympathetic afferent fibers that pass through the inferior hypogastric plexus and travel with the sacral splanchnic nerves

3. Arterial supply is from the superior rectal artery, a branch of the inferior mesenteric artery

4. Venous drainage is into the superior rectal vein, which drains into the inferior mesenteric vein, a tributary of the portal venous system; varicosities of superior rectal vein tributaries within the anal canal are referred to as internal hemorrhoids

5. Lymphatics drain to inferior mesenteric nodes

6. The characteristics of the anal canal above the pectinate line are also true of the rectum

b. Anal canal below the pectinate line

1. Lined by nonkeratinized stratified squamous epithelium

2. Sensory innervation to the mucosa is provided by somatic afferent fibers from the inferior rectal nerve, a branch of the pudendal nerve

3. Arterial supply is from the inferior rectal artery, a branch of the internal pudendal artery

4. Venous drainage is into the inferior rectal vein, which drains into the internal pudendal vein, a tributary of the systemic venous system; varicosities of inferior rectal vein tributaries within the anal canal are referred to as external hemorrhoids

5. Lymphatics drain to superficial inguinal lymph nodes

6. The characteristics of the anal canal below the pectinate line are also true of the perianal skin, except that the stratified squamous epithelium of the perianal skin is keratinized

c. Clinical notes

1. The part of the anal canal below the pectinate line is supplied by a somatic nerve and is thus very sensitive and responds to touch, pain, and thermal stimuli like skin; consequently, external hemorrhoids and anal fissures in this region are very painful, in contrast to internal hemorrhoids or anal fissures above the pectinate line (autonomic afferent fibers have a relatively high pain threshold)

2. Anastomoses between the superior rectal vein of the portal venous system and the inferior rectal vein of the systemic venous system occur in the region of the pectinate line; hemorrhoids or submucosal varicosities may result from an increase in pressure in the valveless portal venous system, for example, as a result of cirrhosis of the liver

3. Carcinomas or infections above the pectinate line will usually spread to inferior mesenteric nodes; carcinomas or infections below the pectinate line will usually spread to superficial inguinal nodes

4. Anal sphincters

a. Sphincteric musculature forms a series of rings around the anal canal; the tone of the anal sphincters keeps the anal canal closed, that is, it maintains anal continence

b. Internal anal sphincter

1. Formed by a thickened ring of the circular smooth muscle layer of the muscularis externa (the longitudinal smooth muscle layer

of the muscularis externa is replaced by a sleeve of connective tissue that surrounds the internal anal sphincter); extends from the anorectal junction to the white line, encircling the superior part of the anal canal

2. Controlled involuntarily by pelvic splanchnic nerves and postganglionic sympathetic fibers from the inferior hypogastric plexus; they cause relaxation and contraction, respectively

c. External anal sphincter

1. Composed of three parts, that is, three adjacent rings of skeletal muscle; together, they surround the whole length of the anal canal

2. Subcutaneous part

a. Lies deep to the perianal skin and surrounds the anal orifice; located inferior to the internal anal sphincter and superficial part of the external anal sphincter

b. The sleeve of connective tissue that replaced the longitudinal smooth muscle layer of the muscularis externa extends between the subcutaneous part of the external anal sphincter and internal anal sphincter to attach to the white line; this accounts for the relative avascularity of the white line

3. Superficial part: lies deep to the subcutaneous part and surrounds the inferior part of the internal anal sphincter

4. Deep part: lies deep to the superficial part and surrounds the superior part of the internal anal sphincter; its deepest fibers merge with those of the puborectalis muscle

5. Attaches anteriorly to the perineal body and posteriorly to the anococcygeal ligament and coccyx (the anococcygeal ligament is a mass of fibromuscular tissue between the anal canal and coccyx)

6. Controlled voluntarily by somatic fibers from the inferior rectal nerve

B. Ischioanal (ischiorectal) fossae

1. Two wedge-shaped, fat-filled spaces on either side of the anal canal

2. Walls

a. Lateral wall

1. Formed by the obturator fascia covering the inferior part of obturator internus

2. Pudendal (Alcock's) canal: lies within the obturator fascia medial to the ischial tuberosity and ischial ramus; contains the pudendal nerve and internal pudendal vessels

b. Roof: pelvic diaphragm

c. Medial wall: external anal sphincter

d. Floor: skin

e. Recesses

   1. Anterior recesses (two): pyramidal extensions of the ischioanal fossae into the urogenital triangle; they lie between the pelvic diaphragm superiorly, the urogenital diaphragm inferiorly, and the obturator fascia laterally

   2. Posterior recesses (two): lie deep to the inferior portions of the gluteus maximus muscles

f. Clinical note: posterior to the anal canal, the ischioanal fossae communicate with each other above and below the attachment of the external anal sphincter to the anococcygeal ligament and coccyx; infections may spread via this route from one ischioanal fossa to the other

3. Contents

   a. Inferior rectal nerve: arises from the pudendal nerve in the pudendal canal and courses medially across the ischioanal fossa to supply motor fibers to the external anal sphincter and sensory fibers to the mucosa of the anal canal below the pectinate line

   b. Inferior rectal artery: branches from the internal pudendal artery in the pudendal canal and courses medially across the ischioanal fossa with the inferior rectal nerve to supply the anal canal below the pectinate line

   c. Inferior rectal vein: drains the anal canal below the pectinate line and courses laterally across the ischioanal fossa with the inferior rectal artery to join the internal pudendal vein in the pudendal canal

The Urogenital Triangle

I. Urogenital Diaphragm

    A. Located within the urogenital triangle, inferior to the anterior part of the pelvic diaphragm, and penetrated by the membranous urethra as well as the vagina in the female; its fasciae and muscles are noted below

    B. Superior and inferior fasciae of the urogenital diaphragm

        1. Attached to the pubic arch and fused posteriorly, enclosing the deep perineal pouch and its contents

        2. The superior fascia of the urogenital diaphragm consists of a thin layer of loose connective tissue inferior to the pelvic diaphragm; the inferior fascia of the urogenital diaphragm, or perineal membrane, is a thick sheet of connective tissue

    C. Muscles

        1. Lie within the deep perineal pouch, between the superior and inferior fasciae of the urogenital diaphragm

        2. Sphincter urethrae

            a. Surrounds and compresses the membranous urethra, and thus maintains urinary continence

            b. In the male, the bulbourethral (Cowper's) glands lie within the deep perineal pouch on each side of the membranous urethra

3. Deep transverse perineal muscle

    a. Fibers run transversely attaching on each side to the pubic arch; some posterior fibers attach to the perineal body

    b. Supports the pelvic viscera, especially through its attachment to the perineal body

4. Innervation: perineal nerves, branches of the pudendal nerves

II. Superficial Perineal Pouch

  A. Associated fasciae

    1. Bounded deeply by the inferior fascia of the urogenital diaphragm or perineal membrane

    2. Bounded superficially by the deep perineal fascia

      a. The deep perineal fascia is comparable to the deep fascia covering the external abdominal oblique and rectus abdominis; it attaches to the pubic arch and posterior margin of the urogenital diaphragm

      b. The deep perineal fascia continues into the penis as the deep penile fascia as far as the glans; it does not extend into the scrotum

  B. Contents

    1. In the female, the superficial perineal pouch contains the crura of the clitoris, bulbs of the vestibule, and the greater vestibular (Bartholin's) glands; in the male, it contains the crura and bulb of the penis

    2. Muscles

      a. Superficial transverse perineal muscles

        1. Origin: ischial tuberosities

        2. Insertion: perineal body

        3. Action: support the pelvic viscera

      b. Ischiocavernosus muscles

        1. Origin: ischial tuberosities, rami of the ischia, and perineal membrane

  2. Insertion: crura of the penis/clitoris

  3. Action: may play a role in maintaining erection by compressing the crura and impeding venous return

 c. Bulbospongiosus (bulbocavernosus) muscles

  1. Origin: female—perineal body; male—perineal body and the midline raphe on the ventral surface of the penis

  2. Insertion: female—bulbs of the vestibule; male—dorsal aspect of the bulb and body of the penis

  3. Action: female—diminish the orifice of the vagina; male—help to expel urine and semen

 d. Innervation: perineal nerves, branches of the pudendal nerves

III. Potential Space

 A. Associated fasciae

  1. Bounded deeply by the deep perineal fascia

  2. Bounded superficially by the superficial perineal fascia (Colles' fascia)

   a. The superficial perineal fascia is continuous with the membranous layer of the superficial fascia of the anterior abdominal wall (Scarpa's fascia); attaches to the pubic arch and posterior margin of the urogenital diaphragm and descends into the scrotum as the dartos fascia

   b. Continues into the penis as the superficial penile fascia, which extends into the prepuce and then reflects back on itself to attach at the junction of the glans and body

 B. Contents: none

 C. Clinical notes

  1. The urethra in the male may be ruptured inferior to the perineal membrane, perhaps as the result of the faulty insertion of a catheter or a perineal straddling injury; if the deep perineal fascia is not torn, extravasated urine may be limited to the superficial perineal pouch, distending the perineum within the pubic arch as well as the body of the penis (urine cannot pass posteriorly into the anal triangle because the deep perineal fascia attaches to the posterior margin of the urogenital diaphragm)

2. If the deep perineal fascia is also torn, extravasated urine may accumulate in the potential space between the superficial and deep perineal fasciae, distending the perineum as far posteriorly as the posterior margin of the urogenital diaphragm, as well as the body of the penis, prepuce, scrotum, and anterior abdominal wall (urine cannot pass into the thighs because Scarpa's fascia fuses with the deep fascia of the thigh just distal to the inguinal ligament)

IV. Perineal Body

A. Substantial fibromuscular mass lying midway along the posterior margin of the urogenital diaphragm, between the anus and vagina in the female and the anus and scrotum in the male; it is also referred to as the central tendon of the perineum or the perineum

B. Serves as a central point of attachment for the deep transverse perineal muscle, superficial transverse perineal muscles, bulbospongiosus muscles, external anal sphincter, and pubococcygeus muscles; through these attachments it provides important support for the pelvic viscera

C. Clinical notes

1. To prevent uncontrolled tearing of the perineal body during childbirth and possibly a difficult sutural repair, a clean incision from the vagina toward the anus may be performed; this surgical procedure is referred to as an episiotomy

2. Failure to repair a torn perineal body following childbirth may result in prolapse or downward displacement of pelvic viscera

V. Penis

A. Regions

1. Root: composed of the two crura and bulb of the penis

2. Body: extends from the pubic symphysis to the glans; composed of the two corpora cavernosa and the corpus spongiosum

3. Glans: mushroomlike, terminal enlargement of the corpus spongiosum

B. Erectile tissue

1. Composed of connective tissue containing large venous spaces

2. Corpora cavernosa

   a. Commence as the two crura attached to each side of the pubic arch and perineal membrane; they fuse at the pubic symphysis

   b. Their rounded distal ends are covered by the glans

3. Corpus spongiosum

   a. Bulb of the penis

      1. Proximal enlargement of the corpus spongiosum

      2. The membranous urethra penetrates its superior surface and bends anteriorly at almost a right angle to run in the corpus spongiosum as the penile (spongy) urethra; the ducts of the bulbourethral glands pass through the bulb of the penis and empty into the proximal end of the penile urethra

      3. Clinical note: because of the abrupt change in direction of the penile urethra in the bulb of the penis, it is prone to injury here during insertion of a catheter

   b. In the body of the penis, the narrow intermediate portion of the corpus spongiosum fuses to the ventromedial grooved surfaces of the corpora cavernosa; distally, the corpus spongiosum expands to form the glans

4. The corpora cavernosa are responsible for producing penile erection; the erectile tissue of the corpus spongiosum does not contribute significantly to an erection

C. Fasciae and ligaments

1. Superficial penile fascia

   a. Located between the skin and deep penile fascia; it is continuous with the superficial perineal fascia (Colles' fascia), the membranous layer of the superficial fascia of the anterior abdominal wall (Scarpa's fascia), and the dartos fascia of the scrotum

   b. Extends into the prepuce and then reflects back on itself to attach at the junction of the glans and body

2. Deep penile fascia

   a. Located between the superficial penile fascia and tunica albuginea; it is continuous with the deep perineal fascia

      b. It does not continue into the prepuce, extending only as far as the glans

  3. Tunica albuginea

      a. Thick, dense connective tissue layer deep to the deep penile fascia; it binds together the corpora cavernosa and corpus spongiosum in the body of the penis

      b. The deep dorsal vein of the penis, the dorsal arteries of the penis, and the dorsal nerves of the penis course between the deep penile fascia and tunica albuginea

  4. Suspensory ligament of the penis: attaches the deep penile fascia at the proximal, dorsal end of the body of the penis to the pubic symphysis; it is derived from the deep fascia covering the rectus abdominis

  5. Fundiform ligament of the penis

      a. Descends from the inferior part of the linea alba and blends with the superficial penile fascia, forming a sling around the proximal part of the body of the penis

      b. Derived from the membranous layer of the superficial fascia of the anterior abdominal wall (Scarpa's fascia)

VI. Female External Genitalia (Vulva)

  A. Labia majora: wide folds of skin and subcutaneous fat; they contain the round ligaments of the uterus

  B. Labia minora

    1. Thin, fat-free folds of skin medial to the labia majora

    2. The cleft between the labia minora is the vestibule of the vagina

      a. Anteriorly, the vestibule of the vagina receives the external urethral orifice

      b. The vaginal orifice opens posterior to the external urethral orifice; the hymen is a semilunar fold of mucous membrane forming the posterior border of the vaginal orifice

3. Anteriorly, each labium minus divides into two folds; the anterior folds pass to the dorsal side of the clitoris and fuse to form the prepuce of the clitoris and the posterior folds fuse to form the frenulum of the clitoris on the ventral side of the clitoris

C. Clitoris

1. Its body is composed of the two fused corpora cavernosa; they are the distal continuations of the two crura of the clitoris which lie along the sides of the pubic arch

2. The proximal, dorsal end of the body is attached to the pubic symphysis by the suspensory ligament of the clitoris; the clitoris ends distally at the glans

D. Bulbs of the vestibule

1. Oval masses of erectile tissue on each side of the vaginal orifice; they lie within the superficial perineal pouch, deep to the labia minora

2. The mucus-secreting greater vestibular (Bartholin's) glands lie at the posterior ends of the vestibular bulbs; their ducts open into the vestibule of the vagina on each side of the vaginal orifice

VII. Pudendal Nerve

A. Branch of the sacral plexus; formed by contributions from ventral rami of spinal nerves S2 to S4

B. After giving off the inferior rectal nerve within the pudendal canal, the pudendal nerve divides into its terminal branches, the perineal nerve and dorsal nerve of the penis/clitoris, as it exits the pudendal canal near the posterior border of the urogenital diaphragm

1. Perineal nerve: motor branches supply the muscles within the deep and superficial perineal pouches; the posterior scrotal/labial nerves are sensory branches that supply the skin of the posterior portion of the scrotum/labium majus

2. Dorsal nerve of the penis/clitoris: passes anteriorly along the medial surface of the crus and then pierces the suspensory ligament of the penis/clitoris to run lateral to the dorsal artery of the penis/clitoris on the dorsum of the penis/clitoris; provides cutaneous innervation to the body, glans, and prepuce of the penis/clitoris

VIII. Vessels

    A. Arteries

        1. Perineal artery

            a. Arises from the internal pudendal artery as it exits the pudendal canal near the posterior border of the urogenital diaphragm; its branches are noted below

            b. Transverse branch: passes medially along the superficial transverse perineal muscle to the perineal body

            c. Posterior scrotal/labial arteries: accompany the posterior scrotal/labial nerves to the posterior portion of the scrotum/labium majus

        2. Artery of the bulb: arises from the internal pudendal artery distal to the perineal artery; supplies the bulb of the penis, corpus spongiosum, and glans in the male, and the bulb of the vestibule and greater vestibular (Bartholin's) gland in the female

        3. The internal pudendal artery continues anteriorly along the medial surface of the crus; here, it divides into its terminal branches, the deep artery of the penis/clitoris and the dorsal artery of the penis/clitoris

            a. Deep artery of the penis/clitoris: enters the erectile tissue of the crus of the penis/clitoris to supply it and its continuation, the corpus cavernosum

            b. Dorsal artery of the penis/clitoris

                1. Continues anteriorly along the medial surface of the crus; pierces the suspensory ligament of the penis/clitoris and courses distally on the dorsum of the penis/clitoris, between the deep dorsal vein of the penis/clitoris and the dorsal nerve of the penis/clitoris

                2. Supplies the skin, fasciae, prepuce, and glans of the penis/clitoris

    B. Veins

        1. Veins in the region of the urogenital triangle traveling with branches of the internal pudendal artery join the internal pudendal vein

        2. Deep dorsal vein of the penis/clitoris

            a. Courses proximally in the midline on the dorsal surface of the body of the penis/clitoris between the dorsal arteries of the penis/clitoris; drains the erectile tissue of the penis/clitoris

b. Pierces the suspensory ligament of the penis/clitoris to course inferior to the pubic symphysis to join the prostatic venous plexus in the male or the vesical venous plexus in the female

C. Lymphatics

1. Deep perineal pouch: lymphatics drain along the internal pudendal vessels to internal iliac nodes

2. Superficial perineal pouch: lymphatics drain to superficial inguinal nodes

The Pelvis

I. Bones and Bony Landmarks

    A. Pelvic (hip) bone

        1. Composed of three bones, the ilium, ischium, and pubis; they meet in the acetabulum (a cup-shaped cavity that receives the head of the femur) and fuse at about age 16

        2. Ilium

           a. Ala

               1. Upper, flat, expanded, winglike part; its bony landmarks are noted below

               2. Auricular surface: medial, ear-shaped, articular region; forms a synovial sacroiliac joint with an auricular surface of the sacrum

               3. Iliac fossa: anterior, shallow concavity

               4. Iliac crest: convex, superior border; its highest point is on a level with the spinous process of vertebra L4

               5. Anterior superior iliac spine: prominence at the anterior end of the iliac crest; palpable at the junction of the anterolateral abdominal wall and thigh

           b. Body: lower, bulky portion that forms the superior part of the acetabulum; medially, it is divided from the ala by a ridge, the arcuate line

3. Ischium

    a. Body: bulky, superior portion that forms the posteroinferior part of the acetabulum; medially, it exhibits a pointed projection, the ischial spine

    b. Ramus: inferior, curved part that exhibits a posterior, bony mass, the ischial tuberosity

    c. Greater sciatic notch: concavity superior to the ischial spine

    d. Lesser sciatic notch: concavity between the ischial spine and ischial tuberosity

4. Pubis

    a. Body

        1. Wide, medial part; its bony landmarks are noted below

        2. Pubic crest: superior border

        3. Pubic tubercle: rounded projection at the lateral end of the pubic crest

        4. Symphysial surface: oval, medial surface

    b. Superior ramus

        1. Upper part that bounds the obturator foramen superiorly and forms the anteroinferior part of the acetabulum; its bony landmarks are noted below

        2. Pecten pubis: ridge extending posteriorly from the pubic tubercle; continuous anteriorly and posteriorly with the pubic crest and arcuate line, respectively

        3. Iliopubic eminence: rounded elevation between the superior ramus of the pubis and iliac fossa

    c. Inferior ramus: flat, lower part; with the ramus of the ischium, it bounds the obturator foramen inferiorly

B. Sacrum

    1. Triangular bone formed by the fusion of the five sacral vertebrae; its ventral surface faces inferiorly

2. Promontory: anteriorly projecting edge of the superior surface of the body of vertebra S1

3. Ala: lateral, winglike extensions on each side of the body of vertebra S1

4. Auricular surfaces: lateral, ear-shaped, articular regions that form the synovial sacroiliac joints with the auricular surfaces of the ilia

5. Sacral canal: central canal transmitting the dorsal and ventral roots of spinal nerves S1 to S5 and the coccygeal spinal nerve

6. Ventral and dorsal sacral foramina (four pairs each): transmit the ventral and dorsal rami of spinal nerves S1 to S4, respectively

C. Coccyx: small, triangular bone formed by three to five rudimentary coccygeal vertebrae; may occur in two or three separate parts

D. Orientation of the bony pelvic ring: in the anatomical position, the anterior superior iliac spines and pubic tubercles are in the same coronal plane

E. Pelvic inlet and outlet

1. Pelvic inlet

a. Defined by the pelvic brim

   1. Bounded on each side by the pubic crest, pecten pubis, arcuate line, anterior border of the ala of the sacrum, and promontory

   2. The lesser or true pelvis lies below the pelvic brim; the greater or false pelvis lies above the pelvic brim, bounded on each side by an ala of an ilium

b. Diameters

   1. Conjugate or anteroposterior diameter: measured from the superior border of the pubic symphysis to the midpoint of the sacral promontory

   2. Transverse diameter: maximum side-to-side distance between corresponding points of the pelvic brim

2. Pelvic outlet

a. Bordered anterolaterally by the pubic arch and posterolaterally by the sacrotuberous ligaments; the coccyx projects into the pelvic outlet posteriorly

b. Diameters

    1. Conjugate or anteroposterior diameter: measured from the inferior border of the pubic symphysis to the tip of the coccyx

    2. Transverse diameter: distance between the ischial tuberosities

c. Sex difference: in the female the pubic arch has an angle of about 90°; in the male the angle is about 60°

II. Joints and Ligaments

  A. Pubic symphysis: fibrocartilaginous joint between the symphysial surfaces of the bodies of the pubic bones

  B. Sacroiliac joint

    1. Synovial joint between an auricular surface of an ilium and an auricular surface of the sacrum; permits a small amount of movement

    2. Ventral and dorsal sacroiliac ligaments: transversely oriented ligaments ventral and dorsal to a sacroiliac joint, respectively

  C. Sacrotuberous and sacrospinous ligaments

    1. Extend from the sacrum to the ischial tuberosity and ischial spine, respectively; stabilize the sacroiliac joints by resisting forward movement of the promontory

    2. The sacrotuberous ligament forms the inferior boundary of the lesser sciatic foramen; the sacrospinous ligament divides the lesser sciatic foramen from the greater sciatic foramen

  D. Obturator membrane: dense connective tissue sheet closing the obturator foramen, except superiorly, where the obturator nerve and vessels pass through the obturator canal; provides attachment for obturator internus and obturator externus on its internal and external surfaces, respectively

  E. Clinical note: a loosening of the ligaments of the bony pelvic ring occurs during pregnancy to facilitate the passage of the fetus through the pelvic inlet and pelvic outlet

III. Muscles

  A. Pelvic wall

    1. Piriformis

      a. Origin: ventral surface of the sacrum

b. Insertion: emerges from the pelvis through the greater sciatic foramen and inserts on the medial aspect of the greater trochanter

c. Action: lateral rotation of the hip

d. Innervation: nerve to the piriformis

2. Obturator internus

a. Origin: internal surface of the obturator membrane and the surrounding bone

b. Insertion: emerges from the pelvis through the lesser sciatic foramen, turns at an acute angle over the ischium, and inserts on the medial aspect of the greater trochanter

c. Action: lateral rotation of the hip

d. Innervation: nerve to the obturator internus

e. The thick obturator fascia covers its upper pelvic and lower perineal surfaces

B. Pelvic diaphragm

1. Levator ani

a. Pubococcygeus

   1. Origin: anterior part of the arcus tendineus or tendinous arch; the tendinous arch is a linear thickening of the obturator fascia extending from the body of the pubis to the ischial spine

   2. Insertion: perineal body, anococcygeal ligament, and coccyx

   3. Puborectalis muscle: U-shaped, muscular sling that loops behind the anorectal junction; formed by medial fibers of the pubococcygeus muscles (within the urogenital triangle, the midline gap delimited by the puborectalis muscle is termed the urogenital hiatus; it transmits the urethra as well as the vagina in the female)

b. Iliococcygeus

   1. Origin: posterior part of the tendinous arch

   2. Insertion: anococcygeal ligament and coccyx

   3. May be mostly aponeurotic

    c. Action: supports the pelvic viscera; the puborectalis portion of the pubococcygeus muscles plays an important sphincteric role in maintaining anal continence

    d. Innervation: nerve to the levator ani

  2. Coccygeus (ischiococcygeus)

    a. Origin: ischial spine

    b. Insertion: sacrum and coccyx

    c. Action: supports the pelvic viscera

    d. Innervation: nerve to the coccygeus

IV. Viscera

  A. Urinary bladder

    1. Reservoir whose size, shape, and position changes as it fills with urine

      a. When empty, it lies within the lesser pelvis behind the bodies of the pubic bones; when distended, it assumes an ovoid shape and may extend to the umbilicus

      b. An empty urinary bladder has the shape of a three-sided pyramid with two inferolateral surfaces, a superior surface, and a posterior surface or base

        1. The pointed, anterior end is the apex and the narrow inferior part is the neck; the superior and inferolateral surfaces define the body

        2. The triangular base is often called the trigone

          a. Its angles are marked posterolaterally by the orifices of the ureters and inferiorly by the internal urethral orifice

          b. Its mucosal surface remains smooth and does not stretch or contract as the urinary bladder fills and empties

    2. The interlacing smooth muscle of the urinary bladder wall is collectively known as the detrusor muscle; the oblique course of the ureters through the detrusor muscle serves to compress the ureter as the urinary bladder fills, thus preventing backflow of urine into the ureter

3. Peritoneal relations

   a. Parietal peritoneum from the posterior surface of the anterior abdominal wall becomes visceral peritoneum as it continues inferiorly onto the superior surface of the urinary bladder; peritoneum extends laterally from the urinary bladder to line the paravesical fossae, depressions on either side of the urinary bladder

   b. In the male, the peritoneum descends onto the posterior surface of the urinary bladder, covers the seminal vesicles, and is then reflected onto the anterior surface of the rectum forming the rectovesical pouch; in the female, the peritoneum reflects from the urinary bladder onto the uterus, lining the vesicouterine pouch

   c. Clinical note: the urinary bladder may be surgically approached superior to the bodies of the pubic bones, without incising the peritoneum

4. Ligaments

   a. In the male and female, the neck of the urinary bladder is attached to the pubic symphysis by the puboprostatic and pubovesical ligaments, respectively

   b. The median umbilical ligament, the remains of the embryonic urachus, extends from the apex of the urinary bladder to the umbilicus

5. Clinical note: cystitis or inflammation of the bladder is more common in females because of the relatively short distance between the urinary bladder and the external environment (via the urethra)

B. Male urethra

1. Divided into three parts; from proximal to distal, they are termed the prostatic, membranous, and penile (spongy) urethrae

2. Prostatic urethra

   a. Descends through the substance of the prostate

   b. Urethral crest

      1. Median mucosal ridge on the posterior wall of the prostatic urethra

      2. Expands at about its middle into an oval elevation, the colliculus seminalis

         a. The prostatic utricle, a vestigial, blind-ending diverticulum representing the male homologue of the uterus, opens near the center of the colliculus seminalis

　　　b. Two tiny, ejaculatory ducts open onto the colliculus seminalis on each side of the prostatic utricle

　　3. On either side of the urethral crest there is a shallow depression, the prostatic sinus; receive the numerous prostatic ducts

　3. Membranous urethra: short, intermediate part; encircled by the sphincter urethrae as it passes through the urogenital diaphragm

　4. Penile urethra: enters the bulb of the penis and then bends anteriorly at almost a right angle to run within the corpus spongiosum; terminates at the external urethral orifice on the glans

C. Prostate

　1. Cone-shaped; its base contacts the neck of the bladder, its apex is in contact with the superior fascia of the urogenital diaphragm, and, on each side, it is supported by the pubococcygeus muscles

　2. Bound to the pubic symphysis by the puboprostatic ligament; its whitish secretion contains enzymes that liquify semen and buffers that neutralize the acid pH of the vagina

　3. Clinical notes

　　　a. Benign enlargement of the prostate commonly occurs after the age of 50 and may result in narrowing of the prostatic urethra and impedence of urine flow; the prostate is also a frequent site of malignancy

　　　b. An enlarged prostate may be detected by digital rectal examination

D. Ductus (vas) deferens

　1. After ascending through the inguinal canal, the ductus deferens descends into the lesser pelvis; at the base of the urinary bladder, it courses superior, then medial to the ureter

　2. Its distal, dilated portion, the ampulla, narrows before joining the duct of the seminal vesicle to form the ejaculatory duct; the ureter penetrates the urinary bladder wall between the ampulla of the ductus deferens and seminal vesicle

E. Seminal vesicle

1. Blind-ending, sacculated tube; located lateral to the ampulla of the ductus deferens on the posterior surface of the bladder

2. Its yellowish secretion contains fructose, which is nutritive to spermatozoa; spermatozoa are stored in the epididymis, ductus deferens, and ampulla of the ductus deferens, but not in the seminal vesicle

F. Ejaculatory duct: formed by the union of the ductus deferens and the duct of the seminal vesicle near the base of the prostate; passes through the posterior portion of the prostate and opens onto the colliculus seminalis lateral to the prostatic utricle

G. Ovary

1. Suspensory ligament of the ovary: fold of peritoneum suspending the ovary from the pelvic brim; contains the ovarian vessels, which descend over the pelvic brim adjacent to the ureter

2. Ligament of the ovary: band of connective tissue and smooth muscle extending from the ovary to the lateral margin of the uterus, below the uterotubal junction

H. Uterine (Fallopian) tube or oviduct

1. Extends from the ovary to the uterus; serves as a conduit for ova and spermatozoa

2. Parts

a. Infundibulum

   1. Funnellike, lateral end; its rim has a fringe of fingerlike processes called fimbriae that embrace the ovary

   2. Opens into the peritoneal cavity and thus provides for communication between the peritoneal cavity and the external environment (via the uterine tube, uterus, cervix, and vagina)

b. Ampulla: wide part medial to the infundibulum; comprises about half of the uterine tube

c. Isthmus: narrow part between the ampulla and intramural part; comprises approximately one-third of the uterine tube

d. Intramural (uterine) part: passes through the wall of the uterus and opens into the uterine cavity

3. Clinical notes

   a. The uterine tube is where fertilization usually occurs and is a common site of ectopic pregnancy; tubal rupture is a medical emergency and must be considered as a possible cause of acute abdominal pain in women

   b. Peritonitis or inflammation of the peritoneal cavity is more frequent in females because the peritoneal cavity is in communication with the external environment

I. Uterus

1. General remarks

   a. Thick-walled, muscular organ shaped like an inverted pear; it is flattened anteroposteriorly and has a narrow triangular lumen

   b. Located within the lesser pelvis, posterior to the urinary bladder and anterior to the rectum

2. Parts

   a. Fundus: upper, rounded part above the entrance of the uterine tubes

   b. Body: tapering, intermediate part

   c. Cervix: cylindrical, lower part of the uterus whose inferior part projects into the vagina; the cavity of the cervix, or cervical canal, communicates with the uterine cavity and vagina through its internal os and external os, respectively

3. Peritoneal relations

   a. The anterior surface of the uterus is covered with peritoneum as far inferiorly as the superior part of the cervix; it then reflects forward onto the posterior surface of the urinary bladder to form the vesicouterine pouch

   b. The posterior surface of the uterus is covered with peritoneum which extends as far inferiorly as the superior part of the vagina; it then reflects backward onto the anterior surface of the rectum to form the rectouterine pouch or pouch of Douglas

4. Orientation: the body of the uterus is angled forward, or anteflexed, on the cervix; the cervix is also angled forward, or anteverted, in relation to the vagina (the longitudinal axes of the body of the uterus and vagina form a right angle)

5. Ligaments

   a. Broad ligament

      1. Formed by the two layers of peritoneum that come together along the lateral margin of the body of the uterus and extend to the lateral pelvic wall; supports the uterus in the pelvic cavity

      2. Parts

         a. Mesovarium: fold of the posterior layer of the broad ligament that suspends the ovary

         b. Mesosalpinx: portion of the broad ligament superior to the mesovarium; it contains the uterine tube in its upper free margin

         c. Mesometrium: portion of the broad ligament inferior to the mesovarium

   b. Round ligament

      1. Continuation of the musculofibrous ovarian ligament; both the ovarian ligament and round ligament of the uterus are derivatives of the genitoinguinal ligament of the embryo

      2. Commences below the uterotubal junction and courses forward to the deep inguinal ring; traverses the inguinal canal and ends in the labium majus

   c. Cardinal (transverse cervical) ligament

      1. Thick mass of extraperitoneal connective tissue within the base of the mesometrium; extends from the cervix to the lateral pelvic wall and supports the uterus in the pelvic cavity

      2. The uterine vessels course along its superior aspect

      3. Clinical note: stretching of the cardinal ligaments during childbirth may contribute to prolapse or downward displacement of the uterus into the vagina

d. Uterosacral ligament

1. Condensation of extraperitoneal connective tissue extending from the cervix to the sacrum; lateral to the rectum, it forms a fold of peritoneum, the rectouterine fold

2. Functions to support the uterus in the pelvic cavity and helps maintain its anteflexed and anteverted position

J. Vagina

1. Highly distensible, fibromuscular tube; descends anteroinferiorly from the cervix

2. The upper end of the vagina forms a circular gutter around the inferior part of the cervix; the different regions of the gutter are designated the anterior, posterior, and lateral fornices of the vagina

3. The urethra commences at the internal urethral orifice and descends within the anterior wall of the vagina; it terminates at the external urethral orifice anterior to the vaginal orifice, in the vestibule of the vagina

4. The upper, anterior wall of the vagina contacts the bladder; its posterior wall contacts the rectum and anal canal

5. Clinical note: in certain procedures, the peritoneal cavity is entered through the posterior fornix of the vagina

K. Rectum

1. The part of the large intestine between the sigmoid colon and anal canal; extends from the third sacral vertebra to the tip of the coccyx, and measures about 15 centimeters in length

2. External anatomy

a. The sigmoid mesocolon ends

b. The taeniae coli blend to form a complete longitudinal smooth muscle layer around the rectum, thus, there are no haustra; epiploic appendages are also absent

c. As the rectum descends along the ventral surface of the sacrum and coccyx, it exhibits a curvature that is concave anteriorly and called the sacral flexure

d. Its dilated, distal portion is the rectal ampulla

e. Peritoneal relations

   1. Superior one-third: peritoneum covers its anterior and lateral surfaces; peritoneum that extends laterally from the rectum lines the pararectal fossae, depressions on either side of the rectum

   2. Middle one-third: peritoneum covers only the anterior surface from which it is reflected onto the bladder in the male forming the rectovesical pouch; in the female it is reflected onto the upper part of the vagina, cervix, and uterus forming the rectouterine pouch or pouch of Douglas

   3. Inferior one-third: lies inferior to the parietal peritoneum, and thus has no peritoneal relation

f. Puborectalis

   1. Medial part of the pubococcygeus muscles; forms a U-shaped muscular sling behind the anorectal junction, pulling it forward, producing the perineal flexure of the rectum

   2. Clinical notes

      a. The puborectalis plays an important sphincteric role, such that if it is torn or severed, anal incontinence results

      b. With the deep part of the external anal sphincter, the puborectalis forms the anorectal ring, a circumferential ridge which protrudes into the lumen at the anorectal junction and is palpable in digital rectal examination

3. Internal anatomy: three, shelflike, transverse rectal folds (valves of Houston) are found in the rectum; they may serve to support fecal material within the rectum

4. Vessels: the rectum is supplied primarily by the superior rectal artery, a branch of the inferior mesenteric artery, and is drained by the superior rectal vein, a tributary of the inferior mesenteric vein; lymphatics drain to inferior mesenteric nodes

5. Nerves: pelvic splanchnic nerves and postganglionic sympathetic fibers from the inferior hypogastric plexuses supply the rectum; they increase and inhibit peristaltic and secretory activity, respectively

6. Clinical notes: structures palpable in digital rectal examination

   a. Male

      1. Anteriorly: prostate, seminal vesicles, and base of the bladder

2. Posteriorly: coccyx and sacrum

3. Laterally: ischial tuberosity, sacrotuberous ligament, and ischial spine

4. Circumferentially

    a. Intersphincteric groove and its bordering subcutaneous part of the external anal sphincter and internal anal sphincter

    b. The protruding anorectal ring at the anorectal junction; formed by the puborectalis and the deep part of the external anal sphincter (somewhat deficient anteriorly due to the absence of the U-shaped puborectalis)

    b. Female: same as the male, except anteriorly, where the vagina, cervix, and uterus are palpable

V. Vessels

  A. Internal iliac artery

    1. Arises at the bifurcation of the common iliac artery near the sacroiliac joint and descends over the pelvic brim; divides into an anterior and a posterior trunk, whose branches supply most of the pelvic structures

    2. Anterior trunk

        a. Exhibits a highly variable pattern of branching; branches are often best identified on the basis of their area of termination

        b. Umbilical artery

            1. Its patent, proximal portion courses anteriorly along the lateral wall of the pelvis and gives off two or three superior vesical arteries to the superior surface of the bladder; the artery of the ductus deferens usually arises from one of the superior vesical arteries

            2. Its obliterated, distal portion continues to the umbilicus as the medial umbilical ligament

        c. Inferior vesical artery: supplies the inferior part of the bladder; in the male, it also supplies the prostate and seminal vesicle

        d. Middle rectal artery: courses medially to the rectum; may arise from the inferior vesical or internal pudendal artery or may be absent

e. Uterine artery (female only)

　　1. Courses medially, superior to the ureter, along the superior aspect of the cardinal ligament; near the lateral fornix of the vagina it gives off branches to the upper part of the vagina and cervix, and then courses superiorly along the lateral margin of the uterus

　　2. Near the uterotubal junction it gives off its tubal and ovarian branches

　　3. Clinical note: during a hysterectomy the ureter is liable to injury when severing the uterine vessels near the lateral fornix of the vagina

f. Vaginal artery (female only): courses inferior to the ureter to supply the lower part of the vagina; often arises from the uterine artery

g. Internal pudendal artery

　　1. Exits the pelvis through the greater sciatic foramen between the piriformis and coccygeus

　　2. After crossing the back of the ischial spine, it enters the lesser sciatic foramen and then the pudendal canal; supplies perineal structures

h. Inferior gluteal artery: usually descends between the first and second sacral ventral rami before exiting the pelvis through the greater sciatic foramen between the piriformis and coccygeus; supplies structures of the gluteal region

i. Obturator artery

　　1. Exits the pelvis through the obturator canal with the obturator vein and nerve; supplies the obturator externus muscle in the thigh

　　2. Clinical note: in about 25 percent of individuals, the obturator artery originates from the inferior epigastric artery and descends posterior to the superior ramus of the pubis to enter the obturator canal; one needs to be aware of this abnormal origin during hernia repairs in this region

3. Posterior trunk

a. Superior gluteal artery: usually descends between the lumbosacral trunk and first sacral ventral ramus before exiting the pelvis through the greater sciatic foramen superior to the piriformis; supplies structures of the gluteal region

b. Iliolumbar artery: ascends into the greater pelvis anterior to the sacroiliac joint; supplies the iliacus and psoas major muscles

c. Lateral sacral artery: descends on the ventral surface of the sacrum; branches enter the ventral sacral foramina to supply the contents of the sacral canal

B. Internal iliac vein

1. Tributaries parallel corresponding branches of the internal iliac artery, however, there is no umbilical vein; also, they receive the prostatic and vesical venous plexuses and anastomose with the external and internal vertebral venous plexuses

2. Clinical note: metastases of neoplasms from pelvic viscera may become widely dispersed via anastomoses of pelvic veins with the vertebral venous plexuses

C. Lymphatics drain to internal iliac nodes

VI. Nerves

A. Somatic nerves

1. Derived from the sacral plexus, which is formed on the ventral surface of the piriformis by ventral rami L4 to S4 (L4 and L5 contributions are from the lumbosacral trunk)

2. Sciatic nerve (L4, 5, S1, 2, 3): supplies muscles and skin of the lower limb

3. Pudendal nerve (S2, 3, 4): accompanies the internal pudendal vessels; supplies perineal structures

4. Nerve to the piriformis (S2): innervates piriformis

5. Nerves to the levator ani and coccygeus (S4): innervate the levator ani and coccygeus

6. Superior gluteal nerve (L4, 5, S1): accompanies superior gluteal vessels; innervates gluteus medius, gluteus minimus, and tensor fasciae latae

7. Inferior gluteal nerve (L5, S1, 2): accompanies the inferior gluteal vessels; innervates gluteus maximus

8. Nerve to the obturator internus (L5, S1, 2): innervates the obturator internus and superior gemellus

9. Nerve to the quadratus femoris (L4, 5, S1): innervates the quadratus femoris and inferior gemellus

10. Posterior femoral cutaneous nerve (S1, 2, 3): supplies the skin of the lower limb

B. Autonomic nerves

1. Hypogastric nerves: formed by the splitting of the superior hypogastric plexus, an inferior extension of the intermesenteric plexus between the inferior mesenteric artery and aortic bifurcation (like the intermesenteric plexus, the superior hypogastric plexus is composed of preganglionic sympathetic fibers from the greater, lesser, least, and lumbar splanchnic nerves); descend into the pelvis medial to the internal iliac arteries and terminate in the inferior hypogastric plexuses

2. Inferior hypogastric plexuses: formed by the comingling of the hypogastric nerves, sacral splanchnic nerves, pelvic splanchnic nerves, and clusters of sympathetic postganglionic cell bodies; located in the extraperitoneal connective tissue on each side of the rectum

3. Sympathetic trunks

a. Descend on the ventral surface of the sacrum medial to the ventral sacral foramina

b. Sacral sympathetic ganglia

1. Give off postganglionic gray rami communicantes to ventral rami of sacral spinal nerves for distribution to the sweat glands, arrector pili muscles, and blood vessels of the lower limb

2. Give off preganglionic sacral splanchnic nerves to the inferior hypogastric plexus for synapse on its postganglionic sympathetic cell bodies; postganglionic sympathetic fibers from the inferior hypogastric plexus are distributed along branches of the internal iliac artery to pelvic and perineal structures

4. Pelvic splanchnic nerves (nervi erigentes)

a. Formed by fibers of preganglionic parasympathetic cell bodies located in nuclei within the lateral horns of spinal cord segments S2 to S4; they exit the spinal cord in their respective ventral roots and spinal nerves and emerge from corresponding ventral rami to join the inferior hypogastric plexuses

b. Fibers leave the inferior hypogastric plexuses and are distributed along branches of the internal iliac artery to postganglionic para-sympathetic cell bodies within pelvic and perineal structures

5. In the male and female, the pelvic splanchnic nerves are responsible for the engorgement of erectile tissue with blood; in the male, postganglionic sympathetic fibers from the inferior hypogastric plexuses are responsible for the smooth muscle contractions that expel semen during ejaculation

part **V**

The
Head
and Neck

The Skull

I. Cranial and Facial Bones

    A. Cranial bones

        1. Encase the brain

        2. Paired: parietal and temporal

        3. Unpaired: frontal, ethmoid, sphenoid, and occipital

    B. Facial bones

        1. Paired: maxilla, zygomatic, nasal, lacrimal, inferior nasal concha, and palatine

        2. Unpaired: mandible and vomer

II. Calvaria or Skullcap

    A. Frontal bone

    B. Parietal bones

    C. Occipital bone

    D. Coronal suture: articulation between the frontal and two parietal bones

    E. Sagittal suture: articulation between the parietal bones

F. Bregma: site of junction of the sagittal and coronal sutures

G. Lambdoid suture: articulation between the occipital and two parietal bones

H. Lambda: site of junction of the sagittal and lambdoid sutures

I. Parietal foramina (inconstant): openings on either side of the posterior part of the sagittal suture

J. Sutural or Wormian bones (inconstant): supernumerary bones that usually occur along the lambdoid suture

K. Parietal tuber: region of maximum convexity anterolateral to the lambda

L. Vertex: highest part of the skull; lies near the middle of the sagittal suture

M. Outer table: outer layer of compact bone

N. Inner table: inner layer of compact bone

O. Diploë: spongy bone between the outer and inner tables

P. Sulcus for the superior sagittal sinus: midline groove on the intracranial surface

Q. Foveolae granulares (depressions for the arachnoid granulations): pits located lateral to the sulcus for the superior sagittal sinus

R. Grooves for branches of the middle meningeal artery: arborizing recesses on the intracranial surface

III. Anterior View

A. Maxilla

1. Piriform aperture: anterior opening of the nasal cavities; bordered by the maxillae and nasal bones

2. Anterior nasal spine: midline projection along the inferior border of the piriform aperture

3. Intermaxillary suture: articulation between the maxillae

4. Infraorbital foramen: aperture within the anterior surface of the maxilla; located inferior to the orbital aperture, the anterior opening of the bony orbit

5. Canine eminence: elevation formed by the root of the canine tooth

6. Canine fossa: depression lateral to the canine eminence and inferior to the infraorbital foramen

7. Incisive fossa: depression medial to the canine eminence and superior to the incisor teeth

8. Zygomatic process: lateral extension; articulates with the zygomatic bone at the zygomaticomaxillary suture

B. Vomer: forms the inferior part of the bony nasal septum

C. Inferior nasal concha: curved bone draping from the inferior part of the lateral nasal wall

D. Ethmoid

1. Perpendicular plate: forms the superior part of the bony nasal septum

2. Middle nasal concha: curved bony process; drapes from the lateral nasal wall, superior to the inferior nasal concha

E. Nasal bones: bound the piriform aperture superiorly; the articulation between them is the internasal suture

F. Frontal bone

1. Squamous part: extends from the orbital apertures to the coronal suture

2. Supraorbital margin: superior border of the orbital aperture

3. Superciliary arch: smooth ridge superior to the medial part of the supraorbital margin

4. Glabella: midline elevation between the superciliary arches

5. Frontal tuber: rounded bulge superior to the superciliary arch

6. Supraorbital foramen or notch: aperture or groove within the medial part of the supraorbital margin

7. Frontal notch or foramen: groove or aperture within the supraorbital margin, medial to the supraorbital foramen or notch

8. Zygomatic process: forms the lateral part of the supraorbital margin; descends to articulate with the zygomatic bone at the frontozygomatic suture

9. Nasal part: inferior, median extension; articulates with the nasal bones at the frontonasal suture

10. Nasion: site of junction of the internasal and frontonasal sutures

IV. Lateral View

  A. Zygomatic bone

    1. Lateral surface: forms the prominence of the cheek

    2. Zygomaticofacial foramen: opening on the lateral surface

    3. Temporal surface: forms the anterior wall of the temporal fossa, a shallow depression on the side of the skull

    4. Zygomaticotemporal foramen: opening on the temporal surface

    5. Frontal process: forms the lateral border of the orbital aperture

    6. Temporal process: posterior extension; articulates with the zygomatic process of the temporal bone at the zygomaticotemporal suture

  B. Maxilla

    1. Alveolar process: ridge containing the sockets or alveoli for the teeth

    2. Maxillary tuber: rounded eminence posterior to the third upper molar

    3. Frontal process: forms the medial border of the orbital aperture

    4. Anterior lacrimal crest: vertical ridge of the frontal process; borders the fossa for the lacrimal sac anteriorly

  C. Sphenoid

    1. Greater wing: forms the anteroinferior part of the temporal fossa; articulates with the parietal bone at the sphenoparietal suture

    2. Pterion: a reference point midway along the sphenoparietal suture

    3. Lateral pterygoid plate: broad, lateral leaflet of the pterygoid process; lies posterior to the maxilla

    4. Pterygomaxillary fissure: slit between the lateral pterygoid plate and maxilla

5. Pterygopalatine fossa

   a. Lies within the depth of the pterygomaxillary fissure and is bounded anteriorly by the maxilla, posteriorly by the pterygoid process of the sphenoid, medially by the perpendicular plate of the palatine bone, and superiorly by the body of the sphenoid; inferiorly, it narrows and becomes continuous with the greater palatine canal

   b. Contents: maxillary nerve and artery, the nerve of the pterygoid canal, and pterygopalatine ganglion

   c. Communicates with the nasal cavity through the sphenopalatine foramen, an aperture between the superior end of the perpendicular plate of the palatine bone and the body of the sphenoid; the pterygoid canal and foramen rotundum open onto its posterior wall inferomedially and superolaterally, respectively

D. Temporal bone

   1. Squamous part: forms the posteroinferior part of the temporal fossa

   2. Squamosal suture: articulation between the squamous part of the temporal bone and the parietal bone and greater wing of the sphenoid

   3. Zygomatic process: anterior extension; articulates with the temporal process of the zygomatic bone at the zygomaticotemporal suture

   4. Zygomatic arch: formed by the zygomatic process of the temporal bone and the temporal process of the zygomatic bone

   5. External acoustic (auditory) meatus: canal posterior to the temporomandibular joint

   6. Suprameatal spine (inconstant): spicule posterosuperior to the external acoustic meatus

   7. Tympanic part: forms the anterior wall, floor, and part of the posterior wall of the external acoustic meatus

   8. Mastoid process: rounded projection posterior to the external acoustic meatus

   9. Parietomastoid suture: articulation between the mastoid process and parietal bone

   10. Occipitomastoid suture: articulation between the mastoid process and occipital bone

11. Asterion: site of junction of the parietomastoid, occipitomastoid, and lambdoid sutures

12. Temporal fossa: shallow depression on the side of the skull, between the superior temporal line and zygomatic arch

E. Parietal bone: with the squamous part of the frontal bone, it forms the superior part of the temporal fossa; the superior and inferior temporal lines arch posteriorly from the zygomatic process of the frontal bone across the frontal and parietal bones

V. Posterior View

A. Occipital bone

1. Squamous part: portion posterior to foramen magnum

2. External occipital protuberance (inion): midline eminence about midway between foramen magnum and lambda

3. External occipital crest: midline ridge between the external occipital protuberance and foramen magnum

4. Supreme nuchal line (inconstant): arched ridge extending laterally from the external occipital protuberance

5. Superior nuchal line: ridge extending laterally from the external occipital protuberance, inferior to the supreme nuchal line

6. Inferior nuchal line: ridge extending laterally about midway along the external occipital crest

B. Temporal bone: the mastoid foramen is an opening on the posterior aspect of the mastoid process

C. Maxilla

1. Infratemporal surface: convex surface posterior to the first upper molar

2. Alveolar foramina: openings near the middle of the infratemporal surface

D. Choanae: posterior apertures of the nasal cavities; separated by the vomer

VI. External Surface of the Base of the Skull

A. Occipital bone

1. Foramen magnum: large, midline aperture

2. Occipital condyle: oblong eminence lateral to the anterior half of foramen magnum

3. Condylar fossa (inconstant): depression posterior to the occipital condyle

4. Condylar canal (inconstant): opening within the condylar fossa

5. Jugular foramen: aperture lateral to the occipital condyle

6. Basilar part: portion anterior to foramen magnum

7. Pharyngeal tubercle: small, midline eminence on the basilar part, approximately 1 centimeter anterior to foramen magnum

8. Lateral part: portion lateral to foramen magnum; includes the occipital condyle and jugular process

9. Jugular process: extends laterally from the posterior part of the occipital condyle

10. Jugular notch: anterior indentation of the jugular process; bounds the jugular foramen posteriorly

B. Temporal bone

1. Petrous part: portion lateral to the basilar part of the occipital bone

2. Apex of the petrous part: pointed, anterior end of the petrous part

3. Foramen lacerum: serrated aperture anterior to the apex of the petrous part; for the most part, it is filled with cartilage in the living

4. Styloid process: long, pointed process lateral to the jugular foramen; it is usually broken off

5. Stylomastoid foramen: opening between the styloid and mastoid processes

6. Mastoid canaliculus: tiny canal whose external opening is located on the lateral wall of the jugular foramen, near the base of the styloid process

7. Tympanic canaliculus: tiny canal whose external opening is on the bony ridge between the jugular foramen and carotid canal

8. Carotid canal: passageway within the petrous part of the temporal bone; its external opening lies anterior to the jugular foramen

9. Mandibular fossa: depression anterior to the external acoustic meatus

10. Tympanosquamous fissure: slit located laterally in the mandibular fossa, between the tympanic and squamous parts of the temporal bone

11. Petrosquamous fissure: anterior slit located medially in the mandibular fossa, between the petrous and squamous parts of the temporal bone; the petrous part of the temporal bone is represented medially in the mandibular fossa by a tiny spicule of bone insinuated between the tympanic and squamous parts of the temporal bone

12. Petrotympanic fissure: posterior slit located medially in the mandibular fossa, between the petrous and tympanic parts of the temporal bone

13. Articular tubercle: rounded, transverse elevation anterior to the mandibular fossa

14. Musculotubal canal: passageway whose external opening lies anterior to the external opening of the carotid canal; it is divided into two semicanals by a thin bony septum

15. Mastoid notch: groove medial to the mastoid process

16. Groove for the occipital artery: shallow furrow medial to the mastoid notch

17. Jugular fossa: smooth depression roofing the jugular foramen

18. Tympanic part: portion anterior to the styloid process; medially, it is fused to the petrous part

C. Sphenoid

1. Greater wing: located lateral to the lateral pterygoid plate

2. Foramen ovale: oval opening near the superior end of the lateral pterygoid plate

3. Foramen spinosum: small, round opening posterolateral to foramen ovale

4. Sphenoid spine: inferiorly projecting process posterolateral to foramen spinosum

5. Pterygoid canal: passageway extending from the anterior wall of foramen lacerum to the pterygopalatine fossa

6. Pterygoid process: bileaflet projection medial to the greater wing of the sphenoid

7. Medial pterygoid plate: narrow, medial leaflet of the pterygoid process

8. Lateral pterygoid plate: broad, lateral leaflet of the pterygoid process

9. Pterygoid fossa: depression between the medial and lateral pterygoid plates

10. Scaphoid fossa: fusiform depression lateral to the superior end of the medial pterygoid plate

11. Pterygoid hamulus: fingerlike, inferior extension of the posterior border of the medial pterygoid plate

12. Groove of the pterygoid hamulus: lateral furrow at the junction of the pterygoid hamulus and medial pterygoid plate

13. Infratemporal fossa

    a. Walls: anterior wall—infratemporal surface of the maxilla; roof—greater wing of the sphenoid; medial wall—lateral pterygoid plate; lateral wall—ramus and coronoid process of the mandible; inferior wall—absent; posterior wall—absent

    b. Contents: medial and lateral pterygoid muscles, pterygoid venous plexus, maxillary artery, chorda tympani nerve, and the mandibular nerve and its branches

    c. Communicates with the orbit through the inferior orbital fissure and with the pterygopalatine fossa through the pterygomaxillary fissure

14. Infratemporal crest: ridge between the infratemporal and temporal fossae

15. Vaginal process of the medial pterygoid plate: thin, medial plate inferior to the body of the sphenoid

16. Palatovaginal canal: tiny passageway between the perpendicular plate of the palatine bone and vaginal process of the medial pterygoid plate

D. Palatine bone

1. Perpendicular plate: vertical plate forming the posterior part of the lateral nasal wall

2. Greater palatine canal: lies between the perpendicular plate of the palatine bone and maxilla; extends from the pterygopalatine fossa to the greater and lesser palatine foramina

3. Horizontal plate: with its fellow of the opposite side, it forms the posterior one-third of the hard palate

4. Greater palatine foramen: opening in the horizontal plate, medial to the third upper molar

5. Lesser palatine foramina: openings posterior to the greater palatine foramen

6. Posterior nasal spine: pointed, midline projection along the posterior border of the hard palate

7. Pyramidal process: pointed, bony extension insinuated between the inferior portions of the medial and lateral pterygoid plates; may be difficult to discern

8. Median palatine suture: articulation between the horizontal plates of the palatine bones

9. Palatomaxillary suture: articulation between the horizontal plates of the palatine bones and the palatine processes of the maxillae

E. Maxilla

1. Palatine process: shelflike plate that forms the anterior two-thirds of the hard palate with its fellow of the opposite side

2. Intermaxillary suture: articulation between the maxillae

3. Torus palatinus (inconstant): bony ridge along the intermaxillary suture, near the middle of the hard palate

4. Incisive fossa: midline depression posterior to the central incisors

5. Incisive canal: passageway between the incisive fossa and a nasal cavity

6. Dental arch: consists of two medial incisors, two lateral incisors, two canines, four premolars, and six molars

VII. Internal Surface of the Base of the Skull

A. Arranged in three tiers; from anterior to posterior (and from superior to inferior), they are the anterior, middle, and posterior cranial fossae

B. Anterior cranial fossa

1. Cribriform plate: central, perforated region

2. Crista galli: small, midline partition extending superiorly from the cribriform plate

3. Foramen cecum: opening anterior to the crista galli

4. Frontal crest: midline ridge anterior to foramen cecum

5. Orbital part of the frontal bone: thin, convex plate forming most of the lateral part of the anterior cranial fossa; its ridges conform to the sulci of the cerebrum

6. Lesser wing of the sphenoid: forms the lateral, posterior ridge separating the anterior cranial fossa from the middle cranial fossa

7. Anterior clinoid process: projects posteriorly from the medial end of the lesser wing of the sphenoid

8. Jugum: portion of the body of the sphenoid between the lesser wings of the sphenoid

C. Middle cranial fossa

1. Body of the sphenoid: central, cubical part between the greater and lesser wings; the portion posterior to the jugum is associated with the middle cranial fossa

2. Optic canal: aperture between the lesser wing and body of the sphenoid

3. Prechiasmatic sulcus: groove between the optic canals

4. Tuberculum sellae: elevation posterior to the prechiasmatic sulcus

5. Hypophyseal fossa: depression posterior to the tuberculum sellae

6. Dorsum sellae: inclined, posterior plate of the body of the sphenoid; located posterior to the hypophyseal fossa

7. Posterior clinoid processes: tubercles at the superolateral angles of the dorsum sellae

8. Sella turcica (Turkish saddle): composed of the tuberculum sellae, hypophyseal fossa, and dorsum sellae

9. Carotid sulcus: groove on the lateral aspect of the body of the sphenoid

10. Middle clinoid process (inconstant): projection medial to the tip of the anterior clinoid process

11. Greater wing of the sphenoid: forms the floor of the middle cranial fossa anteriorly

12. Superior orbital fissure: crescentic opening between the greater and lesser wings of the sphenoid

13. Foramen rotundum: round opening inferior to the medial end of the superior orbital fissure

14. Foramen ovale: oval opening posterolateral to foramen rotundum

15. Foramen spinosum: small, round opening posterolateral to foramen ovale

16. Groove for the middle meningeal artery: indentation extending laterally from foramen spinosum

17. Petrous part of the temporal bone: forms the floor of the middle cranial fossa posteriorly; its petrous ridge borders the posterior cranial fossa

18. Apex of the petrous part of the temporal bone: pointed, anterior end of the petrous part of the temporal bone

19. Foramen lacerum: serrated aperture anterior to the apex of the petrous part of the temporal bone; for the most part, it is filled with cartilage in the living

20. Trigeminal impression: slight depression posterolateral to the apex of the petrous part of the temporal bone

21. Hiatus for the greater petrosal nerve: tiny opening near the center of the petrous part of the temporal bone

22. Sulcus for the greater petrosal nerve: groove extending from the hiatus for the greater petrosal nerve to foramen lacerum

23. Hiatus for the lesser petrosal nerve: tiny opening lateral to the hiatus for the greater petrosal nerve

24. Sulcus for the lesser petrosal nerve: groove extending from the hiatus for the lesser petrosal nerve to foramen ovale

25. Arcuate eminence: rounded elevation anterior to the middle of the petrous ridge

26. Tegmen tympani: slight elevation anterolateral to the arcuate eminence

27. Sulcus for the superior petrosal sinus: groove along the petrous ridge

D. Posterior cranial fossa

1. Foramen magnum: large, midline aperture

2. Jugular foramen: aperture lateral to foramen magnum, between the petrous part of the temporal bone and lateral part of the occipital bone

3. Internal acoustic (auditory) meatus: canal within the petrous part of the temporal bone; lies superior to the jugular foramen

4. Vestibular aqueduct: tiny canal within the petrous part of the temporal bone; opens into the posterior cranial fossa posteroinferior to the internal acoustic meatus, beneath a thin process of bone

5. Cochlear canaliculus: tiny canal within the petrous part of the temporal bone; opens onto the roof of the jugular foramen, inferior to the internal acoustic meatus

6. Sulcus for the sigmoid sinus: S-shaped groove between the asterion and jugular foramen

7. Jugular tubercle: rounded elevation medial to the jugular foramen

8. Hypoglossal canal: opening inferior to the jugular tubercle

9. Condylar canal (inconstant): aperture posterolateral to the hypoglossal canal; opens into the sulcus for the sigmoid sinus

10. Clivus: sloping surface anterior to foramen magnum; formed by the basilar part of the occipital bone and dorsum sellae

11. Sulcus for the inferior petrosal sinus: groove between the petrous part of the temporal bone and basilar part of the occipital bone

12. Internal occipital protuberance: midline eminence about midway between foramen magnum and lambda

13. Sulcus for the transverse sinus: groove between the internal occipital protuberance and asterion

14. Cerebral fossa: depression superior to the sulcus for the transverse sinus

15. Cerebellar fossa: depression inferior to the sulcus for the transverse sinus and lateral to the internal occipital crest

16. Internal occipital crest: midline ridge between the internal occipital protuberance and foramen magnum

VIII. Mandible

    A. Body

        1. Anterior, teeth-bearing, U-shaped portion; its bony landmarks are noted below

        2. Mental protuberance: midline ridge on the external surface

        3. Mental tubercle: elevation extending inferolaterally from the mental protuberance

        4. Oblique line: slight ridge extending from the mental tubercle to the anterior border of the ramus

        5. Mental foramen: opening on the external surface, inferior to the second premolar

        6. Incisive fossa: depression on the external surface, inferior to the incisor teeth

        7. Mental spines (two superior and two inferior): bony spicules on the internal surface near the midline

        8. Digastric fossa: depression inferolateral to the mental spines

        9. Mylohyoid line: oblique ridge on the internal surface between the digastric fossa and third molar

      10. Sublingual fossa (fovea): depression superior to the anterior part of the mylohyoid line

      11. Submandibular fossa (fovea): depression inferior to the posterior part of the mylohyoid line

      12. Alveolar process: ridge containing the sockets or alveoli for the teeth

      13. Dental arch: consists of two medial incisors, two lateral incisors, two canines, four premolars, and six molars

    B. Ramus

        1. Vertical, posterior portion; its bony landmarks are noted below

        2. Angle: region of junction of the ramus and body

        3. Coronoid process: pointed projection at the superior end of the anterior border of the ramus

4. Condylar process: projection at the superior end of the posterior border of the ramus; its head is the wide, superior part, its neck is the constricted part inferior to the head, and the pterygoid fovea is the pit on the anterior surface of the neck

5. Mandibular notch: concavity between the coronoid and condylar processes

6. Mandibular foramen: opening on the internal surface of the ramus, near its middle; it is the entrance to the mandibular canal

7. Mandibular canal: tunnel within the ramus and body of the mandible

8. Lingula: tongue-shaped process anterior to the mandibular foramen

9. Mylohyoid groove: slight indentation descending anteriorly from the mandibular foramen

IX. Fetal Skull

A. Frontal (metopic) suture: median articulation between the two frontal bones; usually obliterated by age 8

B. Anterior, posterior, mastoid (posterolateral), and sphenoidal (anterolateral) fontanelles: membranous "soft spots" located at the future sites of the bregma, lambda, asterion, and pterion, respectively

C. Clinical note: during parturition, the skull bones of the fetus partially overlap one another, or undergo molding, to facilitate passage of the head through the birth canal

The Face

I. Superficial Fascia

  A. Cutaneous nerves

    1. Cutaneous innervation of the face is provided by branches of the ophthalmic, maxillary, and mandibular nerves, the three divisions of the trigeminal nerve (see also The Cranial Nerves, p. 275)

    2. Branches of the ophthalmic nerve

      a. Supraorbital nerve: emerges from the supraorbital foramen and ascends to supply the forehead and the scalp as far posteriorly as the vertex

      b. Supratrochlear nerve: emerges from the frontal notch medial to the supraorbital nerve and ascends to supply the forehead near the midline

      c. Infratrochlear nerve: emerges from the orbit inferior to the supratrochlear nerve and supplies the medial part of the upper eyelid

      d. External nasal nerve: emerges inferior to the nasal bone to supply the dorsum and tip of the nose

      e. Lacrimal nerve: emerges along the superolateral border of the orbital aperture to supply the lateral part of the upper eyelid

    3. Branches of the maxillary nerve

      a. Infraorbital nerve: emerges from the infraorbital foramen and supplies the lower eyelid, side of the nose, upper lip, and the skin overlying the anterior surface of the maxilla

b. Zygomaticofacial nerve: emerges from the zygomaticofacial foramen to supply the skin overlying the lateral surface of the zygomatic bone

c. Zygomaticotemporal nerve: emerges from the zygomaticotemporal foramen to supply the anterior part of the temple

4. Branches of the mandibular nerve

a. Mental nerve: emerges from the mental foramen to supply the lower lip and chin

b. Buccal nerve: emerges from the deep face and supplies the cheek

c. Auriculotemporal nerve: emerges posterior to the neck of the mandible and ascends anterior to the auricle to supply the posterior part of the temple

B. Muscles

1. Depressor anguli oris

a. Origin: anterior part of the oblique line of the mandible

b. Insertion: corner of the mouth

c. Action: draws the corner of the mouth inferiorly and laterally

d. Innervation: marginal mandibular branch of the facial nerve

2. Depressor labii inferioris

a. Origin: anterior part of the oblique line of the mandible, deep to depressor anguli oris

b. Insertion: lower lip

c. Action: draws the lower lip inferiorly and laterally

d. Innervation: marginal mandibular branch of the facial nerve

3. Mentalis

a. Origin: incisive fossa of the mandible

b. Insertion: descends to insert into the skin of the chin

c. Action: elevation and protrusion of the lower lip

d. Innervation: marginal mandibular branch of the facial nerve

4. Orbicularis oris

   a. Encircles the mouth within the substance of the lips

   b. Action: closure of the mouth; protrusion of the lips

   c. Innervation: marginal mandibular and buccal branches of the facial nerve

5. Risorius

   a. Origin: fascia covering the parotid gland

   b. Insertion: corner of the mouth

   c. Action: draws the corner of the mouth posteriorly

   d. Innervation: buccal branches of the facial nerve

6. Buccinator

   a. Origin: external surfaces of the posterior aspects of the alveolar processes of the maxilla and mandible and the pterygomandibular raphe; the pterygomandibular raphe extends from the pterygoid hamulus to the posterior end of the mylohyoid line and represents the region of interdigitation of muscle fibers of the buccinator and superior pharyngeal constrictor

   b. Insertion: corner of the mouth

   c. Action: compression of the cheek; this action positions food between the teeth

   d. Innervation: buccal branches of the facial nerve

   e. The buccal fat pad lies between the buccinator and masseter

7. Zygomaticus major

   a. Origin: lateral surface of the zygomatic bone

   b. Insertion: corner of the mouth

   c. Action: draws the corner of the mouth superiorly and laterally

   d. Innervation: buccal branches of the facial nerve

8. Zygomaticus minor

   a. Origin: lateral surface of the zygomatic bone, anterior to zygomaticus major

   b. Insertion: upper lip

   c. Action: elevation of the upper lip

   d. Innervation: buccal branches of the facial nerve

9. Levator labii superioris

   a. Origin: inferior border of the orbital aperture

   b. Insertion: upper lip

   c. Action: elevation of the upper lip

   d. Innervation: buccal branches of the facial nerve

10. Levator labii superioris alaeque nasi

   a. Origin: frontal process of the maxilla

   b. Insertion: medial part—ala of the nose; lateral part—upper lip

   c. Action: medial part—dilation of the nostril; lateral part—elevation of the upper lip

   d. Innervation: buccal branches of the facial nerve

11. Levator anguli oris

   a. Origin: canine fossa of the maxilla (inferior to the infraorbital foramen)

   b. Insertion: corner of the mouth

   c. Action: elevation of the corner of the mouth

   d. Innervation: buccal branches of the facial nerve

12. Platysma

   a. Origin: deep fascia covering the upper part of pectoralis major

b. Insertion: inferior border of the mandible and corner of the mouth

c. Action: depression of the mandible; draws the corner of the mouth inferiorly and laterally, producing ridges in the skin of the anterior neck

d. Innervation: cervical branch of the facial nerve

e. The platysma as well as other muscles inserting into the corner of the mouth interdigitate with each other and with fibers of the orbicularis oris; the convergence of these muscle fibers forms a palpable swelling, the modiolus, lateral to the corner of the mouth

13. Depressor septi

a. Origin: maxilla, superior to the central incisor

b. Insertion: nasal septum

c. Action: depression of the nasal septum

d. Innervation: buccal branches of the facial nerve

14. Nasalis

a. Origin: transverse part—canine eminence; alar part—maxilla, superior to the lateral incisor

b. Insertion: transverse part—side of the nose; alar part—ala of the nose

c. Action: transverse part—compression of the nostril; alar part—dilation of the nostril

d. Innervation: buccal branches of the facial nerve

15. Procerus

a. Origin: nasal bone

b. Insertion: skin overlying the glabella

c. Action: depresses the medial end of the eyebrow, producing transverse wrinkles at the bridge of the nose

d. Innervation: buccal branches of the facial nerve

16. Orbicularis oculi

    a. Orbital part

        1. Origin: nasal part of the frontal bone and medial palpebral ligament; the medial palpebral ligament extends from the frontal process of the maxilla to the medial ends of the free margins of the upper and lower eyelids

        2. Insertion: muscle fibers make complete loops around the orbital aperture and insert on the frontal process of the maxilla and medial palpebral ligament

    b. Palpebral part

        1. Origin: frontal process of the maxilla and medial palpebral ligament

        2. Insertion: fibers course laterally within each eyelid and interdigitate with one another lateral to the lateral angle of the eye at the lateral palpebral raphe

    c. Lacrimal part

        1. Origin: posterior lacrimal crest and lacrimal sac

        2. Insertion: fibers course laterally within each eyelid and interdigitate with one another at the lateral palpebral raphe

    d. Action: orbital part—closes the eyelids tightly; palpebral part—closes the eyelids in normal blinking; lacrimal part—closes the eyelids in normal blinking and pulls on the lacrimal sac, creating suction for removal of lacrimal fluid from the medial angle of the eye

    e. Innervation: zygomatic and temporal branches of the facial nerve

17. Corrugator supercilii

    a. Origin: medial end of the superciliary arch

    b. Insertion: skin above the medial half of the supraorbital margin

    c. Action: draws the eyebrow medially, producing vertical wrinkles at the bridge of the nose

    d. Innervation: temporal branches of the facial nerve

18. Auricularis anterior

   a. Origin: galea aponeurotica, above the zygomatic arch; the galea aponeurotica is the deep fascia of the scalp

   b. Insertion: anterior part of the auricle

   c. Action: draws the auricle anteriorly

   d. Innervation: temporal branches of the facial nerve

19. Auricularis superior

   a. Origin: galea aponeurotica, posterior to the auricularis anterior

   b. Insertion: superior part of the auricle

   c. Action: elevation of the auricle

   d. Innervation: temporal branches of the facial nerve

20. Auricularis posterior

   a. Origin: mastoid process

   b. Insertion: posterior part of the auricle

   c. Action: draws the auricle posteriorly

   d. Innervation: posterior auricular branch of the facial nerve

21. Occipitalis

   a. Origin: lateral part of the supreme nuchal line

   b. Insertion: galea aponeurotica

   c. Action: tenses the galea aponeurotica

   d. Innervation: posterior auricular branch of the facial nerve

22. Frontalis

   a. Origin: anteriorly, its muscle fibers interdigitate with those of the procerus, corrugator supercilii, and orbicularis oculi

b. Insertion: galea aponeurotica

c. Action: elevation of the eyebrows

d. Innervation: temporal branches of the facial nerve

II. Deep Fascia: Absent

III. Facial Nerve

A. Emerges from the skull through the stylomastoid foramen and gives off its posterior auricular branch, which ascends behind the auricle to supply the auricularis posterior and occipitalis muscles; here, it also gives off branches to the posterior belly of the digastric and stylohyoid, and receives postganglionic parasympathetic secretomotor fibers from the otic ganglion via the auriculotemporal nerve

B. The facial nerve then enters the parotid gland, supplying it with postganglionic parasympathetic secretomotor fibers as it forms a plexus within its substance; its major branches emerge along the borders of the parotid gland and are named according to their region of distribution

1. Temporal branches (two or three): ascend superficial to the zygomatic arch and supply orbicularis oculi, corrugator supercilii, auricularis anterior, auricularis superior, and frontalis

2. Zygomatic branches (two or three): course toward the prominence of the cheek and supply orbicularis oculi

3. Buccal branches (two or three): course toward the corner of the mouth and supply orbicularis oris, risorius, buccinator, zygomaticus major, zygomaticus minor, levator labii superioris, levator labii superioris alaeque nasi, levator anguli oris, depressor septi, nasalis, and procerus

4. Marginal mandibular branch: courses anteriorly above the inferior border of the mandible and supplies depressor anguli oris, depressor labii inferioris, mentalis, and orbicularis oris

5. Cervical branch: descends anteriorly, inferior to the angle of the mandible, and supplies the platysma

C. Within the superficial fascia of the face, branches of the facial nerve anastomose with each other and with cutaneous branches of the ophthalmic, maxillary, and mandibular nerves

IV. Vessels

    A. Facial artery

        1. Arises in the neck from the external carotid artery and appears along the inferior border of the mandible, anterior to the masseter (its pulse can be felt here); it then ascends deep to the facial musculature, coursing near the corner of the mouth and along the side of the nose toward the medial angle of the eye

        2. Branches

            a. Inferior labial artery: arises inferior to the corner of the mouth and courses medially within the lower lip

            b. Superior labial artery: arises superior to the corner of the mouth and courses medially within the upper lip

            c. Lateral nasal artery: arises distal to the superior labial artery and courses forward on the side of the nose; distal to the lateral nasal artery, the facial artery is sometimes called the angular artery

    B. Ophthalmic artery

        1. Arises from the internal carotid artery within the cranial cavity and courses forward within the orbit; branches that emerge from the orbit to supply the face are noted below

        2. Supraorbital artery: emerges from the supraorbital foramen and courses with the supraorbital nerve

        3. Supratrochlear artery: emerges from the frontal notch and courses with the supratrochlear nerve

        4. Dorsal nasal artery: emerges from the orbit with the infratrochlear nerve and anastomoses with the angular artery

        5. Medial and lateral palpebral arteries: supply the medial and lateral parts of the eyelids, respectively

    C. Maxillary artery

        1. Arises from the external carotid artery posterior to the neck of the mandible and courses within the deep face; its branches to the face are noted below

2. Infraorbital artery: emerges from the infraorbital foramen and courses with the infraorbital nerve

3. Mental artery: emerges from the mental foramen and courses with the mental nerve

4. Buccal artery: emerges from the deep face and courses with the buccal nerve (do not confuse the buccal nerve, a branch of the mandibular nerve, with the buccal branches of the facial nerve)

D. Superficial temporal artery: arises from the external carotid artery posterior to the neck of the mandible and ascends anterior to the auricle with the auriculotemporal nerve; one of its branches, the transverse facial artery, courses anteriorly on the face, inferior to the zygomatic arch, with a zygomatic branch of the facial nerve

E. Facial vein

1. Descends from the medial angle of the eye, lateral to the facial artery, and superficial to the facial musculature; its tributaries are noted below

2. Superior ophthalmic vein: emerges from the orbit and drains into the facial vein near the medial angle of the eye; since it is valveless, it may also drain posteriorly through the orbit and into the cavernous sinus, a dural venous sinus within the cranial cavity

3. Deep facial vein: extends from the pterygoid venous plexus in the deep face to the facial vein near the corner of the mouth

4. Superior and inferior labial veins: course with their corresponding arteries and drain into the facial vein superior and inferior to the corner of the mouth, respectively; above the superior labial vein, the facial vein is sometimes called the angular vein

5. Clinical note: if infectious material enters the facial vein through one of its tributaries, perhaps from squeezing a pimple, it may spread to the superior ophthalmic vein, through the orbit, and into the cavernous sinus within the cranial cavity; through the communicating system of intracranial dural venous sinuses, there may be widespread dispersion of the infectious material to the meninges and brain

F. Other veins that drain the face accompany corresponding branches of the ophthalmic, maxillary, and superficial temporal arteries

G. Lymphatics: drain to submental, submandibular, superficial and deep parotid, and superficial and deep cervical nodes

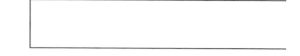

The Scalp

I. Layers

A. As noted below, the first letters of the layers of the scalp, from superficial to deep, spell SCALP

B. Skin

C. Connective tissue

1. Fibrous superficial fascia between the skin and galea aponeurotica; it contains nerves and vessels

2. Clinical note: bleeding from wounds in this layer is often profuse and sustained because the vessels are held open by the surrounding fibrous connective tissue

D. Aponeurosis or galea aponeurotica: tough membranous sheet connecting the frontalis and occipitalis muscles; represents the deep fascia of the scalp

E. Loose connective tissue

1. Lies between the galea aponeurotica and pericranium and allows movement of the first three layers over the skull

2. Clinical notes

a. Infections can spread easily within this layer and emissary veins traversing it can serve to channel extracranial infectious material into the communicating system of intracranial dural venous sinuses

b. Traumatic scalping occurs within this layer

F. Pericranium: periosteum covering the outer table of the skull

II. Nerves

    A. Anterior nerve: supraorbital nerve—supplies the scalp as far posteriorly as the vertex

    B. Lateral nerves: auriculotemporal nerve—ascends anterior to the auricle and supplies the scalp in the temporal region; lesser occipital nerve—ascends on the side of the neck and supplies the scalp posterior to the auricle

    C. Posterior nerves: greater occipital nerve—emerges from the trapezius inferolateral to the external occipital protuberance and ascends to supply the scalp as far anteriorly as the vertex; third occipital nerve (dorsal ramus of the third cervical spinal nerve)—supplies a small portion of the scalp on the back of the neck, near the midline

III. Vessels

    A. Anterior artery: supraorbital artery—accompanies the supraorbital nerve

    B. Lateral artery: superficial temporal artery—accompanies the auriculo-temporal nerve and divides into an anterior and a posterior branch which supply the lateral part of the scalp

    C. Posterior arteries: posterior auricular artery—arises from the external carotid artery posterior to the ramus of the mandible and ascends posterior to the auricle to supply the scalp posterior and superior to the auricle; occipital artery—arises from the external carotid artery in the neck and ascends posteriorly across the back of the neck to course with the greater occipital nerve

    D. Veins: accompany their respective arteries

    E. Lymphatics: drain directly or indirectly to deep cervical nodes; in the latter instance, lymph first passes through either occipital, retroauricular, superficial parotid, or deep parotid nodes

    F. Clinical note: since arteries and nerves ascend into the scalp, surgical flaps are left attached from below

The Cranial Meninges and Dural Venous Sinuses

I. Cranial Meninges

  A. Dura mater

    1. Dense connective tissue covering consisting of two layers, a superficial periosteal layer attached to the intracranial surface of the skull and a deep meningeal layer which, in certain locations, gives rise to partitions that project into the cranial cavity

    2. Dural partitions

      a. Falx cerebri: midline, sickle-shaped partition between the cerebral hemispheres; attaches to the crista galli, frontal crest, sulcus for the superior sagittal sinus, and superior surface of the tentorium cerebelli

      b. Tentorium cerebelli

        1. Tentlike partition attaching to the sulci for the transverse sinuses, sulci for the superior petrosal sinuses, posterior clinoid processes, and anterior clinoid processes; its U-shaped, anterior free edge forms the tentorial notch and, with the dorsum sellae, transmits the brainstem

        2. Separates the cerebrum from the cerebellum

      c. Falx cerebelli: small, midline, sickle-shaped partition between the cerebellar hemispheres; attaches to the inferior surface of the tentorium cerebelli and to the internal occipital crest

      d. Diaphragma sellae: horizontal partition attaching to the anterior and posterior clinoid processes; forms a roof for the hypophyseal fossa, except for a central aperture which transmits the pituitary stalk

3. Epidural space

   a. In contrast to spinal dura mater, cranial dura mater is not surrounded by an epidural space; however, there is a potential epidural space between the cranial dura mater and intracranial surface of the skull

   b. Clinical note: the potential epidural space may become a real space if, for example, there is a hemorrhage (epidural hematoma) between the cranial dura mater and intracranial surface of the skull; this may result from rupture of the middle meningeal artery following a skull fracture

B. Arachnoid

   1. Translucent connective tissue membrane deep to the cranial dura mater and separated from it by only a slitlike, potential subdural space

   2. From its deep surface, thin, anastomosing connective tissue strands extend through the cerebrospinal fluid within the subarachnoid space and merge with the pia mater covering the brain

   3. Arachnoid villi are tiny, fingerlike diverticula of the arachnoid that protrude through the cranial dura mater into the superior sagittal sinus (or its lateral lacunae); they are sites of resorption of cerebrospinal fluid into the venous system and, when they form aggregations called arachnoid granulations, they may induce resorption of bone on the inner table of the skull, producing foveolae granulares

C. Pia mater: microscopic connective tissue layer covering the surface of the brain

D. Vessels

   1. Middle meningeal artery

   a. Arises from the maxillary artery, enters the skull through foramen spinosum, and courses laterally within the groove for the middle meningeal artery; although it lies within and supplies the cranial dura mater, its major function is to supply the skull (tiny foramina can be observed in the depth of its grooves)

   b. Divides into an anterior and a posterior branch which course near the pterion and toward the lambda, respectively

2. Accessory meningeal artery: arises from the maxillary artery and enters the skull through foramen ovale; supplies the trigeminal ganglion and adjacent dura mater

3. Anterior meningeal arteries: arise from the ophthalmic artery and pass posteriorly through the superior orbital fissure to supply the dura mater and bone of the middle cranial fossa

4. Posterior meningeal arteries: arise from the occipital artery and enter the skull through the jugular foramen to supply the dura mater and bone of the posterior cranial fossa

5. Meningeal veins: accompany the meningeal arteries and drain into dural venous sinuses

E. Nerves: sensory innervation of the cranial dura mater is provided primarily by meningeal branches of the ophthalmic, maxillary, and mandibular divisions of the trigeminal nerve

II. Dural Venous Sinuses

A. Venous channels within the cranial dura mater; they receive cerebral and meningeal veins and drain into the internal jugular and emissary veins

B. Superior sagittal sinus

1. Courses posteriorly within the attached superior margin of the falx cerebri; receives many cerebral veins and drains into the confluence of the sinuses, the site of junction of the superior sagittal, straight, and occipital sinuses, anterior to the internal occipital protuberance

2. Laterally, it exhibits several diverticula called lateral lacunae

3. Clinical note: in head trauma, the brain may move abruptly, tearing cerebral veins at the site of their entry into the superior sagittal sinus; blood from torn cerebral veins may accumulate between the cranial dura mater and arachnoid, forming a subdural hematoma, which converts the potential subdural space into a real subdural space

C. Inferior sagittal sinus: courses posteriorly within the inferior free margin of the falx cerebri; joins the great cerebral vein at the anterior margin of the tentorium cerebelli to form the straight sinus (the great cerebral vein drains deep structures of the brain)

D. Straight sinus: courses posteriorly within the tentorium cerebelli along its site of attachment to the falx cerebri; drains into the confluence of the sinuses

E. Transverse sinus: courses laterally from the confluence of the sinuses within the attachment of the tentorium cerebelli to the sulcus for the transverse sinus

F. Sigmoid sinus: represents the continuation of the transverse sinus after it leaves the tentorium cerebelli near the asterion to course within the sulcus for the sigmoid sinus; becomes continuous with the internal jugular vein at the jugular foramen

G. Occipital sinus: ascends to the confluence of the sinuses within the attachment of the falx cerebelli to the internal occipital crest

H. Cavernous sinus

   1. Located in the middle cranial fossa lateral to the body of the sphenoid; extends from the superior orbital fissure to the apex of the petrous part of the temporal bone

   2. Anteriorly, it receives the superior ophthalmic vein and sphenoparietal sinus; posteriorly, it drains into the superior and inferior petrosal sinuses (it also communicates with its fellow of the opposite side via the intercavernous sinus within the diaphragma sellae)

   3. Traversed by the oculomotor, trochlear, abducens, and ophthalmic nerves, and the internal carotid artery; also, numerous fibrous bands traverse its lumen, giving it a cavernous or labyrinthlike structure

   4. Clinical note: a fracture of the base of the skull may tear the internal carotid artery within the cavernous sinus; the arteriovenous fistula thus created may produce a throbbing mass in the orbit as the superior ophthalmic vein and its tributaries become distended with pulsatile arterial blood

I. Superior petrosal sinus: from the cavernous sinus, it courses posteriorly within the attachment of the tentorium cerebelli to the sulcus for the superior petrosal sinus (along the petrous ridge); drains into the junction of the transverse and sigmoid sinuses

J. Inferior petrosal sinus: from the cavernous sinus, it descends within the sulcus for the inferior petrosal sinus between the petrous part of the temporal bone and the basilar part of the occipital bone; exits the skull through the jugular foramen and drains into the internal jugular vein

K. Basilar plexus: network of venous channels within the cranial dura mater covering the clivus; connects the inferior petrosal sinuses

L. Marginal sinus: lies within the cranial dura mater lateral to foramen magnum; anastomoses with the basilar plexus, internal vertebral venous plexus, and occipital sinus

M. Sphenoparietal sinus: courses medially on the inferior surface of the lesser wing of the sphenoid and drains into the cavernous sinus

N. Emissary veins

    1. Anastomotic channels between intracranial dural venous sinuses and extracranial veins; some emissary veins are noted below

    2. Mastoid emissary vein: traverses the mastoid foramen; connects the sigmoid sinus with the occipital and posterior auricular veins

    3. Parietal emissary vein: traverses the parietal foramen; connects the superior sagittal sinus and occipital vein

    4. Emissary vein of the foramen cecum: present in the child, but often absent in the adult; connects the superior sagittal sinus with veins of the nose

    5. Condylar emissary vein (inconstant): traverses the condylar canal; connects the sigmoid sinus and external vertebral venous plexus

    6. Emissary veins also traverse foramen ovale and foramen lacerum; they connect the cavernous sinus with the pterygoid venous plexus

The Orbit

I. Eyelid and Lacrimal Apparatus

   A. Eyelid

      1. Palpebral conjunctiva: mucosa covering the posterior surface of the eyelid; it turns back on itself at a region called the conjunctival fornix and becomes continuous with the bulbar conjunctiva covering the anterior part of the sclera or "white of the eye"

      2. Tarsus: semilunar plate of dense connective tissue between the palpebral conjunctiva and superficial fascia; borders the free margin of the eyelid and attaches to the medial and lateral walls of the orbit, just inside the orbital margin, via the medial and lateral palpebral ligaments, respectively

      3. Tarsal glands: modified sebaceous glands within a tarsus; their ducts open on the free margin of the eyelid and their oily secretion forms a surface film that reduces evaporation of lacrimal fluid

      4. Tarsal muscles

         a. Superior tarsal muscle: smooth muscle within the tendon of levator palpebrae superioris that attaches to the tarsus of the upper eyelid; receives sympathetic innervation from the internal carotid plexus and contracts reflexly to elevate the upper eyelid

         b. Inferior tarsal muscle: smooth muscle extending from the tarsus of the lower eyelid to the fascial sheath of the inferior rectus muscle; its function is unknown

5. Orbital septum

    a. Fibrous membrane extending from the orbital margin to the tarsus; it is continuous with the pericranium

    b. Clinical note: the orbital septum acts as a "fire wall" by preventing the spread of fluid or infectious material from the superficial fascia of the eyelid to the interior of the orbit and perhaps into the cranial cavity

B. Lacrimal apparatus

1. Lacrimal gland

    a. Located just inside the superolateral orbital margin and indented medially by the tendon of levator palpebrae superioris; the part of the lacrimal gland superior to the tendon of levator palpebrae superioris lies in the fossa for the lacrimal gland on the roof of the bony orbit, and the part of the lacrimal gland inferior to the tendon of levator palpebrae superioris lies in association with the conjunctival fornix of the upper eyelid

    b. Several ducts extend from the inferior part of the gland and open into the lateral part of the conjunctival fornix; from here, blinking moves lacrimal fluid toward the medial angle of the eye for drainage

2. Lacus lacrimalis: triangular depression at the medial angle of the eye; collects excess lacrimal fluid

3. Lacrimal papilla: tiny projection along the free margin of each eyelid at the medial angle; at its apex is a tiny opening, the lacrimal punctum, which drains lacrimal fluid from the lacus lacrimalis into a lacrimal canaliculus

4. Lacrimal canaliculus: small duct draining lacrimal fluid from the lacrimal punctum to the lacrimal sac

5. Lacrimal sac: membranous reservoir within the fossa for the lacrimal sac, just inside the medial orbital margin; it is continuous inferiorly with the nasolacrimal duct which transports lacrimal fluid to the nasal cavity (thus, excessive lacrimation is accompanied by a "runny" nose)

II. Bony Orbit

A. Shaped like a four-sided pyramid

1. Base or orbital margin: anterior perimeter formed by the frontal bone

superiorly, the zygomatic bone laterally and inferolaterally, and the maxilla medially and inferomedially

2. Apex: narrow, posterior region penetrated by the superior orbital fissure and optic canal

B. Roof

1. Formed primarily by the orbital part of the frontal bone (separates the orbit from the anterior cranial fossa); the lesser wing of the sphenoid forms a small part of the roof posteriorly

2. The fossa for the lacrimal gland forms a shallow, anterolateral depression and the trochlear fovea forms a slight, anteromedial depression; the latter may contain a bony spicule, the trochlear spine

C. Medial wall

1. The orbital lamina of the ethmoid bone forms most of the medial wall; honeycomblike ethmoidal air cells can be seen through its thin wall

2. The frontoethmoidal suture represents the articulation between the orbital lamina of the ethmoid bone and the orbital part of the frontal bone; the anterior and posterior ethmoidal foramina are openings near the anterior and posterior parts of the frontoethmoidal suture, respectively

3. The lacrimal bone forms part of the medial wall, anterior to the orbital lamina of the ethmoid bone; it exhibits a vertical ridge, the posterior lacrimal crest, which borders the fossa for the lacrimal sac posteriorly

4. The frontal process of the maxilla forms part of the medial wall, anterior to the lacrimal bone; it also exhibits a vertical ridge, the anterior lacrimal crest, which borders the fossa for the lacrimal sac anteriorly

5. The fossa for the lacrimal sac is a depression between the anterior and posterior lacrimal crests, and contains the lacrimal sac; the fossa for the lacrimal sac is continuous inferiorly with the nasolacrimal canal, which opens into the nasal cavity and contains the nasolacrimal duct

D. Floor

1. The orbital surface of the maxilla forms most of the floor; from posterior to anterior, it exhibits an infraorbital groove and infraorbital canal which extend forward from the inferior orbital fissure

2. The inferior orbital fissure is located posteriorly between the orbital surface of the maxilla and greater wing of the sphenoid; it opens poste-

riorly into the pterygopalatine fossa, at its middle into the infratemporal fossa, and anteriorly into the temporal fossa

3. The orbital surface of the zygomatic bone forms the anterolateral part of the floor and the orbital process of the palatine bone comprises a tiny portion of the floor anterior to the posterior end of the inferior orbital fissure

E. Lateral wall

1. The greater wing of the sphenoid forms the posterior part of the lateral wall and separates the orbit from the middle cranial fossa; the orbital surface of the zygomatic bone forms the anterior part of the lateral wall and separates the orbit from the temporal fossa

2. The zygomatico-orbital foramina are openings on the lateral wall in the orbital surface of the zygomatic bone

III. Muscles

A. Levator palpebrae superioris

1. Origin: lesser wing of the sphenoid, superior to the optic canal

2. Insertion: ends in an aponeurotic tendon that splits into a superior and an inferior lamella; the superior lamella inserts into the skin of the upper eyelid and the inferior lamella attaches to the tarsus of the upper eyelid and contains the superior tarsal muscle

3. Action: elevation of the upper eyelid

4. Innervation: superior branch of the oculomotor nerve

B. Superior oblique

1. Origin: body of the sphenoid, medial to the optic canal

2. Insertion: its tendon passes through a fibrocartilaginous trochlea or pulley, which is attached to the trochlear fovea; it then bends posteriorly and courses laterally, inferior to the superior rectus, to insert into the sclera of the superolateral quadrant of the posterior half of the eye

3. Action: moves the pupil inferiorly and laterally

4. Innervation: trochlear nerve

C. Lateral rectus

    1. Origin: lateral part of the common annular tendon (the common annular tendon is a ring-shaped tendon located anterior to the superior orbital fissure and optic canal; it attaches medially to the body of the sphenoid, laterally to the greater wing of the sphenoid, and provides origin for the lateral rectus, medial rectus, inferior rectus, and superior rectus muscles)

    2. Insertion: sclera on the lateral aspect of the eye

    3. Action: moves the pupil laterally

    4. Innervation: abducens nerve

D. Superior rectus

    1. Origin: superior part of the common annular tendon

    2. Insertion: sclera on the superior aspect of the eye

    3. Action: moves the pupil superiorly and medially

    4. Innervation: superior branch of the oculomotor nerve

E. Medial rectus

    1. Origin: medial part of the common annular tendon

    2. Insertion: sclera on the medial aspect of the eye

    3. Action: moves the pupil medially

    4. Innervation: inferior branch of the oculomotor nerve

F. Inferior rectus

    1. Origin: inferior part of the common annular tendon

    2. Insertion: sclera on the inferior aspect of the eye

    3. Action: moves the pupil inferiorly and medially; the superior and inferior rectus muscles move the pupil medially because the longitudinal axis of the orbit, from the base to the apex, slants medially

    4. Innervation: inferior branch of the oculomotor nerve

G. Inferior oblique

  1. Origin: orbital surface of the maxilla, lateral to the fossa for the lacrimal sac

  2. Insertion: courses laterally and posteriorly, between the inferior rectus and floor of the orbit, and inserts into the sclera of the inferolateral quadrant of the posterior half of the eye

  3. Action: moves the pupil superiorly and laterally

  4. Innervation: inferior branch of the oculomotor nerve

H. Fasciae

  1. Periorbita: periosteum covering the walls of the orbit; it is continuous at the orbital margin with the orbital septum and pericranium

  2. Intermuscular membrane: composed of four fascial sheets interposed between, and continuous with, the fascial sheaths of the four recti muscles; the intermuscular membrane and fascial sheaths of the recti muscles enclose the retrobulbar space

  3. Bulbar sheath (Tenon's capsule)

    a. Fascial covering of the posterior, unexposed part of the sclera; an episcleral space lies between the bulbar sheath and sclera

    b. The tendons of the recti and oblique muscles pass through the episcleral space to reach their insertions on the sclera; as they pierce the bulbar sheath, their own fascial sheaths become continuous with it

  4. Medial and lateral check ligaments: medial and lateral horizontal extensions of the fascial sheaths of the medial rectus and lateral rectus, respectively; they attach to the lacrimal and zygomatic bones, respectively, and restrict eye movements

  5. Suspensory ligament of the eye (Lockwood's ligament)

    a. Formed by medial and lateral extensions of the fascial sheath of the inferior rectus; they attach to the medial and lateral check ligaments, respectively, forming a fascial sling below the eyeball

    b. Clinical note: entrapment of the suspensory ligament of the eye when reducing a fracture of the floor of the orbit may render the eye immobile

IV. Nerves

A. Nerves which course between the periorbita and retrobulbar space after entering the orbit through the superior orbital fissure, superior to the common annular tendon

1. Frontal nerve: branches from the ophthalmic nerve near the superior orbital fissure and courses anteriorly, superior to levator palpebrae superioris; near the middle of the orbit it divides into the supraorbital and supratrochlear nerves, which emerge through the supraorbital foramen and frontal notch, respectively, and provide cutaneous innervation to the forehead and scalp

2. Lacrimal nerve

a. Branches from the ophthalmic nerve near the superior orbital fissure and courses anteriorly, superior to the lateral rectus

b. Receives a branch from the zygomaticotemporal nerve containing postganglionic parasympathetic secretomotor fibers from the pterygopalatine ganglion for the lacrimal gland; after supplying the lacrimal gland with postganglionic parasympathetic secretomotor fibers, the lacrimal nerve pierces the orbital septum to provide cutaneous innervation to the lateral part of the upper eyelid

3. Trochlear nerve: courses medially, superior to the posterior end of levator palpebrae superioris; penetrates the superior aspect of the superior oblique and innervates it

B. Nerves entering the retrobulbar space through the superior orbital fissure and common annular tendon

1. Superior branch of the oculomotor nerve: the oculomotor nerve divides into a superior and an inferior branch near the superior orbital fissure; the superior branch courses superiorly to innervate the superior rectus and levator palpebrae superioris

2. Inferior branch of the oculomotor nerve

a. Gives off the oculomotor root of the ciliary ganglion and then courses anteriorly to innervate the medial rectus, inferior rectus, and inferior oblique; the oculomotor root of the ciliary ganglion contains preganglionic parasympathetic fibers from the Edinger-Westphal nucleus in the brainstem for synapse on postganglionic parasympathetic cell bodies in the ciliary ganglion (branches of the nasociliary nerve and internal carotid plexus form the nasociliary and sympathetic roots of the ciliary ganglion, respectively; they pass through the ciliary ganglion without synapse)

    b. The ciliary ganglion is about 2 millimeters in diameter and located between the optic nerve and lateral rectus about 1 centimeter anterior to the apex of the orbit

    c. From the ciliary ganglion, postganglionic parasympathetic fibers course anteriorly via the short ciliary nerves and enter the eye near the optic nerve; they supply the ciliary and sphincter pupillae muscles which focus the lens and constrict the pupil, respectively

3. Abducens nerve: courses anteriorly on the medial surface of the lateral rectus, innervating it

4. Nasociliary nerve

    a. Arises from the ophthalmic nerve near the superior orbital fissure; its branches are noted below

    b. Long ciliary nerves: given off as the nasociliary nerve courses medially, superior to the optic nerve; they enter the sclera near the optic nerve and provide general sensory innervation to the eye

    c. Posterior ethmoidal nerve: arises as the nasociliary nerve courses anteriorly between the superior oblique and medial rectus; enters the posterior ethmoidal foramen and provides sensory innervation to the sphenoidal sinus and posterior ethmoidal air cells

    d. Anterior ethmoidal nerve (terminal branch): enters the anterior ethmoidal foramen and provides sensory innervation to the anterior and middle ethmoidal air cells; it then emerges above the cribriform plate, descends through it into the nasal cavity, and divides into the internal nasal and external nasal nerves which provide sensory innervation to the nasal cavity and nose, respectively

    e. Infratrochlear nerve (terminal branch): emerges from the orbit inferior to the trochlea and supplies the medial part of the upper eyelid

C. Optic nerve: actually, not a nerve, but an extension of the brain covered by meninges; emerges from the posterior aspect of the eye, courses posteriorly within the retrobulbar space, and exits the orbit through the common annular tendon and optic canal

D. Maxillary nerve

1. Exits the skull through foramen rotundum and emerges into the pterygo-

palatine fossa; here, it gives off the infraorbital and zygomatic nerves which enter the orbit through the inferior orbital fissure

2. Infraorbital nerve: courses forward along the floor of the orbit in the infraorbital groove and infraorbital canal; emerges onto the face through the infraorbital foramen

3. Zygomatic nerve: upon entering the orbit, the zygomatic nerve divides into the zygomaticotemporal and zygomaticofacial nerves, which penetrate the zygomatico-orbital foramina and emerge onto the face through the zygomaticotemporal and zygomaticofacial foramina, respectively; before entering its zygomatico-orbital foramen, the zygomaticotemporal nerve gives off a branch to the lacrimal nerve containing postganglionic parasympathetic secretomotor fibers from the pterygopalatine ganglion for the lacrimal gland

V. Vessels

A. Ophthalmic artery

1. Arises within the cranial cavity from the internal carotid artery, traverses the optic canal inferior to the optic nerve, enters the retrobulbar space lateral to the optic nerve, and then turns medially, superior to the optic nerve, to course with the nasociliary nerve; its branches are noted below

2. Central artery of the retina: arises as the ophthalmic artery emerges from the optic canal; penetrates the meninges of the optic nerve, courses forward in the center of the optic nerve and, upon entering the eye, supplies the retina

3. Lacrimal artery: arises lateral to the optic nerve and ascends out of the retrobulbar space to course with the lacrimal nerve; supplies the lacrimal gland and then gives rise to lateral palpebral arteries for the lateral parts of the upper and lower eyelids

4. Posterior ciliary arteries: given off as the ophthalmic artery courses medially, superior to the optic nerve; they enter the eye near the optic nerve and, with the anterior ciliary arteries, supply most of the eye (anterior ciliary arteries enter the anterior part of the eye and are derived from the variable muscular branches of the ophthalmic artery)

5. Supraorbital artery: given off after the ophthalmic artery has passed medially across the optic nerve; courses with the supraorbital nerve

6. Anterior and posterior ethmoidal arteries: given off as the ophthalmic artery courses anteriorly between the superior oblique and medial rec-

tus; they pass into the anterior and posterior ethmoidal foramina with their respective nerves and supply the sphenoidal sinus, ethmoidal air cells, and nasal cavity

7. Medial palpebral arteries: arise distal to the anterior ethmoidal artery and supply the medial parts of the upper and lower eyelids

8. The terminal branches of the ophthalmic artery, the supratrochlear and dorsal nasal arteries, accompany the supratrochlear and infratrochlear nerves, respectively; the dorsal nasal artery anastomoses with the angular artery

B. Ophthalmic veins

1. Superior ophthalmic vein: courses posteriorly within the retrobulbar space and receives tributaries corresponding to branches of the ophthalmic artery; ascends out of the retrobulbar space, exits the orbit through the superior orbital fissure above the common annular tendon, and drains into the cavernous sinus

2. Inferior ophthalmic vein: arises from a network of veins on the floor of the orbit and drains into the superior ophthalmic vein

The Neck

I. Superficial Fascia

   A. Anteriorly, the superficial fascia contains a thin, sheetlike muscle, the platysma

   B. Cutaneous nerves

      1. Emerge into the superficial fascia midway along the posterior border of the sternocleidomastoid; derived from the cervical plexus, which is formed from ventral rami of spinal nerves C1 to C4

      2. Lesser occipital nerve (C2): ascends along the posterior border of the sternocleidomastoid and supplies the skin and scalp posterior to the auricle

      3. Great auricular nerve (C2, 3): ascends on the sternocleidomastoid toward the auricle and supplies the auricle and skin overlying the parotid gland

      4. Transverse cervical nerve (C2, 3): courses anteriorly across the sternocleidomastoid and supplies the skin of the anterior neck

      5. Supraclavicular nerves (C3, 4)

         a. May arise as a single nerve, which then divides into the medial, intermediate, and lateral supraclavicular nerves; they descend deep to the platysma

         b. The medial supraclavicular nerve supplies the skin near the sternoclavicular joint, the intermediate supraclavicular nerve supplies the skin along the shaft of the clavicle, and the lateral supraclavicular nerve supplies the skin of the shoulder

C. Superficial veins

1. External jugular vein

   a. Formed posterior to the angle of the mandible by the union of the posterior auricular vein and posterior division of the retromandibular vein

   b. Descends posteriorly on the sternocleidomastoid adjacent to the great auricular nerve; penetrates the deep fascia posterior to the sternocleidomastoid and drains into the subclavian vein

2. Anterior jugular vein

   a. Formed by the coalescence of veins under the chin; descends near the anterior cervical midline, pierces the deep fascia, and drains into the external jugular vein posterior to the sternocleidomastoid

   b. Superior to the jugular notch, the anterior jugular veins may communicate via a jugular venous arch

II. Deep Fascia

A. Composed of five separate cylindrical connective tissue sleeves termed the investing, prevertebral, and pretracheal fasciae, and the two carotid sheaths

B. Investing fascia: lies deep to the superficial fascia; originates in the posterior cervical midline and, from posterior to anterior, invests the trapezius, forms the roof of the posterior triangle of the neck (region between the trapezius and sternocleidomastoid), invests the sternocleidomastoid and infrahyoid muscles, and then becomes continuous with the investing fascia of the opposite side in the anterior cervical midline

C. Prevertebral fascia

1. Lies deep to the investing fascia

2. Originates in the posterior cervical midline and, from posterior to anterior, ensheaths the semispinalis capitis, splenius capitis, levator scapulae, scalenus posterior, scalenus medius, scalenus anterior, longus capitis, and longus colli, and then becomes continuous with the prevertebral fascia of the opposite side in the anterior cervical midline

3. Anterior to the vertebral column, the prevertebral fascia splits into two layers separated by loose connective tissue; the anterior layer or alar fascia ends inferiorly by fusing with the posterior wall of the esophagus at about vertebral level T3 and the posterior layer continues inferiorly on the anterior surface of thoracic vertebral bodies

4. Clinical note: a "danger space" exists between the two layers of the prevertebral fascia that lie anterior to the vertebral column; an infection within this space can spread essentially unimpeded between the base of the skull and thorax

D. Pretracheal fascia: ensheaths the larynx, trachea, and thyroid gland

E. Carotid sheaths: lie deep to the sternocleidomastoids and extend from the base of the skull to the root of the neck; each contains an internal jugular vein, common/internal carotid artery, vagus nerve, some deep cervical lymph nodes, and the inferior root of an ansa cervicalis

F. Clinical note: deep fascia of the neck, as well as deep fascia in other parts of the body, serves as a retaining barrier and helps prevent the spread of infectious material

III. Triangles of the Neck

A. Anterior triangle

1. Bounded by the anterior cervical midline, inferior border of the mandible, and sternocleidomastoid; it is subdivided into the triangles noted below

2. Submandibular triangle

a. Bordered by the anterior and posterior bellies of the digastric and the inferior border of the mandible

b. Contains submandibular lymph nodes and the part of the submandibular gland that lies superficial to the mylohyoid; the facial vein courses superficial to the submandibular gland and the lingual and facial arteries and hypoglossal nerve course deep to the submandibular gland

3. Carotid triangle

a. Bordered by the posterior belly of the digastric, superior belly of the omohyoid, and the upper part of sternocleidomastoid

b. Contains the external carotid artery and proximal portions of the superior thyroid, ascending pharyngeal, lingual, occipital, and facial arteries; it also contains the portion of the hypoglossal nerve that gives off the superior root of an ansa cervicalis

4. Muscular triangle: bordered by the superior belly of the omohyoid, anterior cervical midline, and the lower part of sternocleidomastoid; contains the sternohyoid, sternothyroid, and thyrohyoid muscles

5. Submental triangle

a. Unpaired; bordered by the anterior bellies of the digastric and body of the hyoid

b. Contains submental lymph nodes and veins that coalesce to form the anterior jugular veins; its floor is formed by the medial portions of the mylohyoid muscles

B. Posterior triangle

1. Bounded by the sternocleidomastoid, clavicle, and anterior border of trapezius; it is subdivided into the triangles noted below

2. Occipital triangle

a. Bordered by the upper part of sternocleidomastoid, the inferior belly of the omohyoid, and the anterior border of trapezius; from superior to inferior, its floor is formed by splenius capitis, levator scapulae, scalenus posterior, and scalenus medius, and their covering of prevertebral fascia

b. The accessory nerve descends across the triangle on levator scapulae; the nerves to levator scapulae (ventral rami C3 and C4), the dorsal scapular nerve, and the long thoracic nerve may emerge into the triangle through scalenus medius

c. The occipital and transverse cervical arteries course posteriorly in the superior and inferior regions of the triangle, respectively

3. Subclavian triangle: bordered by the lower part of sternocleidomastoid, the inferior belly of the omohyoid, and clavicle; contains the subclavian artery, brachial plexus, and the lower part of scalenus anterior

IV. Muscles

A. Sternocleidomastoid

1. Origin: manubrium of the sternum and sternal end of the clavicle

2. Insertion: mastoid process and lateral part of the superior nuchal line

3. Action: laterally flexes the head and neck and rotates the head and neck to the opposite side; both muscles acting together flex the head and neck

4. Innervation: accessory nerve

B. Infrahyoid muscles

1. Hyoid bone

   a. The infrahyoid and suprahyoid muscles suspend the U-shaped hyoid bone at the angle between the chin and neck; it has no bony articulation

   b. The hyoid has a wide, anterior body from which greater cornua extend posteriorly on each side; lesser cornua project superiorly at the junctions of the body and greater cornua

2. Sternohyoid

   a. Origin: manubrium

   b. Insertion: body of the hyoid

3. Omohyoid

   a. Origin (superior belly): body of the hyoid, lateral to the sternohyoid

   b. An intermediate tendon is located posterior to the sternocleidomastoid and is bound to the clavicle by a fascial sling

   c. Insertion (inferior belly): superior border of the scapula, medial to the scapular notch

4. Sternothyroid

   a. Origin: manubrium

   b. Insertion: oblique line of the thyroid cartilage of the larynx

5. Thyrohyoid

   a. Origin: oblique line of the thyroid cartilage of the larynx

   b. Insertion: body and greater cornu of the hyoid

6. Action: depression of the hyoid and elevation and depression of the larynx and pharynx, motions used in vocalization and deglutition

7. Innervation: ansa cervicalis, a motor nerve loop derived from the cervical plexus

C. Suprahyoid muscles

1. Stylohyoid

   a. Origin: lateral side of the styloid process

   b. Insertion: body of the hyoid

   c. Innervation: facial nerve

2. Digastric

   a. Origin (posterior belly): mastoid notch

   b. An intermediate tendon passes through the stylohyoid insertion and is bound to the body of the hyoid by a fascial sling

   c. Insertion (anterior belly): digastric fossa

   d. Innervation: posterior belly—facial nerve; anterior belly—nerve to the mylohyoid, a branch of the mandibular division of the trigeminal nerve

3. Mylohyoid

   a. Origin: mylohyoid line

   b. Insertion: midline raphe and body of the hyoid

   c. Innervation: nerve to the mylohyoid

   d. The C-shaped submandibular gland wraps around its posterior free border

4. Geniohyoid

   a. Origin: inferior mental spine

   b. Insertion: body of the hyoid

c. Innervation: fibers from the ventral ramus of C1 that travel with the hypoglossal nerve

d. Lies deep to the mylohyoid

5. Action: elevation of the hyoid, larynx, and pharynx, motions used in vocalization and deglutition; assist in opening the mouth when the hyoid is fixed by the infrahyoid muscles and, when acting with the infrahyoid muscles, the suprahyoid muscles stabilize the hyoid so that it affords a stable base for movements of the tongue

D. Deep neck muscles

1. Scalenus anterior

   a. Origin: anterior tubercles of the transverse processes of vertebrae C3, 4, 5, and 6

   b. Insertion: tubercle for the scalenus anterior on the superior surface of the first rib (located anterior to the groove for the subclavian artery and posterior to the groove for the subclavian vein)

   c. Action: lateral flexion of the neck, rotation of the head and neck to the opposite side, and elevation of the first rib; both muscles acting together flex the neck

   d. Innervation: ventral rami C4, 5, and 6

2. Scalenus medius

   a. Origin: transverse processes of the atlas and axis and the posterior tubercles of the transverse processes of vertebrae C3, 4, 5, 6, and 7

   b. Insertion: first rib, posterior to the groove for the subclavian artery

   c. Action: lateral flexion of the neck and elevation of the first rib

   d. Innervation: ventral rami C3, 4, 5, 6, 7, and 8

   e. Clinical note: the interscalene triangle is formed by scalenus anterior, scalenus medius, and the first rib, and is traversed by the subclavian artery and brachial plexus; narrowing of the interscalene triangle, perhaps as a result of hypertrophy of scalenus anterior or scalenus medius, may compress the subclavian artery and brachial plexus, producing vascular and neurologic impairment in the upper limb, a condition known as scalenus anticus syndrome

3. Scalenus posterior

    a. Origin: posterior tubercles of the transverse processes of vertebrae C4, 5, and 6

    b. Insertion: second rib

    c. Action: lateral flexion of the neck and elevation of the second rib

    d. Innervation: ventral rami C6, 7, and 8

4. Scalenus minimus

    a. Origin: anterior tubercle of the transverse process of vertebra C7

    b. Insertion: first rib, posterior to the subclavian artery, and the suprapleural membrane

    c. Action: lateral flexion of the neck and elevation of the first rib

    d. Innervation: ventral ramus of C7

    e. Absent in about 70 percent of individuals

    f. Clinical note: since scalenus minimus lies between scalenus anterior and scalenus medius, it is located within the interscalene triangle and may contribute to scalenus anticus syndrome

5. Longus capitis

    a. Origin: anterior tubercles of the tranverse processes of vertebrae C3, 4, 5, and 6

    b. Insertion: basilar part of the occipital bone, posterior to the pharyngeal tubercle

    c. Action: flexion of the head

    d. Innervation: ventral rami C1, 2, and 3

6. Longus colli

    a. Origin: inferior oblique part—bodies of vertebrae T1, 2, and 3; superior oblique part—anterior arch of the atlas; vertical part—bodies of vertebrae C2, 3, and 4

    b. Insertion: inferior oblique part—anterior tubercles of the transverse processes of vertebrae C5 and C6; superior oblique part—anterior tubercles of the transverse processes of vertebrae C3, 4, and 5; vertical part—bodies of vertebrae C5, 6, 7, T1, 2, and 3

   c. Action: flexion of the neck; inferior oblique part—rotation of the head and neck to the opposite side

   d. Innervation: ventral rami C2, 3, 4, 5, and 6

7. Rectus capitis anterior

   a. Origin: transverse process of the atlas

   b. Insertion: basilar part of the occipital bone, posterior to longus capitis

   c. Action: flexion of the head

   d. Innervation: ventral rami C1 and C2

8. Rectus capitis lateralis

   a. Origin: transverse process of the atlas, lateral to the rectus capitis anterior

   b. Insertion: jugular process of the occipital bone

   c. Action: lateral flexion of the head

   d. Innervation: ventral rami C1 and C2

V. Nerves

  A. Vagus nerve

    1. Emerges from the jugular foramen and descends within the carotid sheath, behind and between the internal jugular vein and internal/common carotid artery; from superior to inferior, its branches are noted below

    2. Auricular branch: enters the mastoid canaliculus on the lateral wall of the jugular foramen; its branches provide general sensory innervation to the auricle, external acoustic meatus, and tympanic membrane

    3. Pharyngeal branch: contributes to the pharyngeal plexus and provides motor innervation to muscles of the pharynx and palate

    4. Superior laryngeal nerve

      a. Descends lateral to the pharynx; divides into the internal laryngeal and external laryngeal nerves posterosuperior to the tip of the greater cornu of the hyoid, medial to the external carotid artery

    b. Internal laryngeal nerve: penetrates the thyrohyoid membrane deep to the thyrohyoid muscle; provides general sensory innervation to the mucosa of the larynx and pharynx, and general sensory and taste innervation to the very posterior part of the tongue and epiglottis

    c. External laryngeal nerve: descends inferior to the oblique line of the thyroid cartilage, deep to the sternothyroid and superficial to the inferior pharyngeal constrictor; innervates the cricothyroid and part of the inferior pharyngeal constrictor

5. Nerves to the carotid body: provide sensory innervation to the carotid body, a sensor of the oxygen content of the blood

6. Recurrent laryngeal nerves

    a. The right and left recurrent laryngeal nerves loop posteriorly around the right subclavian artery and aortic arch, respectively; they ascend in the grooves between the trachea and esophagus on their respective sides

    b. As they ascend posterior to the lobes of the thyroid gland, they enter the larynx and provide general sensory innervation to the mucosa of the larynx and pharynx and motor innervation to all the muscles of the larynx, except the cricothyroids (which are innervated by the external laryngeal nerves)

B. Accessory nerve: emerges from the jugular foramen and descends posteriorly on the deep surface of sternocleidomastoid, innervating it; passes across the posterior triangle of the neck on levator scapulae and then descends on the deep surface of trapezius, innervating it

C. Hypoglossal nerve

1. Emerges from the hypoglossal canal, descends anteriorly in the neck, and appears along the inferior border of the posterior belly of the digastric; here, it hooks around the sternocleidomastoid branch of the occipital artery, gives off the superior root of the ansa cervicalis, and then the branch of the ansa cervicalis to the thyrohyoid

2. It subsequently courses anteriorly, deep to the posterior belly of the digastric and submandibular gland

D. Ansa cervicalis

1. Motor nerve loop derived from the cervical plexus; consists of a superior and an inferior root

2. Superior root: formed by fibers from the ventral ramus of C1; courses with the hypoglossal nerve before branching off to join the inferior root

3. Inferior root: formed by fibers from ventral rami C2 and C3; descends in the carotid sheath and then emerges to form a loop with the superior root, anterior to the common carotid artery

4. Branches from the ansa cervicalis innervate the sternohyoid, omohyoid, and sternothyroid; the branch to the thyrohyoid continues with the hypoglossal nerve for a short distance

E. Phrenic nerve

1. Motor nerve of the cervical plexus; derived from ventral rami C3, 4, and 5, especially C4

2. Descends medially on the anterior surface of scalenus anterior, deep to the prevertebral fascia; from superior to inferior, it is crossed anteriorly by the transverse cervical artery, suprascapular artery, and subclavian vein

3. Passes between the subclavian artery and vein medial to scalenus anterior and then descends into the thorax

4. If the contribution from ventral ramus C5 descends lateral to the phrenic nerve, it is referred to as the accessory phrenic nerve; it usually joins the phrenic nerve above the first rib

F. Brachial plexus: formed by ventral rami C5, 6, 7, 8, and T1, which emerge from between scalenus anterior and scalenus medius with the subclavian artery

G. Sympathetic trunk

1. Descends posterior to the carotid sheath and anterior to the longus capitis, longus colli, and prevertebral fascia; although there are eight cervical spinal nerves there are only three cervical sympathetic ganglia, as noted below

2. Superior cervical ganglion

a. Large, oblong, flattened structure lying on the longus capitis, anterior to the transverse processes of the upper three cervical vertebrae; postganglionic sympathetic fibers emerge from the superior cervical ganglion and are distributed to the head and neck along branches of the internal and external carotid arteries as the internal and external carotid plexuses, respectively

b. Some postganglionic sympathetic fibers from the superior cervical ganglion form gray rami communicantes which join ventral rami of spinal nerves C1 to C4 for distribution to blood vessels as well as arrector pili muscles and sweat glands in the skin; other postganglionic sympathetic fibers from the superior cervical ganglion form the superior cervical cardiac nerves that descend into the thorax to supply the heart

3. Middle cervical ganglion

   a. Located anterior to the transverse process of vertebra C6; some fibers from the middle cervical ganglion form the ansa subclavia by passing in front of the subclavian artery and looping posteriorly to join the inferior cervical ganglion

   b. Some postganglionic sympathetic fibers from the middle cervical ganglion form gray rami communicantes which join ventral rami of spinal nerves C5 and C6 for distribution to blood vessels as well as arrector pili muscles and sweat glands in the skin; other postganglionic sympathetic fibers from the middle cervical ganglion form the middle cervical cardiac nerves that descend into the thorax to supply the heart

4. Inferior cervical ganglion

   a. Often fuses with the first thoracic ganglion to form the stellate or cervicothoracic ganglion; lies between the vertebral artery and transverse process of vertebra C7

   b. Some postganglionic sympathetic fibers from the inferior cervical ganglion form gray rami communicantes which join ventral rami of spinal nerves C7 and C8 for distribution to blood vessels as well as arrector pili muscles and sweat glands in the skin; other postganglionic sympathetic fibers from the inferior cervical ganglion form the inferior cervical cardiac nerves that descend into the thorax to supply the heart

VI. Vessels

A. Common carotid artery

1. On the right side, the common carotid artery arises from the brachiocephalic trunk and, on the left side, it arises from the aortic arch; ascends in the carotid sheath medial to the internal jugular vein

2. Its distal end is dilated, forming the carotid sinus, a sensor of blood pressure that receives sensory innervation from the glossopharyngeal nerve

3. Bifurcates into the internal and external carotid arteries at the superior border of the thyroid cartilage; the carotid body, a tiny vascular structure within the angle formed by the internal and external carotid arteries, is a sensor of the oxygen content of the blood and is innervated by sensory branches from the glossopharyngeal and vagus nerves

B. Internal carotid artery: ascends in the carotid sheath medial to the internal jugular vein and enters the skull through the carotid canal to supply the brain; it has no branches in the neck

C. External carotid artery

1. Ascends anterior to the internal carotid artery; its branches are noted below

2. Superior thyroid artery: arises inferior to the tip of the greater cornu of the hyoid, descends with the external laryngeal nerve deep to the sternothyroid, and supplies the thyroid gland; gives rise to the superior laryngeal artery which penetrates the thyrohyoid membrane with the internal laryngeal nerve

3. Ascending pharyngeal artery: slender branch arising from the medial side of the external carotid artery; ascends between the internal carotid artery and lateral wall of the pharynx

4. Lingual artery: arises posterior to the tip of the greater cornu of the hyoid; ascends deep to the posterior belly of the digastric and submandibular gland

5. Occipital artery

a. Arises from the posterior side of the external carotid artery, opposite the origin of the lingual artery; the hypoglossal nerve hooks around its branch to the sternocleidomastoid

b. Ascends posteriorly, deep to the posterior belly of the digastric and within the groove for the occipital artery, medial to the mastoid process; traverses the superior part of the posterior triangle of the neck and emerges through the trapezius inferolateral to the external occipital protuberance

6. Facial artery

a. Arises superior to the tip of the greater cornu of the hyoid; courses deep to the submandibular gland and gives rise to the branches noted below

b. Ascending palatine artery: ascends deep to the medial pterygoid on the lateral aspect of the superior pharyngeal constrictor; arches over the superior border of the superior pharyngeal constrictor and descends to the soft palate

    c. Tonsillar artery: perforates the superior pharyngeal constrictor to supply the palatine tonsil

    d. Submental artery: courses anteriorly on the inferior surface of the mylohyoid accompanied by the nerve to the mylohyoid

    e. In about 40 percent of individuals the facial and lingual arteries arise from a common stem, the linguofacial trunk

  7. Posterior auricular artery: arises deep to the posterior belly of the digastric and ascends posteriorly between the auricle and mastoid process

  8. Maxillary and superficial temporal arteries: terminal branches of the external carotid artery; arise posterior to the neck of the mandible

D. Subclavian artery

  1. On the right side, the subclavian artery arises from the brachiocephalic trunk and, on the left side, it arises from the aortic arch; its first part extends from the origin to the medial border of scalenus anterior, the second part lies posterior to scalenus anterior, and the third part extends from the lateral border of scalenus anterior to the outer border of the first rib where it becomes continuous with the axillary artery (its branches, which originate from the first part of the subclavian artery, are noted below—their first letters spell VIT C)

  2. Vertebral artery: ascends to the angle between scalenus anterior and longus colli, and then traverses the transverse foramina of the upper six cervical vertebrae

  3. Internal thoracic artery: passes into the thorax and descends posterior to the costal cartilages

  4. Thyrocervical trunk

    a. Ascends along the medial border of scalenus anterior; its branches are noted below

    b. Suprascapular artery: passes laterally, anterior to scalenus anterior, and then posterior to the clavicle to course with the suprascapular nerve; often arises from the third part of the subclavian artery

    c. Transverse cervical artery

      1. Courses laterally, anterior to scalenus anterior and superior to the suprascapular artery; passes across the posterior triangle of the neck and divides into a superficial and deep branch

2. The superficial branch descends on the deep surface of the trapezius with the accessory nerve and the deep branch descends deep to levator scapulae, rhomboideus minor, and rhomboideus major with the dorsal scapular nerve

3. The deep branch of the transverse cervical artery arises independently from the second or third part of the subclavian artery in about 70 percent of individuals; in this case, it is then called the dorsal scapular artery, and the remaining artery is referred to as the superficial cervical artery

d. Inferior thyroid artery: ascends along the medial border of scalenus anterior, posterior to the carotid sheath, and then loops inferiorly to the thyroid gland; gives rise to the ascending cervical artery, which ascends between scalenus anterior and longus capitis, and the inferior laryngeal artery, which enters the larynx with the recurrent laryngeal nerve

5. Costocervical trunk: arises from the dorsal side of the subclavian artery; divides into the supreme intercostal artery, which gives rise to the first two posterior intercostal arteries, and the deep cervical artery, which passes posteriorly and ascends deep to semispinalis capitis

E. Internal jugular vein: descends within the carotid sheath lateral to the internal/common carotid artery; receives the superior thyroid, middle thyroid, pharyngeal, lingual, occipital, and common facial veins

F. Subclavian vein: receives the external jugular vein which, in turn, receives the suprascapular and transverse cervical veins; the vertebral, internal thoracic, inferior thyroid, and deep cervical veins drain into the brachiocephalic vein

G. Lymphatics

1. Deep cervical nodes: located within and around the carotid sheath and receive lymphatic drainage from the head and neck via submental, submandibular, retropharyngeal, occipital, retroauricular, superficial and deep parotid, and superficial cervical nodes; inferiorly, they drain into the jugular lymphatic trunk

2. Superficial cervical nodes: lie along the external jugular vein; receive lymphatic drainage from occipital, retroauricular, and superficial and deep parotid nodes, and drain to deep cervical nodes

3. Thoracic duct: courses laterally, anterior to the left vertebral artery, and

empties into the angle of junction of the left subclavian and left internal jugular veins; near its termination it receives the left jugular, left subclavian, and left bronchomediastinal trunks

4. Right lymphatic duct: formed by the union of the right jugular, right subclavian, and right bronchomediastinal trunks; immediately after its formation it empties into the angle of junction of the right subclavian and right internal jugular veins

VII. Thyroid and Parathyroid Glands

A. Thyroid gland

1. Lobes: located anterolaterally, between the oblique line of the thyroid cartilage of the larynx and fifth tracheal ring; an isthmus extends across the second to fourth tracheal rings and unites the lobes

2. Pyramidal lobe: conical process extending superiorly from the isthmus; present in about 40 percent of individuals

3. Vessels

a. Superior and inferior thyroid arteries: arise from the external carotid artery and thyrocervical trunk, respectively (see pp. 217 and 219, respectively)

b. Thyroidea ima artery (inconstant): unpaired artery; usually arises from the brachiocephalic trunk and ascends to the thyroid gland on the anterior surface of the trachea

c. Superior thyroid vein: courses with its corresponding artery; drains into the internal jugular vein

d. Middle thyroid vein: has no corresponding artery; drains into the internal jugular vein

e. Inferior thyroid vein: drains inferiorly into its respective brachiocephalic vein; the two inferior thyroid veins may unite into a single vein which drains into the left brachiocephalic vein

f. Lymphatics: drain to deep cervical nodes

4. Clinical note: tracheostomy surgery is usually performed inferior to the thyroid isthmus; sources of hemorrhage may include the isthmus of the thyroid, inferior thyroid veins, jugular venous arch, or the thyroidea ima artery, if present

B. Parathyroid glands: consist of four small glands (two superior and two inferior), each about 5 millimeters in diameter; usually lie on the posterior surfaces of the lobes of the thyroid gland in their respective positions

VIII. Trachea and Esophagus

A. Trachea

1. Inferior continuation of the larynx; lies posterior to the sternohyoid and sternothyroid muscles and anterior to the esophagus

2. Supported anteriorly and laterally by a series of horseshoe-shaped, cartilaginous bars united by ligaments; its posterior wall is completed by a musculofibrous membrane

B. Esophagus: inferior continuation of the pharynx; descends anterior to the vertebral column

The Parotid Gland

I. General Remarks

    A. Extends inferiorly from the zygomatic arch to the angle of the mandible; extends anteriorly from the upper part of the sternocleidomastoid to the middle of the external surface of the masseter (a deep portion of the parotid gland extends between the ramus of the mandible and mastoid process)

    B. Ensheathed by parotid fascia, a superior continuation of the investing fascia of the neck; a thickening of the parotid fascia on the deep surface of the gland forms the stylomandibular ligament, which extends from the styloid process to the angle of the mandible and separates the parotid gland from the submandibular gland

II. Associated Structures

    A. Parotid (Stensen's) duct

        1. Emerges from the anterior border of the parotid gland and courses anteriorly on the external surface of the masseter about 1 centimeter inferior to the zygomatic arch; it is palpable when the masseter is tensed

        2. Anterior to the masseter, the parotid duct bends medially, pierces the buccinator, and opens on the parotid papilla on the mucosal surface of the cheek opposite the second upper molar; a separate accessory parotid gland may lie along the superior aspect of the parotid duct

    B. Vessels

        1. External carotid artery: ascends within a groove on the deep surface of

the parotid gland; divides into its terminal branches, the superficial temporal and maxillary arteries, posterior to the neck of the mandible

2. Retromandibular vein

    a. Formed within the substance of the parotid gland by the union of the superficial temporal and maxillary veins; descends within the parotid gland and divides into an anterior and a posterior division near its inferior border

    b. The posterior division of the retromandibular vein joins the posterior auricular vein to form the external jugular vein, which descends posteriorly on the sternocleidomastoid and drains into the subclavian vein; the anterior division joins the facial vein to form the common facial vein which drains into the internal jugular vein

3. Lymphatics: deep and superficial parotid nodes lie in relation to their respective surfaces of the gland; they drain to superficial and deep cervical nodes

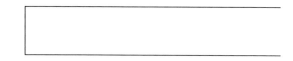

The Deep Face

I. Muscles

    A. Masseter

        1. Origin: zygomatic arch

        2. Insertion: external surface of the ramus and angle of the mandible

        3. Action: elevation of the mandible

        4. Innervation: masseteric nerve, a branch of the mandibular nerve

    B. Temporalis

        1. Origin: temporal fossa and overlying temporal fascia

        2. Insertion: coronoid process of the mandible

        3. Action: elevation and retraction of the mandible

        4. Innervation: anterior and posterior deep temporal nerves, branches of the mandibular nerve

    C. Lateral pterygoid

        1. Origin: superior head—infratemporal surface of the greater wing of the sphenoid; inferior head—lateral surface of the lateral pterygoid plate

        2. Insertion: articular disc of the temporomandibular joint and pterygoid fovea of the mandible

3. Action: protraction and depression of the mandible; deviation of the mandible to the opposite side

4. Innervation: nerve to the lateral pterygoid, a branch of the mandibular nerve

D. Medial pterygoid

1. Origin: superficial head—maxillary tuber; deep head—medial surface of the lateral pterygoid plate (the two heads embrace the anterior portion of the inferior head of the lateral pterygoid)

2. Insertion: internal surface of the ramus and angle of the mandible

3. Action: elevation of the mandible

4. Innervation: nerve to the medial pterygoid, a branch of the mandibular nerve

II. Temporomandibular Joint

A. Bony components include the condyle of the mandible and the mandibular fossa and articular tubercle of the temporal bone; a fibrous capsule attaches near the margins of the articular surfaces

B. Ligaments

1. Lateral temporomandibular ligament: reinforces the lateral aspect of the fibrous capsule between the articular tubercle and neck of the mandible

2. Sphenomandibular ligament: fibrous band extending from the sphenoid spine to the lingula of the mandible; it stands clear of the temporomandibular joint

C. An articular disc attaches to the circumference of the fibrous capsule and divides the joint into an upper and a lower synovial cavity; protraction and retraction of the mandible occur in the upper synovial joint and depression and elevation occur in the lower synovial joint

III. Nerves

A. Mandibular nerve

1. Emerges from foramen ovale deep to the lateral pterygoid and immediately breaks up into the sensory and motor branches noted below (it is the only division of the trigeminal nerve with motor branches)

2. Nerve to the medial pterygoid: penetrates the deep surface of the medial pterygoid, innervating it; gives rise to the nerve to the tensor tympani and the nerve to the tensor veli palatini

3. Masseteric nerve: emerges superior to the lateral pterygoid and passes through the mandibular notch to supply the masseter

4. Deep temporal nerves: the anterior deep temporal and posterior deep temporal nerves emerge between the two heads of the lateral pterygoid and superior to the lateral pterygoid, respectively; they ascend in the temporal fossa and innervate the temporalis

5. Nerve to the lateral pterygoid: penetrates the deep surface of the lateral pterygoid, innervating it

6. Buccal nerve: emerges between the two heads of the lateral pterygoid; some branches supply the skin of the cheek and others penetrate the buccinator to provide sensory innervation to the mucosa of the cheek

7. Auriculotemporal nerve

   a. Courses posteriorly, deep to the lateral pterygoid; emerges posterior to the neck of the mandible and gives off postganglionic parasympathetic secretomotor fibers from the otic ganglion to the facial nerve

   b. Ascends between the auricle and superficial temporal artery and provides sensory innervation to the auricle, external acoustic meatus, and posterior part of the temple

8. Lingual nerve

   a. Descends deep to the lateral pterygoid and appears along its inferior border; after coursing anteriorly on the lateral surface of the medial pterygoid, the lingual nerve provides general sensory innervation to the anterior two-thirds of the tongue

   b. Proximally, it is joined on its posterior aspect by the chorda tympani nerve, a branch of the facial nerve which contains taste fibers for the anterior two-thirds of the tongue and preganglionic parasympathetic fibers for synapse in the submandibular ganglion

9. Inferior alveolar nerve

   a. Descends deep to the lateral pterygoid and appears along its inferior border, posterior to the lingual nerve; it then courses toward the mandibular foramen on the lateral surface of the medial pterygoid, inferior to the lingual nerve

b. Before entering the mandibular foramen, the inferior alveolar nerve gives off the nerve to the mylohyoid, which runs in the mylohyoid groove and then on the inferior surface of the mylohyoid muscle; the nerve to the mylohyoid innervates the mylohyoid and anterior belly of the digastric

c. Within the mandibular canal the inferior alveolar nerve provides sensory innervation to the lower teeth and gums; at the second premolar it gives off the mental nerve, which emerges from the mental foramen and provides cutaneous innervation to the lower lip and chin

d. Clinical note: dentists often anesthetize the lower teeth and gums with an injection into mucosa adjacent to the inferior alveolar nerve, near its point of entry into the mandibular foramen (perhaps using the lingula as a palpable landmark); since the mental nerve is a branch of the inferior alveolar nerve, the lower lip and chin are also anesthetized, and, if the nearby lingual nerve is also affected, the anterior two-thirds of the tongue will be anesthetized as well

B. Maxillary nerve

1. Traverses foramen rotundum and emerges into the pterygopalatine fossa; its branches to the upper teeth and gums are noted below

2. Posterior superior alveolar nerve: its branches enter the alveolar foramina on the infratemporal surface of the maxilla and supply the upper molars

3. Middle superior alveolar nerve: arises from the infraorbital nerve as it courses forward in the infraorbital canal; descends within the lateral wall of the maxillary sinus and supplies the upper premolars

4. Anterior superior alveolar nerve: arises from the infraorbital nerve just before it emerges from the infraorbital foramen; descends within the anterior wall of the maxillary sinus and supplies the upper canine and incisors

IV. Vessels

A. Maxillary artery

1. Courses anteriorly, deep to the neck of the mandible, and then deep or superficial to the lateral pterygoid, before entering the pterygomaxillary fissure and pterygopalatine fossa; its branches are noted below

2. Deep auricular artery: supplies the temporomandibular joint and then

penetrates the external acoustic meatus, supplying it and the tympanic membrane

3. Anterior tympanic artery: enters the petrotympanic fissure to supply the tympanic cavity and tympanic membrane

4. Middle meningeal artery: ascends deep to the lateral pterygoid and pierces the auriculotemporal nerve; enters the skull through foramen spinosum and supplies the skull and cranial dura mater

5. Accessory meningeal artery: ascends deep to the lateral pterygoid, anterior to the middle meningeal artery; traverses foramen ovale and supplies the trigeminal ganglion and cranial dura mater

6. Inferior alveolar artery: before entering the mandibular foramen with the inferior alveolar nerve, it gives off the mylohyoid artery, which courses with the nerve to the mylohyoid; after entering the mandibular foramen, it traverses the mandibular canal, supplies the lower teeth and gums, and gives off the mental artery, which exits the mental foramen with the mental nerve

7. Masseteric artery: passes through the mandibular notch with the masseteric nerve and supplies the masseter

8. Anterior and posterior deep temporal arteries: ascend in the temporal fossa with the anterior and posterior deep temporal nerves, respectively, and supply the temporalis

9. Pterygoid arteries: supply the medial and lateral pterygoids

10. Buccal artery: courses anteriorly with the buccal nerve and supplies the mucosa and skin of the cheek

11. Posterior superior alveolar artery: arises as the maxillary artery enters the pterygomaxillary fissure; its branches enter the alveolar foramina with branches of the posterior superior alveolar nerve and supply the upper molars and premolars

12. Infraorbital artery: enters the orbit through the inferior orbital fissure and courses anteriorly within the infraorbital groove and infraorbital canal with the infraorbital nerve; gives off anterior superior alveolar arteries to the upper canine and incisors and then emerges through the infraorbital foramen to supply the face

13. Descending palatine artery (terminal branch): leaves the pterygopalatine fossa and descends within the greater palatine canal; divides into the greater and lesser palatine arteries, which emerge through the greater

and lesser palatine foramina to supply the hard and soft palates, respectively

14. Sphenopalatine artery (terminal branch): passes from the pterygopalatine fossa into the nasal cavity through the sphenopalatine foramen; supplies the lateral wall of the nasal cavity and nasal septum

B. Maxillary vein

1. Formed by the coalescence of veins from the pterygoid venous plexus; the pterygoid venous plexus lies within and around the lateral pterygoid and receives veins corresponding to branches of the maxillary artery

2. The maxillary vein courses posteriorly, deep to the neck of the mandible, and unites with the superficial temporal vein within the substance of the parotid gland to form the retromandibular vein

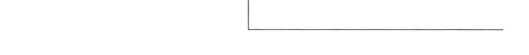

The Craniovertebral Joints

I. Atlanto-occipital Joints

   A. The convex articular surfaces of the occipital condyles and the reciprocally concave superior articular surfaces of the atlas form oblong synovial atlanto-occipital joints that permit flexion, extension, and lateral flexion of the head, but not rotation

   B. The anterior atlanto-occipital membrane is a fibrous joint between the anterior arch of the atlas and anterior margin of foramen magnum; it is reinforced in the midline by the superior end of the anterior longitudinal ligament

   C. The posterior atlanto-occipital membrane is a fibrous joint between the posterior arch of the atlas and posterior margin of foramen magnum; it is penetrated by the vertebral artery and suboccipital nerve

II. Atlantoaxial Joints

   A. Lateral atlantoaxial joints: synovial joints between the superior articular surfaces of the axis and the inferior articular surfaces of the atlas

   B. Median atlantoaxial joints

      1. Anterior joint: synovial joint between the posterior surface of the anterior arch of the atlas and the anterior surface of the dens

      2. Posterior joint: synovial joint between the posterior surface of the dens and the anterior surface of the transverse ligament of the atlas; the trans-

verse ligament of the atlas arches behind the dens and attaches on each side to the atlas

C. Permit rotation of the head, but not flexion, extension, or lateral flexion

III. Fibrous Joints Between the Axis and Occipital Bone

A. Membrana tectoria

1. Represents the superior end of the posterior longitudinal ligament; forms a fibrous joint between the posterior surface of the body of the axis and the superior surface of the basilar part of the occipital bone

2. Lies external to the spinal and cranial dura mater

B. Cruciform ligament of the atlas

1. Formed by the transverse ligament of the atlas and an inferior and a superior longitudinal band

2. The inferior longitudinal band extends from the posterior surface of the body of the axis to the posterior surface of the dens; the superior longitudinal band extends from the posterior surface of the dens to the superior surface of the basilar part of the occipital bone, external to the membrana tectoria

C. Apical ligament of the dens: slender strand extending from the tip of the dens to the anterior margin of foramen magnum; lies between the superior longitudinal band of the cruciform ligament of the atlas and the anterior atlanto-occipital membrane

D. Alar ligaments: stout cords extending like wings from either side of the dens to the medial sides of the occipital condyles; prevent excessive rotation at the atlantoaxial joints

The Pharynx

I. Layers

    A. Mucosa: inner, epithelial-lined coat

    B. Submucosa: connective tissue layer external to the mucosa; in the pharynx it is termed the pharyngobasilar fascia

    C. Muscularis: an inner longitudinal layer along the lateral pharyngeal wall is formed by the palatopharyngeus, salpingopharyngeus, and stylopharyngeus; an outer circular layer, which is deficient anteriorly, is formed by the superior, middle, and inferior pharyngeal constrictors

    D. Buccopharyngeal fascia: outer connective tissue coat containing the pharyngeal plexus of nerves and veins; the retropharyngeal space lies between the buccopharyngeal and prevertebral fasciae

II. Regions and Their Associated Structures

    A. Nasopharynx

        1. Extends from the base of the skull to the soft palate and communicates with the nasal cavities through the choanae; its lateral and posterior walls are formed by the superior pharyngeal constrictors as well as by the pharyngobasilar fascia spanning the gaps between the superior borders of the superior pharyngeal constrictors and base of the skull

        2. Pharyngeal tonsils

            a. Lymphoid tissue within the mucosa of the nasopharynx; prominent in children but involuted in the adult

b. Clinical note: the pharyngeal tonsils are called adenoids when enlarged and may obstruct the nasopharynx, making nasal breathing difficult

3. Pharyngeal ostium of the auditory tube

   a. Opening on the lateral wall of the nasopharynx, superior to the superior border of the superior pharyngeal constrictor

   b. Torus tubarius

      1. Curved eminence superior and posterior to the pharyngeal ostium of the auditory tube; formed by the cartilage of the auditory tube

      2. The salpingopharyngeal fold descends from the posterior part of the torus tubarius and contains the salpingopharyngeus muscle; the pharyngeal recess is the depression posterior to the torus tubarius and salpingopharyngeal fold

   c. Torus levatorius: elevation between the pharyngeal ostium of the auditory tube and soft palate; formed by the levator veli palatini muscle

4. Auditory tube

   a. Canal extending from the pharyngeal ostium of the auditory tube to the tympanic cavity; its anterior two-thirds is cartilaginous and its posterior one-third lies within the inferior semicanal of the musculo-tubal canal

   b. Clinical notes

      1. Respiratory infections may spread from the nasopharynx to the tympanic cavity via the auditory tube

      2. The auditory tube allows for equalization of air pressure between the nasopharynx (outside air) and the tympanic cavity

         a. If air exchange between the nasopharynx and the tympanic cavity is prevented, perhaps by adenoids, the difference in air pressure on the two sides of the tympanic membrane may result in hearing loss due to stretching and decreased sensitivity of the tympanic membrane

         b. Since the salpingopharyngeus, levator veli palatini, and tensor veli palatini attach to the cartilaginous part of the auditory tube, opening of the auditory tube and equalization of air pressure may be achieved by contracting these muscles by swallowing or yawning

B. Oropharynx

1. Extends from the soft palate to the superior border of the epiglottis; its lateral and posterior walls are formed by the pharyngeal constrictors, and its anterior wall is formed by the posterior part of the tongue inferiorly, and opens into the faucial isthmus superiorly

2. Faucial isthmus

a. Region connecting the oropharynx with the oral cavity; it is bounded by the palatopharyngeal and palatoglossal arches and contains the palatine tonsils

b. Palatopharyngeal arch: posterior arch formed by a pair of folds extending from the soft palate to the lateral pharyngeal wall; each fold contains a palatopharyngeus muscle

c. Palatoglossal arch: anterior arch formed by a pair of folds extending from the soft palate to the sides of the tongue; each fold contains a palatoglossus muscle

d. Palatine tonsils: located laterally within the faucial isthmus, between the palatopharyngeal and palatoglossal arches; they are prominent in children but involuted in the adult

C. Laryngopharynx

1. Extends from the superior border of the epiglottis to the esophagus; its lateral and posterior walls are formed by the middle and inferior pharyngeal constrictors and its anterior wall opens into the laryngeal aditus superiorly and, inferiorly, is formed by the mucosa covering the posterior aspect of the larynx and the mucosa lining the piriform recesses, depressions on either side of the larynx

2. Clinical note: bits of food or swallowed foreign objects may lodge in the piriform recesses

III. Muscles

A. Pharyngeal constrictors

1. Superior pharyngeal constrictor

a. Origin: side of the tongue and the pterygomandibular raphe; the pterygomandibular raphe extends from the pterygoid hamulus to the posterior end of the mylohyoid line and represents the region of interdigitation of muscle fibers of the superior pharyngeal constrictor and buccinator

b. Insertion: pharyngeal tubercle and the pharyngeal raphe in the posterior midline; inferiorly, it is overlapped by the middle pharyngeal constrictor

2. Middle pharyngeal constrictor

   a. Origin: greater and lesser cornua of the hyoid bone and the stylohyoid ligament; the stylohyoid ligament extends from the styloid process to the lesser cornu of the hyoid bone

   b. Insertion: fans out from its origin to insert into the pharyngeal raphe; inferiorly, it is overlapped by the inferior pharyngeal constrictor

   c. Laterally, there is a gap between the middle pharyngeal constrictor and superior pharyngeal constrictor and another between the middle pharyngeal constrictor and inferior pharyngeal constrictor

3. Inferior pharyngeal constrictor

   a. Composed of two muscles, the thyropharyngeus and cricopharyngeus; they originate from the oblique line of the thyroid cartilage and the arch of the cricoid cartilage, respectively

   b. Insertion: pharyngeal raphe

4. Action: propel food and drink inferiorly, except for the cricopharyngeus, which relaxes to allow passage into the esophagus

5. Innervation: vagus nerve via the pharyngeal plexus; part of the inferior pharyngeal constrictor is innervated by the external laryngeal nerve

B. Palatopharyngeus

   1. Origin: hard and soft palate

   2. Insertion: lateral wall of the pharynx

   3. Action: elevation of the pharynx

   4. Innervation: vagus nerve via the pharyngeal plexus

C. Salpingopharyngeus

   1. Origin: cartilage of the auditory tube

   2. Insertion: merges with the palatopharyngeus in the lateral pharyngeal wall

   3. Action: elevation of the pharynx

4. Innervation: vagus nerve via the pharyngeal plexus

D. Stylopharyngeus

   1. Origin: medial side of the styloid process

   2. Insertion: passes through the gap in the lateral pharyngeal wall between the superior and middle pharyngeal constrictors and merges with the palatopharyngeus in the lateral pharyngeal wall

   3. Action: elevation of the pharynx

   4. Innervation: glossopharyngeal nerve

E. Deglutition

   1. After the pharynx has been elevated (and thereby shortened and widened) by contraction of the palatopharyngeus, salpingopharyngeus, and stylopharyngeus, the tongue pushes the bolus of food posteriorly into the oropharynx

   2. Elevation of the soft palate by the tensor veli palatini and levator veli palatini closes off the nasopharynx from the oropharynx and successive contractions of the superior and middle pharyngeal constrictors and the thyropharyngeus pass the bolus inferiorly; the cricopharyngeus relaxes to allow the bolus to pass into the esophagus

IV. Nerves

A. Glossopharyngeal nerve

   1. Exits the jugular foramen anterior to the internal jugular vein and descends lateral to the stylopharyngeus

   2. Pharyngeal branches contribute to the pharyngeal plexus and provide sensory innervation to the mucosa of the oropharynx; its only motor branch supplies the stylopharyngeus

B. Vagus nerve

   1. Exits the jugular foramen posterior to the internal jugular vein and medial to the accessory nerve; the hypoglossal nerve exits the hypoglossal canal medial to the vagus nerve and passes laterally, posterior to the vagus nerve, adhering to it

   2. A pharyngeal branch contributes to the pharyngeal plexus and provides motor innervation to the pharyngeal muscles, except the stylopharyn-

geus, which is innervated by the glossopharyngeal nerve; the innervation of the inferior pharyngeal constrictor is supplemented by the external laryngeal nerve

3. The superior laryngeal nerve branches from the vagus nerve, descends lateral to the pharynx, and divides into the internal and external laryngeal nerves; the internal laryngeal nerve penetrates the thyrohyoid membrane and provides sensory innervation to the mucosa of the superior part of the laryngopharynx, and the external laryngeal nerve descends inferior to the oblique line of the thyroid cartilage, deep to the sternothyroid and superficial to the inferior pharyngeal constrictor, and innervates part of the inferior pharyngeal constrictor (as well as the cricothyroid)

4. The recurrent laryngeal nerve ascends posterior to the thyroid gland and, as it enters the larynx between the inferior pharyngeal constrictor and esophagus, it provides sensory innervation to the mucosa of the inferior part of the laryngopharynx

C. Maxillary nerve: its pharyngeal branch courses posteriorly from the pterygopalatine fossa, through the palatovaginal canal, and provides sensory innervation to the mucosa of the nasopharynx

V. Vessels

A. Ascending pharyngeal artery: slender branch arising from the medial side of the external carotid artery; ascends between the lateral wall of the pharynx and internal carotid artery

B. Ascending palatine artery: branch of the facial artery; ascends on the lateral aspect of the superior pharyngeal constrictor, deep to the medial pterygoid

C. Superior thyroid artery: supplies the laryngopharynx as it descends between the sternothyroid and inferior pharyngeal constrictor with the external laryngeal nerve; gives rise to the superior laryngeal artery which supplies the laryngopharynx after penetrating the thyrohyoid membrane with the internal laryngeal nerve

D. Inferior laryngeal artery: branch of the inferior thyroid artery; supplies the laryngopharynx as it ascends between the inferior pharyngeal constrictor and esophagus with the recurrent laryngeal nerve

E. Pharyngeal plexus of veins: venous network within the buccopharyngeal fascia; drains anteriorly on either side of the pharynx into the pterygoid venous plexuses (some pharyngeal veins drain into the internal jugular vein)

F. Lymphatics: drain to retropharyngeal nodes along the posterolateral wall of the pharynx; retropharyngeal nodes drain to deep cervical nodes

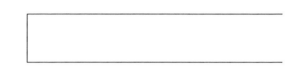

The Nose, Nasal Cavity, and Paranasal Sinuses

I. Nose

    A. Parts: the alae are the flared parts lateral to the nostrils, the dorsum is the ridge between the tip of the nose and forehead, and the bridge of the nose is where the dorsum meets the forehead

    B. Skeleton

        1. Bony components: the nasal part of the frontal bone, the nasal bones, and the portions of the maxillae bordering the piriform aperture provide a firm foundation for the cartilaginous components of the nose

        2. Cartilaginous components

            a. Lateral process of the septal cartilage: triangular plate supporting the side of the nose; articulates superiorly with the nasal bone and fuses to the septal cartilage in the midline

            b. Major alar cartilage: U-shaped plate; composed of a lateral crus that supports the ala and a medial crus which forms the anteroinferior part of the nasal septum with its fellow of the opposite side

II. Nasal Cavity

    A. Regions

        1. Vestibule: dilated region adjacent to the nostril; lined with hairs

2. Olfactory region: narrow region inferior to the cribriform plate (between a superior nasal concha and the nasal septum); lined by a mucosa containing olfactory neurons

3. Respiratory region: comprises most of the nasal cavity; lined by a glandular, vascular mucosa

B. Walls

1. Medial wall

   a. Composed of the nasal septum

   b. Formed posterosuperiorly and posteroinferiorly by the perpendicular plate of the ethmoid bone and vomer, respectively; anteriorly, it is formed by the septal cartilage and the medial crura of the major alar cartilages

   c. Clinical note: a deviated nasal septum is common

2. Lateral wall

   a. Superior, middle, and inferior nasal conchae

      1. Curved bony processes comprising most of the lateral nasal wall; their associated mucosa cleanses, warms, and humidifies the air

      2. The superior and middle nasal conchae are processes of the ethmoid bone; the inferior nasal concha is a separate bone of the skull

      3. The spaces inferior and lateral to the superior, middle, and inferior nasal conchae are the superior, middle, and inferior meatuses, respectively; the space above as well as behind the superior nasal concha is the sphenoethmoidal recess

   b. Ethmoidal bulla

      1. Large, rounded elevation lateral to the middle nasal concha

      2. The semilunar hiatus is the curved slit anterior and inferior to the ethmoidal bulla; anteriorly, it leads into a dilated channel, the ethmoidal infundibulum

   c. Atrium of the middle meatus: expanded region anterior to the middle meatus

   d. Agger nasi: ridge superior to the atrium of the middle meatus; contains some anterior ethmoidal air cells

3. Roof: composed of the cribriform plate anteriorly and body of the sphenoid posteriorly

4. Floor: formed by the hard palate

C. Nerves

1. Olfactory nerve: not a single nerve; nerve processes from olfactory neurons aggregate into numerous olfactory nerves which ascend through the foramina in the cribriform plate and enter the olfactory bulb; the olfactory tract extends posteriorly from the olfactory bulb

2. Anterior ethmoidal nerve: enters the nasal cavity through the cribriform plate and divides into the internal and external nasal nerves; the internal nasal nerve provides sensory innervation to the anterosuperior parts of the lateral nasal wall and nasal septum, and the external nasal nerve exits the nasal cavity between the nasal bone and lateral process of the septal cartilage to supply the dorsum and tip of the nose

3. Maxillary nerve

   a. Traverses foramen rotundum and emerges into the pterygopalatine fossa where the pterygopalatine ganglion is suspended from it; its sensory branches to the nasal cavity are noted below

   b. Posterior superior lateral nasal nerves: enter the nasal cavity through the sphenopalatine foramen, posterior to the middle nasal concha; supply the posterosuperior part of the lateral nasal wall

   c. Posterior superior medial nasal nerves and their largest branch, the nasopalatine nerve: enter the nasal cavity through the sphenopalatine foramen, posterior to the middle nasal concha, and supply the posterosuperior, posteroinferior, and anteroinferior parts of the nasal septum; the nasopalatine nerve continues through the incisive canal and incisive fossa and provides sensory innervation to the hard palate posterior to the upper incisors

   d. Posterior inferior lateral nasal nerves: arise from the greater palatine nerve, a branch of the maxillary nerve, as it descends in the inferior part of the greater palatine canal; supply the posteroinferior part of the lateral nasal wall

   e. Infraorbital nerve: after emerging onto the face through the infraorbital foramen, some of its branches supply the anteroinferior part of the lateral nasal wall

   f. Postganglionic parasympathetic secretomotor fibers from the pterygopalatine ganglion course with branches of the maxillary nerve ; they stimulate secretion of nasal glands

D. Vessels

1. Sphenopalatine artery: arises from the maxillary artery within the pterygopalatine fossa and enters the nasal cavity through the spheno-palatine foramen; divides into posterior lateral nasal arteries and poste-rior septal arteries which supply the posterior parts of the lateral nasal wall and nasal septum, respectively

2. Posterior ethmoidal artery: arises from the ophthalmic artery and emerges through the posterosuperior part of the lateral nasal wall; supplements the blood supply to the posterosuperior parts of the lateral nasal wall and nasal septum

3. Anterior ethmoidal artery: arises from the ophthalmic artery and enters the nasal cavity through the cribriform plate; supplies the anterosuperior parts of the lateral nasal wall and nasal septum

4. Superior labial and greater palatine arteries: arise from the facial and descending palatine arteries, respectively; enter the nasal cavity through the nostril and incisive canal, respectively, and supply the anteroinferior part of the nasal septum

5. Lateral nasal artery: arises from the facial artery; some of its branches supply the anteroinferior part of the lateral nasal wall

6. Veins: course with their corresponding arteries

III. Paranasal Sinuses

A. Mucosal-lined diverticula of the nasal cavity within the frontal, ethmoid, sphenoid, and maxillary bones

B. Frontal sinus: located superomedial to the orbital aperture within the squa-mous and orbital parts of the frontal bone; its frontonasal duct empties in-feriorly into the ethmoidal infundibulum, which, in turn, drains into the nasal cavity through the semilunar hiatus

C. Ethmoidal sinuses

1. Composed of about 10 thin-walled air cells located between the supe-rior and middle nasal conchae and the orbital lamina of the ethmoid bone; they are divided into three groups designated anterior, middle, and posterior

2. Anterior ethmoidal air cells drain into the ethmoidal infundibulum, middle ethmoidal air cells lie within and drain onto the surface of the ethmoidal bulla, and posterior ethmoidal air cells drain into the superior meatus

D. Sphenoidal sinus

1. Located within the body of the sphenoid (a bony septum, which is usually deviated, separates the two sphenoidal sinuses); drains into the sphenoethmoidal recess

2. The pterygoid canal, which transmits the nerve of the pterygoid canal, may produce a posterior-to-anterior ridge along its floor

E. Maxillary sinus

1. Its anterior and posterior walls are formed by the anterior and infratemporal surfaces of the maxilla, respectively; its medial wall forms the inferior part of the lateral nasal wall and the lateral wall extends into the zygomatic bone

2. Its floor is formed by the alveolar process of the maxilla and may exhibit elevations produced by the roots of the upper molar teeth; its roof is the floor of the orbit and may exhibit a posterior-to-anterior ridge formed by the infraorbital groove and infraorbital canal

3. Drains into the nasal cavity through the semilunar hiatus

4. Clinical note: extraction of an upper molar may create a fistula, or abnormal opening, between the maxillary sinus and oral cavity

F. Nerve and blood supply

1. Frontal sinus: supratrochlear and supraorbital nerves and vessels

2. Anterior and middle ethmoidal air cells: anterior ethmoidal nerve and vessels

3. Posterior ethmoidal air cells and sphenoidal sinus: posterior superior lateral nasal nerves, posterior lateral nasal vessels, and the posterior ethmoidal nerve and vessels

4. Maxillary sinus: posterior superior alveolar, middle superior alveolar, anterior superior alveolar, and infraorbital nerves; posterior superior alveolar, anterior superior alveolar, and infraorbital vessels

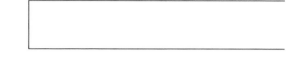

The Oral Cavity, Tongue, and Palate

I. Oral Cavity

    A. Vestibule: U-shaped region between the cheeks and lips and the teeth and gums; contains the labial frenula, midline mucosal folds attaching the lips to the gums, as well as the parotid papillae

    B. Oral cavity proper: region bounded by the teeth and gums, palate, and floor of the mouth; it is continuous posteriorly with the faucial isthmus

II. Tongue

    A. Parts

        1. Root (posterior part)

            a. Joined to the epiglottis by a median and two lateral glossoepiglottic folds; the depressions between the glossoepiglottic folds are called the epiglottic valleculae

            b. Attached to the mandible, hyoid bone, styloid process, and palate by the genioglossus, hyoglossus, styloglossus, and palatoglossus muscles, respectively

        2. Dorsum (superior surface)

            a. Anteriorly, it is covered by slender, filiform papillae and occasional globular, fungiform papillae; posteriorly, large vallate papillae are arranged anterior to the sulcus terminalis, a V-shaped groove exhibiting a pit, the foramen cecum, at its posterior tip (the foramen cecum marks the site of origin of the thyroid gland)

    b. Most posteriorly, it is covered by smooth nodules formed by the lingual tonsil

  3. Inferior surface: the lingual frenulum, a midline mucosal fold, attaches the inferior surface of the tongue to the floor of the mouth

B. Associated structures

  1. Sublingual gland: lies inferior to the tongue within the sublingual fossa; several sublingual ducts empty onto the floor of the mouth along a ridge, the sublingual fold, formed by the subjacent sublingual gland

  2. Submandibular (Wharton's) duct: emerges from the part of the submandibular gland deep to the mylohyoid, courses anteriorly, medial to the sublingual gland, and opens onto the sublingual caruncle, a small mucosal papilla lateral to the lingual frenulum; from proximal to distal, the lingual nerve courses lateral, then inferior, and then medial to the submandibular duct

C. Muscles

  1. A median fibrous septum separates the musculature of each side of the tongue

  2. Extrinsic muscles

    a. Have attachment outside the tongue

    b. Genioglossus

      1. Origin: superior mental spine

      2. Insertion: fibers fan out and insert into the entire tongue

      3. Action: deviation of the tongue to the opposite side; acting together, both muscles protrude the tongue directly forward

    c. Hyoglossus

      1. Origin: body and greater cornu of the hyoid

      2. Insertion: side of the tongue

3. Action: depression of the tongue

4. From superior to inferior, the following structures lie medial to the hyoglossus: glossopharyngeal nerve, stylohyoid ligament, and lingual artery

5. From superior to inferior, the following structures lie lateral to the hyoglossus: lingual nerve, submandibular duct, and hypoglossal nerve

d. Styloglossus

1. Origin: tip of the styloid process

2. Insertion: its fibers intermingle with those of the hyoglossus on the side of the tongue

3. Action: elevation and retraction of the tongue

e. Palatoglossus

1. Origin: soft palate

2. Insertion: side of the tongue

3. Action: elevation of the tongue

3. Intrinsic muscles

a. Have attachment entirely within the tongue; composed of interweaving bundles termed the superior longitudinal, inferior longitudinal, transverse, and vertical muscles

b. Action

1. Superior longitudinal muscles: shorten the tongue and render the dorsum concave

2. Inferior longitudinal muscles: shorten the tongue and render the dorsum convex

3. Transverse muscles: narrow and elongate the tongue

4. Vertical muscles: flatten and widen the tongue

4. Innervation: hypoglossal nerve, except the palatoglossus, which is innervated by the vagus nerve via the pharyngeal plexus

5. Clinical note: following unilateral hypoglossal nerve injury, a protruding tongue deviates to the paralyzed side because of the unopposed action of the functional genioglossus

D. Nerves

1. Lingual nerve

   a. Shortly after branching from the mandibular nerve, the lingual nerve is joined by the chorda tympani nerve; it then descends anteriorly on the lateral surfaces of the medial pterygoid and hyoglossus

   b. The submandibular ganglion is suspended from the lingual nerve opposite the third lower molar and receives preganglionic parasympathetic fibers from the chorda tympani nerve; exiting postganglionic parasympathetic secretomotor fibers supply the adjacent submandibular and sublingual glands

   c. The lingual nerve provides general sensory innervation to the anterior two-thirds of the tongue; taste innervation for the anterior two-thirds of the tongue is provided by the chorda tympani nerve

2. Hypoglossal nerve: courses anteriorly between the mylohyoid and hyoglossus; innervates all the muscles of the tongue, except palatoglossus, which is innervated by the vagus nerve via the pharyngeal plexus

3. Glossopharyngeal nerve

   a. Accompanies the stylopharyngeus through the gap in the lateral pharyngeal wall between the superior and middle pharyngeal constrictors; courses anteriorly, between the palatine tonsil and hyoglossus, and provides general sensory and taste innervation to the posterior one-third of the tongue

   b. Clinical note: as the glossopharyngeal nerve courses deep to the palatine tonsil, it is subject to injury during tonsillectomy; injury may result in loss of general sensation and taste on the posterior one-third of the tongue

4. Internal laryngeal nerve: penetrates the thyrohyoid membrane and provides general sensory and taste innervation to the very posterior part of the tongue and epiglottis

E. Vessels

1. Lingual artery

   a. Arises from the external carotid artery posterior to the tip of the greater cornu of the hyoid and courses anteriorly, deep to the hyoglossus

b. Gives rise to the dorsal lingual arteries, which ascend medial to the hyoglossus and supply the root of the tongue and, near the anterior border of hyoglossus, it divides into its terminal branches, the sublingual and deep lingual arteries; the sublingual artery supplies the adjacent sublingual gland and the deep lingual artery courses forward to the tip of the tongue accompanied by the lingual nerve and deep lingual vein

2. Lingual vein

a. The deep lingual vein unites with the sublingual vein at the anterior border of the hyoglossus to form the vena comitans of the hypoglossal nerve; this vein courses posteriorly with the hypoglossal nerve, lateral to the hyoglossus

b. The vena comitans of the hypoglossal nerve and the dorsal lingual vein unite near the posterior border of the hyoglossus to form the lingual vein, which courses posteriorly to drain into the internal jugular vein

3. Lymphatics: the anterior part of the tongue drains to submental, submandibular, and deep cervical nodes, and the posterior part of the tongue drains to deep cervical nodes; the part of the tongue adjacent to the midline drains into nodes of both sides

III. Palate

A. Separates the oral cavity from the nasal cavities

B. Parts

1. Hard palate: bony, anterior two-thirds; formed anteriorly by the palatine processes of the maxillae and posteriorly by the horizontal plates of the palatine bones

2. Soft palate: nonbony, posterior one-third; a conical projection, the uvula, drapes from the middle of its posterior free border

C. Muscles

1. Levator veli palatini

a. Origin: apex of the petrous part of the temporal bone and the cartilaginous part of the auditory tube

b. Insertion: descends into the soft palate, forming the torus levatorius

c. Action: elevates the soft palate, and thus closes off the oropharynx from the nasopharynx and nasal cavities

2. Tensor veli palatini

a. Origin: scaphoid fossa and the cartilaginous part of the auditory tube

b. Insertion: descends vertically from its origin; its tendon then bends medially, at a right angle, within the groove of the pterygoid hamulus and fans out into the aponeurosis within the soft palate

c. Action: in order for levator veli palatini to elevate the soft palate, the aponeurosis within the soft palate must first be tensed and stabilized by tensor veli palatini

d. Located anterior and lateral to levator veli palatini and medial to the otic ganglion and mandibular nerve

3. Musculus uvulae

a. Origin: posterior nasal spine

b. Insertion: uvula

c. Action: elevation and lateral deviaton of the uvula

4. Innervation: vagus nerve via the pharyngeal plexus, except tensor veli palatini, which is innervated by the nerve to the tensor veli palatini, a branch of the nerve to the medial pterygoid, which, in turn, is a branch of the mandibular nerve

D. Nerves

1. Greater palatine nerve: arises from the maxillary nerve in the pterygopalatine fossa and descends in the greater palatine canal; emerges from the greater palatine foramen and courses anteriorly within the mucosa of the hard palate, providing sensory innervation as far as the incisor teeth

2. Lesser palatine nerves: arise from the maxillary nerve in the pterygopalatine fossa and descend in the greater palatine canal; emerge through the lesser palatine foramina to provide sensory innervation to the soft palate

3. Nasopalatine nerve: largest posterior superior medial nasal nerve given off by the maxillary nerve within the pterygopalatine fossa; enters the

nasal cavity through the sphenopalatine foramen, descends anteriorly on the nasal septum, and passes through the incisive canal and incisive fossa to provide sensory innervation to the hard palate, posterior to the upper incisors

4. Postganglionic parasympathetic secretomotor fibers from the pterygo-palatine ganglion course with the greater palatine, lesser palatine, and nasopalatine nerves and stimulate secretion of palatal glands

E. Vessels

1. Descending palatine artery

   a. Arises from the maxillary artery within the pterygopalatine fossa; descends in the greater palatine canal and divides into the greater and lesser palatine arteries

   b. Greater palatine artery: emerges from the greater palatine foramen and courses anteriorly on the hard palate with the greater palatine nerve; in contrast to the greater palatine nerve, however, the greater palatine artery continues forward, beyond the canine, through the incisive fossa and incisive canal, to supply the anteroinferior part of the nasal septum

   c. Lesser palatine arteries: emerge through the lesser palatine foramina to course with the lesser palatine nerves within the soft palate

2. Ascending palatine artery: branch of the facial artery; ascends on the lateral aspect of the superior pharyngeal constrictor, arches medially over the superior border of the superior pharyngeal constrictor, and descends on the levator veli palatini to supply the soft palate

3. Veins: accompany their corresponding arteries

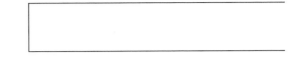

The Larynx

I. Skeleton

   A. Thyroid cartilage

      1. Composed of two laminae and two pairs of cornua

      2. Laminae

         a. Quadrilateral plates that fuse in the anterior midline at an acute angle; superiorly, there is a midline indentation, the superior thyroid notch

         b. Anteriorly descending ridges on the external surfaces of the laminae, the oblique lines, provide attachment for the inferior pharyngeal constrictor, sternothyroid, and thyrohyoid muscles

      3. Cornua

         a. Fingerlike projections

         b. Superior cornua: extend superiorly from the posterior borders of the laminae

         c. Inferior cornua: extend inferiorly from the posterior borders of the laminae; medially, at their tips, they exhibit facets for articulation at synovial cricothyroid joints

      4. Thyrohyoid membrane: connective tissue sheet between the superior border of the thyroid cartilage and hyoid bone; median and lateral thickenings form the median and lateral thyrohyoid ligaments, respectively

5. Clinical note: the thyroid cartilage may calcify and become visible on X-ray

B. Cricoid cartilage

   1. Ring-shaped; consists of a narrow, anterior arch and a broad, posterior lamina

   2. Arch: located on a level with vertebra C6; joined to the thyroid cartilage by the median cricothyroid ligament and to the first tracheal ring by the cricotracheal ligament

   3. Lamina: quadrilateral plate; exhibits facets superiorly and inferolaterally for articulation with the arytenoid cartilages and inferior cornua of the thyroid cartilage, respectively

C. Arytenoid cartilages

   1. Shaped like three-sided pyramids; their bases articulate with the superior surface of the lamina of the cricoid cartilage at synovial cricoarytenoid joints and, atop their apices, reside the corniculate cartilages

   2. A muscular process extends laterally from the base and provides attachment for muscles; a vocal process extends forward from the base and provides attachment for the vocal ligament

   3. The aryepiglottic folds extend between the arytenoid cartilages and the epiglottis, and an interarytenoid fold extends between the arytenoid cartilages themselves

D. Epiglottis: cartilaginous plate shaped like an inverted teardrop; its narrow stalk attaches in the groove formed by the thyroid laminae, about midway along its length

II. Regions and Their Associated Structures

A. Vestibule

   1. Portion of the laryngeal cavity between the laryngeal aditus and rima vestibuli, the slitlike interval between the vestibular folds

   2. The laryngeal aditus is the entrance into the larynx; it is bordered anteriorly by the epiglottis, posteriorly by the interarytenoid fold, and on each side by an aryepiglottic fold

   3. Vestibular folds ("false vocal cords")

a. Prominent mucosal ridges extending from the lateral borders of the arytenoid cartilages to the groove formed by the thyroid laminae, superior to the attachment of the epiglottis

b. The vestibular folds contain the vestibular ligaments, thickenings of the inferior edges of the quadrangular membranes; the quadrangular membranes are supportive, submucosal connective tissue sheets extending between the free borders of the aryepiglottic and vestibular folds

B. Ventricles

1. The portion of the laryngeal cavity between the rima vestibuli and the rima glottidis (the slitlike interval between the vocal folds) expands laterally to form the ventricles, two fusiform chambers between the vestibular and vocal folds; the anterior parts of each ventricle may expand superiorly to form a laryngeal saccule

2. Vocal folds ("true vocal cords")

   a. Prominent mucosal ridges inferior to the vestibular folds; they extend from the vocal processes of the arytenoid cartilages to the groove formed by the thyroid laminae, lateral to the attachment of the epiglottis

   b. The vocal folds contain the vocal ligaments

      1. The vocal ligaments represent thickenings of the superior edge of the conus elasticus, a supportive, submucosal connective tissue sheet similar to the quadrangular membrane; on each side, the conus elasticus extends from the superior border of the arch of the cricoid cartilage to the free border of a vocal fold (it is continuous in the anterior midline with the median cricothyroid ligament)

      2. Vibration of adducted vocal ligaments with expired air produces sound, which can be transformed into speech by the tongue, teeth, and lips; lower-pitched speech in males is primarily a consequence of longer and thicker vocal ligaments

   c. The vocal folds and rima glottidis are sometimes referred to as the glottis

C. Infraglottic cavity: portion of the laryngeal cavity between the rima glottidis and inferior border of the cricoid cartilage; it is continuous inferiorly with the lumen of the trachea

III. Muscles

    A. Cricothyroid

        1. Origin: external surface of the arch of the cricoid cartilage

        2. Insertion: inferior border and inferior cornu of the thyroid cartilage

        3. Action: tilts the thyroid cartilage forward, thereby tensing and adducting the vocal ligaments

    B. Posterior cricoarytenoid

        1. Origin: posterior surface of the lamina of the cricoid cartilage

        2. Insertion: muscular process of the arytenoid cartilage

        3. Action: laterally rotates the arytenoid cartilage, thereby abducting the vocal ligament; since the posterior cricoarytenoids are the only abductors of the vocal ligaments, they assume a vital role in maintaining an open airway

    C. Lateral cricoarytenoid

        1. Origin: superior border of the arch of the cricoid cartilage

        2. Insertion: muscular process of the arytenoid cartilage

        3. Action: medially rotates the arytenoid cartilage, thereby adducting the vocal ligament

    D. Arytenoideus

        1. Transverse part: extends horizontally between the posterior surfaces of the arytenoid cartilages

        2. Oblique part

            a. Lies posterior to the transverse part

            b. Origin: muscular process of the arytenoid cartilage

            c. Insertion: apex of the arytenoid cartilage of the opposite side; some fibers continue forward to the epiglottis within the aryepiglottic fold and comprise the aryepiglotticus muscle

        3. Action: draws the arytenoid cartilages toward one another, thereby ad-

ducting the vocal ligaments; together, the oblique parts of the arytenoideus and the aryepiglotticus muscles close the laryngeal aditus in "purse-string" fashion during deglutition

E. Thyroarytenoideus

   1. Origin: groove formed by the thyroid laminae, lateral to the attachments of the vestibular and vocal folds

   2. Insertion: lateral border of the arytenoid cartilage

   3. Action: adducts the vocal ligament as the muscle thickens during contraction; decreases the tension of the vocal ligament as it draws the arytenoid cartilage toward the thyroid cartilage

   4. Its inferomedial fibers lie within the vocal fold, attach along the vocal ligament, and comprise the vocalis muscle; the vocalis varies the length and tension of the vibrating portion of the vocal ligament to produce variations in pitch

F. Thyroepiglotticus

   1. Origin: groove formed by the thyroid laminae, superior to the thyroarytenoideus

   2. Insertion: lateral margin of the epiglottis

   3. Action: holds the epiglottis against the laryngeal aditus during deglutition

G. Innervation: recurrent laryngeal nerve, except the cricothyroid, which is innervated by the external laryngeal nerve

IV. Nerves

A. Superior laryngeal nerve

   1. Descends lateral to the pharynx; divides into the internal and external laryngeal nerves posterosuperior to the tip of the greater cornu of the hyoid, medial to the external carotid artery

   2. Internal laryngeal nerve: penetrates the thyrohyoid membrane with the superior laryngeal artery, in the gap between the middle and inferior pharyngeal constrictors; descends within the mucosa of the piriform recess and provides sensory innervation to the laryngeal mucosa superior to the vocal folds

3. External laryngeal nerve: descends with the superior thyroid artery, inferior to the oblique line of the thyroid cartilage, deep to the sternothyroid and superficial to the inferior pharyngeal constrictor; innervates the cricothyroid (as well as part of the inferior pharyngeal constrictor)

B. Recurrent laryngeal nerves

1. The right and left recurrent laryngeal nerves loop posteriorly around the right subclavian artery and aortic arch, respectively, and ascend in the grooves between the trachea and esophagus on their respective sides; as they ascend posterior to the lobes of the thyroid gland, they enter the larynx posterior to the cricothyroid articulation, between the inferior pharyngeal constrictor and esophagus

2. Innervate all the muscles of the larynx, except the cricothyroids (which are innervated by the external laryngeal nerves), and provide sensory innervation to the laryngeal mucosa inferior to the vocal folds

C. Clinical notes

1. External laryngeal nerve injury may occur when securing the superior thyroid artery during a thyroidectomy; paralysis of the cricothyroid muscle, and loss of its function in tensing the vocal ligaments, may result in hoarseness

2. Bilateral injury to the recurrent laryngeal nerves, perhaps during a thyroidectomy, produces a narrowing of the rima glottidis as a result of paralysis of the posterior cricoarytenoid muscles and loss of their function as the only abductors of the vocal ligaments; unopposed adduction of the vocal ligaments by the cricothyroid muscles may require surgical intervention to correct respiratory distress

V. Vessels

A. Superior laryngeal artery: arises from the superior thyroid artery; accompanies the internal laryngeal nerve through the thyrohyoid membrane and supplies the superior part of the larynx

B. Inferior laryngeal artery: arises from the inferior thyroid artery; accompanies the recurrent laryngeal nerve into the larynx (between the inferior pharyngeal constrictor and esophagus) and supplies the inferior part of the larynx

C. Veins: accompany their respective arteries

D. Lymphatics: drain to deep cervical nodes

The Ear

I. External Ear

   A. Auricle

      1. Bordered primarily by the rimlike helix, as well as by the pendulous lobule inferiorly, and the pointed tragus anteriorly; its central fossa is termed the concha

      2. Except for the lobule, it is supported by the auricular cartilage

      3. Nerve supply: lesser occipital, great auricular, and auriculotemporal nerves, and the auricular branch of the vagus nerve

      4. Blood supply: posterior auricular and superficial temporal vessels

      5. Function: collects sound waves and channels them into the external acoustic meatus

   B. External acoustic (auditory) meatus

      1. Extends approximately 2.5 centimeters from the concha to the tympanic membrane; its lateral one-third and medial two-thirds are formed by the auricular cartilage and temporal bone, respectively

      2. Parts (from lateral to medial): the first part (pars externa) courses medially, anteriorly, and superiorly, the second part (pars media) courses medially, posteriorly, and superiorly, and the third part (pars interna) courses medially, anteriorly, and inferiorly

3. Ceruminous glands

    a. Modified sweat glands whose secretions combine with secretions of sebaceous glands to form ear wax or cerumen; cerumen prevents maceration of the meatal lining by trapped water and may help repel insects

    b. Clinical note: cerumen may decrease hearing acuity by occluding the external acoustic meatus or by contacting the tympanic membrane and dampening its vibrations

4. Nerve supply: auriculotemporal nerve and the auricular branch of the vagus nerve

5. Blood supply: posterior auricular, superficial temporal, and deep auricular vessels

6. Function: directs sound waves toward the tympanic membrane

II. Middle Ear

A. Tympanic membrane

1. Thin, delicate membrane separating the external acoustic meatus from the tympanic cavity

2. Composed of a middle fibrous layer interposed between a mucosa internally and skin externally; its external surface faces laterally, inferiorly, and anteriorly

3. The manubrium of the malleus attaches to the mucosal side of the tympanic membrane, draws it inward, and gives the tympanic membrane the form of a shallow cone whose apex is called the umbo

    a. Superior to the umbo, the lateral process of the malleus contacts the mucosal surface of the tympanic membrane, producing the anterior and posterior malleolar folds which extend superiorly from the point of contact

    b. The part of the tympanic membrane between the malleolar folds is highly vascular, devoid of a middle fibrous layer, and termed the pars flaccida; the remaining part of the tympanic membrane is called the pars tensa

4. Nerve supply: auriculotemporal nerve, tympanic branch of the glossopharyngeal nerve, and the auricular branch of the vagus nerve

5. Blood supply: deep auricular, anterior tympanic, and stylomastoid vessels (the stylomastoid artery is a branch of the posterior auricular artery and enters the skull through the stylomastoid foramen)

6. Function

   a. Sound consists of alternating waves of gaseous compression and rarefaction; since compressed gas has a higher pressure than rarefied gas, alternating changes in air pressure cause the tympanic membrane to vibrate

   b. Vibration of the tympanic membrane vibrates the malleus, which, in turn, vibrates the incus and then the stapes; through the movements of the auditory ossicles, sound vibrations are transmitted from the tympanic membrane across the tympanic cavity to the fluid of the inner ear

B. Tympanic cavity

   1. Slitlike, air-filled, mucosal–lined space medial to the tympanic membrane; contains the auditory ossicles

   2. Roof: separates the tympanic cavity from the middle cranial fossa; composed of the tegmen tympani, a thin plate of the petrous part of the temporal bone

   3. Floor: formed by the jugular fossa, a smooth depression roofing the jugular foramen; the tympanic branch of the glossopharyngeal nerve arises below the jugular foramen, enters the external opening of the tympanic canaliculus between the carotid canal and jugular foramen, traverses the tympanic canaliculus, and emerges through the internal opening of the tympanic canaliculus on the floor of the tympanic cavity

   4. Anterior wall

      a. Separates the tympanic cavity from the carotid canal; the caroticotympanic nerves, postganglionic sympathetic fibers from the internal carotid plexus, enter the tympanic cavity through its anterior wall

      b. Superiorly, the anterior wall presents the musculotubal canal, which is divided into two parallel semicanals by a thin, bony septum; the inferior semicanal represents the auditory tube, which connects the tympanic cavity to the nasopharynx, and the superior semicanal houses the tensor tympani muscle

      c. The cochleariform process is formed by the pulleylike posterior end of the thin, bony septum separating the semicanals; over this process, the tendon of the tensor tympani bends laterally at a right angle to reach its insertion on the superior part of the manubrium of the malleus

5. Posterior wall

   a. An irregular aperture, the aditus ad antrum, is located superiorly on the posterior wall; it is continuous posteriorly with an expanded chamber, the mastoid antrum, which, in turn, is continuous with the mastoid air cells

   b. The pyramidal eminence, a hollow, volcanolike projection, lies inferior to the aditus ad antrum

6. Medial wall

   a. Promontory

      1. Round bulge located centrally on the medial wall; produced by the basal turn of the cochlea

      2. Within its mucosal covering lies a nerve network, the tympanic plexus, which is formed by the caroticotympanic nerves and the tympanic branch of the glossopharyngeal nerve; the tympanic branch of the glossopharyngeal nerve is composed of preganglionic parasympathetic fibers from the inferior salivatory nucleus in the brainstem as well as general sensory fibers

      3. The tympanic plexus gives rise to the lesser petrosal nerve, which traverses a small canal near the semicanal for the tensor tympani, emerges into the middle cranial fossa through the hiatus for the lesser petrosal nerve, continues anteriorly in the sulcus for the lesser petrosal nerve, and exits the skull through foramen ovale to reach the subjacent otic ganglion; preganglionic parasympathetic fibers within the lesser petrosal nerve synapse in the otic ganglion (postganglionic sympathetic fibers from the caroticotympanic nerves pass through without synapse) and postganglionic parasympathetic secretomotor fibers from the otic ganglion are distributed to the parotid gland via the auriculotemporal and facial nerves

   b. Round window (fenestra cochleae): round opening posteroinferior to the promontory; it is closed in life by the secondary tympanic membrane, which undergoes compensatory movements opposite those of the pistonlike stapes

   c. Oval window (fenestra vestibuli): oval opening superior to the promontory; it is closed in life by the base of the stapes and annular ligament

    d. Prominence of the facial canal: elevation superior to the oval window; produced by the facial nerve as it courses posteriorly from the geniculate ganglion within the facial canal

    e. Prominence of the lateral semicircular canal: elevation superior to the prominence of the facial canal; produced by the ampullary crus of the lateral semicircular canal

7. Lateral wall

    a. Consists primarily of the tympanic membrane; superiorly, it is formed by the lateral wall of the epitympanic recess, a hollowed-out region in the roof, superior to the tympanic membrane

    b. The epitympanic recess contains the head of the malleus and the body and short crus of the incus; it opens posteriorly into the aditus ad antrum

8. Nerve supply: tympanic branch of the glossopharyngeal nerve

9. Blood supply: stylomastoid and anterior tympanic vessels

C. Auditory ossicles

1. Malleus (hammer)

    a. Head: spherical, upper end

    b. Neck: constricted portion inferior to the head

    c. Anterior process: anteriorly directed spicule arising from the neck

    d. Lateral process: conical, lateral projection of the superior end of the manubrium

    e. Manubrium: inferior, elongated projection; its inferior extremity extends to the umbo

2. Incus (anvil)

    a. Body: shaped like a flattened cube; articulates with the head of the malleus at the incudomalleolar joint

    b. Short crus: rounded projection extending posteriorly from the body

c. Long crus: elongated projection descending from the body, parallel and medial to the manubrium of the malleus; its inferior tip bends medially and ends in a nodule, the lenticular process

3. Stapes (stirrup)

   a. Head: laterally directed, apical process; articulates with the lenticular process of the incus at the incudostapedial joint

   b. Neck: constricted part adjoining the head

   c. Crura: an anterior and a posterior crus extend from the neck to the base; the anterior crus is shorter than the posterior crus

   d. Base: flat, oval plate; attached to the margin of the oval window by the annular ligament

4. The auditory ossicles are suspended within the tympanic cavity by delicate ligaments; the mucosa lining the tympanic cavity ensheaths the auditory ossicles and is also continuous with the mucosa lining the mastoid antrum, mastoid air cells, and auditory tube

5. Clinical note: since the incudomalleolar and incudostapedial joints are synovial joints, they are subject to the same diseases, such as arthritis, as other synovial joints

D. Muscles

1. Tensor tympani

   a. Origin: the wall of the superior semicanal of the musculotubal canal

   b. Insertion: its tendon bends laterally at a right angle over the cochleariform process to insert on the medial surface of the superior part of the manubrium of the malleus

   c. Action: contracts reflexly in response to loud sounds, and thus, exerts a protective dampening effect by tensing the tympanic membrane and reducing its sensitivity

   d. Innervation: nerve to the tensor tympani, a branch of the nerve to the medial pterygoid, which, in turn, is a branch of the mandibular nerve

2. Stapedius

   a. Origin: the inner wall of the pyramidal eminence

b. Insertion: its tendon exits the orifice at the apex of the pyramidal eminence and inserts on the posterior aspect of the neck of the stapes

c. Action: contracts reflexly in response to loud sounds, and thus, exerts a protective dampening effect by holding the stapes against the oval window

d. Innervation: nerve to the stapedius, a branch of the facial nerve

e. Clinical note: facial nerve injury and paralysis of the stapedius results in excessive acuteness of hearing or hyperacusia

E. Facial nerve

1. Courses laterally within the internal acoustic (auditory) meatus adjacent to the vestibulocochlear nerve; at the blind, lateral end of the internal acoustic meatus, the facial nerve enters the facial canal within the petrous part of the temporal bone

2. The facial nerve continues laterally within the facial canal along the roof of the vestibule of the inner ear; as it approaches the medial wall of the tympanic cavity, it expands at the geniculate ganglion, which contains the cell bodies of taste fibers that course within the chorda tympani nerve

3. The greater petrosal nerve courses anteriorly from the geniculate ganglion and contains preganglionic parasympathetic fibers from the superior salivatory nucleus in the brainstem

   a. The greater petrosal nerve emerges from the hiatus for the greater petrosal nerve in the middle cranial fossa and continues anteriorly in the sulcus for the greater petrosal nerve

   b. As the greater petrosal nerve passes horizontally across foramen lacerum, it is joined by the deep petrosal nerve from the internal carotid plexus (which contains postganglionic sympathetic fibers), and becomes the nerve of the pterygoid canal; the nerve of the pterygoid canal traverses the pterygoid canal and, when it emerges into the pterygopalatine fossa, its preganglionic parasympathetic fibers from the greater petrosal nerve synapse in the pterygopalatine ganglion, and its postganglionic sympathetic fibers from the deep petrosal nerve pass through without synapse

   c. From the pterygopalatine ganglion, postganglionic, parasympathetic, and sympathetic fibers are distributed to the nasal, palatal, and lacrimal glands via branches of the maxillary nerve

4. The facial nerve continues posteriorly from the geniculate ganglion,

producing the prominence of the facial canal on the medial wall of the tympanic cavity; it then descends within the posterior wall of the tympanic cavity and gives rise to the nerve to the stapedius and the chorda tympani nerve

    a. The chorda tympani nerve enters the tympanic cavity through a posterior canaliculus and courses anteriorly on the medial surface of the superior part of the manubrium, superior to the insertion of tensor tympani; it then exits the tympanic cavity through an anterior canaliculus and emerges from the skull through the petrotympanic fissure to join the lingual nerve

    b. The chorda tympani nerve contains preganglionic parasympathetic fibers from the superior salivatory nucleus in the brainstem as well as taste fibers for the anterior two-thirds of the tongue

  5. The facial nerve exits the skull through the stylomastoid foramen

F. Clinical notes

  1. Infection of the middle ear, otitis media, often spreads to the tympanic cavity from the nasopharynx via the auditory tube; from the tympanic cavity it may spread through the aditus ad antrum into the mastoid antrum and mastoid air cells

  2. Because of the close relationship of the tympanic cavity to the internal jugular vein, internal carotid artery, and subarachnoid space, skull fractures involving the petrous part of the temporal bone may result in leakage of blood or cerebrospinal fluid into the tympanic cavity

  3. Otosclerosis is a condition in which there is hearing loss as a result of ossification of the annular ligament and fixation of the stapes within the oval window; hearing is sometimes restored by surgically replacing the stapes with a prosthesis

III. Inner (Internal) Ear

A. Located within the petrous part of the temporal bone, medial to the middle ear; subserves the functions of balance and hearing

B. Consists of a series of membranous and bony chambers comprising the membranous and bony labyrinths, respectively

  1. The membranous labyrinth is filled with endolymph and is housed within

the bony labyrinth; the membranous and bony labyrinths are separated by a perilymphatic space filled with perilymph

2. Structures comprising the membranous labyrinth include the utricle, saccule, three semicircular ducts, and a cochlear duct; structures comprising the bony labyrinth include the vestibule, three semicircular canals, and the scala vestibuli and scala tympani

C. Vestibule, utricle, and saccule

1. The vestibule is the oval, middle part of the bony labyrinth located posterior to the scala vestibuli and scala tympani and anterior to the semicircular canals; it contains two rounded chambers of the membranous labyrinth, the utricle and saccule

2. The utricle and saccule are joined together by the utriculosaccular duct from which the endolymphatic duct courses posteriorly within the vestibular aqueduct, a tiny canal in the petrous part of the temporal bone; distally, the endolymphatic duct emerges into the posterior cranial fossa on the posterior surface of the petrous part of the temporal bone as a dilatation called the endolymphatic sac

   a. Sensory hair cells within the utricle and saccule sense gravity and initiate reflex contraction of limb and trunk muscles in response to changes in the position of the head

   b. Clinical note: Ménière's disease is characterized by an increase in pressure within the membranous labyrinth, which may damage its sensory hair cells; one form of treatment is to surgically incise the endolymphatic sac in the posterior cranial fossa to allow drainage of excess endolymph into the subarachnoid space

3. Foramina within the medial wall of the vestibule transmit branches of the vestibular division of the vestibulocochlear nerve to the internal acoustic meatus; its lateral wall is perforated by the oval window

D. Semicircular canals and semicircular ducts

1. Each of three tubular, archlike, semicircular canals contains a similarly contoured semicircular duct; each semicircular canal and semicircular duct pair lies in a different plane and, each semicircular canal and duct is composed of two crura, one of which exhibits a terminal dilatation called an ampulla

2. The semicircular canals and semicircular ducts open into the vestibule and utricle, respectively; the ampullae of the semicircular ducts contain

sensory hair cells that sense rotational movements of the head and initiate reflex contraction of eye and neck muscles

3. Anterior semicircular canal

   a. Positioned upright and perpendicular to the petrous ridge; it produces the arcuate eminence in the middle cranial fossa

   b. Its lateral crus opens into the lateral region of the vestibule and exhibits an ampulla; its medial crus joins the anterior crus of the posterior semicircular canal to form the common crus

4. Posterior semicircular canal: positioned upright and parallel to the petrous ridge; its anterior crus forms the common crus with the medial crus of the anterior semicircular canal and its ampullary posterior crus opens into the posterior region of the vestibule

5. Lateral semicircular canal

   a. Positioned horizontally when the chin is tilted downward 30 degrees

   b. Its anterior ampullary crus opens into the vestibule inferior to the ampulla of the anterior semicircular canal and produces the prominence of the lateral semicircular canal on the medial wall of the tympanic cavity; its posterior crus opens into the posterior region of the vestibule near the ampullary posterior crus of the posterior semicircular canal

6. Clinical note: the functional integrity of the semicircular ducts may be tested by revolving an individual; this will cause flow of endolymph in the semicircular ducts that will stimulate their sensory hair cells and produce a nystagmus or oscillation of the eyes

E. Cochlea

1. The cochlea resembles a snail shell that makes two and three-quarter turns from its base to its apex or cupula; the basal turn produces the promontory and the apex points anterolaterally

2. The cochlea consists primarily of two helically arranged chambers of the bony labyrinth, the scala vestibuli and scala tympani, which are continuous with one another at the apex through an opening called the helicotrema; the scala vestibuli is continuous proximally with the vestibule and the scala tympani ends distally at the secondary tympanic membrane within the round window

3. The cochlear duct is also helically arranged and interposed between the

scala vestibuli and scala tympani; it contains the sensory hair cells of the organ of Corti, the organ of hearing, and communicates with the saccule through the ductus reuniens

4. A tiny canal, the aqueduct of the cochlea, extends from the scala tympani to the roof of the jugular foramen and forms a communication between the perilymphatic and subarachnoid spaces

5. Foramina within the region of the cochlea facing the internal acoustic meatus transmit branches of the cochlear division of the vestibulocochlear nerve to the internal acoustic meatus

F. Blood supply: the labyrinthine artery, a branch of the basilar artery, enters the inner ear through the internal acoustic meatus; the accompanying labyrinthine vein drains into the inferior petrosal sinus

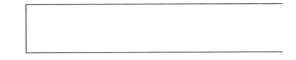

The Autonomic Supply to the Head

I. Sympathetic System

    A. Superior cervical ganglion

        1. Large, oblong, flattened structure lying on the longus capitis, anterior to the transverse processes of the upper three cervical vertebrae

        2. Postganglionic sympathetic fibers emerge from the superior cervical ganglion and are distributed to the head and neck along branches of the external and internal carotid arteries as the external and internal carotid plexuses, respectively; some of the branches of the internal carotid plexus are noted below

        3. Caroticotympanic nerves

            a. Arise from the internal carotid plexus as the internal carotid artery courses in the carotid canal anterior to the tympanic cavity

            b. They penetrate the anterior wall of the tympanic cavity and join the tympanic branch of the glossopharyngeal nerve on the promontory to form the tympanic plexus; they leave the tympanic plexus within the lesser petrosal nerve

            c. The lesser petrosal nerve traverses a small canal near the semicanal for the tensor tympani, emerges into the middle cranial fossa through the hiatus for the lesser petrosal nerve, continues anteriorly in the sulcus for the lesser petrosal nerve, and exits the skull through foramen ovale to reach the subjacent otic ganglion; postganglionic sympathetic fibers from the caroticotympanic nerves pass through the otic ganglion without synapsing and are distributed to the parotid gland via the auriculotemporal and facial nerves and inhibit secretion

4. Deep petrosal nerve

   a. Formed by fibers that leave the internal carotid plexus as the internal carotid artery passes horizontally across foramen lacerum; here, the deep petrosal nerve joins the greater petrosal nerve, a branch of the facial nerve, to form the nerve of the pterygoid canal, which courses anteriorly through the pterygoid canal to the pterygopalatine fossa, where it ends in the pterygopalatine ganglion

   b. Postganglionic sympathetic fibers from the deep petrosal nerve pass through the pterygopalatine ganglion without synapsing and are distributed to the nasal, palatal, and lacrimal glands via branches of the maxillary nerve and inhibit secretion

5. Sympathetic root of the ciliary ganglion: formed by fibers of the internal carotid plexus that leave the ophthalmic artery to join the ciliary ganglion; they pass through the ciliary ganglion without synapsing and course to the eye via the short ciliary nerves to innervate the dilator pupillae muscle within the iris

B. Clinical note: Horner's syndrome results from interruption of sympathetic fibers to the head, perhaps as a result of a tumor compressing the sympathetic trunk in the cervical region; denervation of the superior tarsus and dilator pupillae muscles, as well as the sweat glands of the face, causes drooping of the upper eyelid, pupillary constriction, and lack of sweating on the face, respectively

II. Parasympathetic System

A. Ciliary ganglion

1. Located posteriorly in the orbit between the optic nerve and lateral rectus; receives preganglionic parasympathetic fibers from the Edinger-Westphal nucleus in the brainstem via the oculomotor root of the ciliary ganglion, a branch of the inferior branch of the oculomotor nerve

2. Postganglionic parasympathetic fibers course to the eye via the short ciliary nerves and supply the ciliary and sphincter pupillae muscles, which focus the lens and constrict the pupil, respectively

B. Pterygopalatine ganglion

1. Located in the pterygopalatine fossa, suspended from the maxillary nerve; receives preganglionic parasympathetic fibers from the superior salivatory nucleus in the brainstem which travel, in succession, with the facial nerve, greater petrosal nerve, and nerve of the pterygoid canal

2. Some postganglionic parasympathetic secretomotor fibers from the pterygopalatine ganglion are distributed with nasal and palatal branches of the maxillary nerve to the nasal and palatal glands, respectively; other postganglionic parasympathetic secretomotor fibers from the pterygo-palatine ganglion are distributed to the lacrimal gland

    a. Postganglionic parasympathetic secretomotor fibers destined for the lacrimal gland initially travel with the zygomatic nerve, a branch of the maxillary nerve, and then with one of its branches, the zygoma-ticotemporal nerve

    b. The zygomaticotemporal nerve sends a branch to the lacrimal nerve, a branch of the ophthalmic nerve, which distributes the postgangli-onic parasympathetic secretomotor fibers to the lacrimal gland

C. Otic ganglion

  1. Lies on the medial side of the mandibular nerve, inferior to foramen ovale; receives preganglionic parasympathetic fibers from the inferior saliva-tory nucleus in the brainstem via the lesser petrosal nerve

    a. The lesser petrosal nerve is derived from the tympanic plexus, a nerve network on the promontory on the medial wall of the tympanic cav-ity; the tympanic plexus contains preganglionic parasympathetic fibers from the tympanic branch of the glossopharyngeal nerve (after the glossopharyngeal nerve exits the skull through the jugular foramen, it gives off its tympanic branch, which traverses the tym-panic canaliculus and emerges through the floor of the tympanic cavity to join the tympanic plexus)

    b. The lesser petrosal nerve leaves the tympanic cavity through a small canal near the semicanal for the tensor tympani, emerges into the middle cranial fossa through the hiatus for the lesser petrosal nerve, continues anteriorly in the sulcus for the lesser petrosal nerve, and exits the skull through foramen ovale to reach the subjacent otic gan-glion; preganglionic parasympathetic fibers within the lesser petro-sal nerve synapse in the otic ganglion

  2. Postganglionic parasympathetic secretomotor fibers leave the otic gan-glion and are distributed to the parotid gland via the auriculotemporal and facial nerves

D. Submandibular ganglion

  1. Suspended from the lingual nerve opposite the third lower molar; re-ceives preganglionic parasympathetic fibers from the superior salivatory nucleus in the brainstem via the chorda tympani nerve (as the facial nerve

descends in the facial canal toward the stylomastoid foramen, it gives off the chorda tympani nerve, which enters the tympanic cavity, courses anteriorly, medial to the manubrium of the malleus, and exits the skull through the petrotympanic fissure to join the lingual nerve)

2. Postganglionic parasympathetic secretomotor fibers leave the submandibular ganglion to supply the adjacent submandibular and sublingual salivary glands

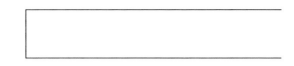

The Cranial Nerves

I. Olfactory Nerve

    A. Olfactory neurons within the mucosa of the olfactory region of the nasal cavity subserve the function of smell

    B. Nerve processes from olfactory neurons aggregate into numerous olfactory nerves, which ascend through the foramina in the cribriform plate and enter the olfactory bulb; the olfactory tract extends posteriorly from the olfactory bulb

II. Optic Nerve

    A. Actually, not a nerve, but an extension of the brain covered by meninges

    B. Emerges from the posterior aspect of the eye, courses posteriorly within the retrobulbar space, and exits the orbit through the common annular tendon and optic canal

III. Oculomotor Nerve

    A. Traverses the cavernous sinus and divides into a superior and an inferior branch, which enter the retrobulbar space through the superior orbital fissure and common annular tendon

    B. Superior branch: courses superiorly to innervate the superior rectus and levator palpebrae superioris

    C. Inferior branch: gives off the oculomotor root of the ciliary ganglion, which contains preganglionic parasympathetic fibers for synapse in the ciliary ganglion, and then proceeds anteriorly to innervate the medial rectus, inferior rectus, and inferior oblique (from the ciliary ganglion postganglionic parasympathetic fibers course to the eye via the short ciliary nerves and supply the ciliary and sphincter pupillae muscles, which focus the lens and constrict the pupil, respectively)

IV. Trochlear Nerve

    A. Traverses the cavernous sinus and enters the orbit through the superior orbital fissure, superior to the common annular tendon

    B. Courses medially, between the periorbita and retrobulbar space, superior to the posterior end of levator palpebrae superioris; penetrates the superior aspect of the superior oblique, innervating it

V. Trigeminal Nerve

    A. Ophthalmic nerve

        1. Traverses the cavernous sinus and then divides into its three sensory branches, the frontal, lacrimal, and nasociliary nerves

        2. Frontal nerve

            a. Enters the orbit through the superior orbital fissure, superior to the common annular tendon, and courses anteriorly, between the periorbita and retrobulbar space, superior to the levator palpebrae superioris; near the middle of the orbit, the frontal nerve divides into the supraorbital and supratrochlear nerves

            b. Supraorbital nerve: emerges through the supraorbital foramen and ascends to supply the forehead and the scalp as far posteriorly as the vertex

            c. Supratrochlear nerve: emerges through the frontal notch and supplies the forehead near the midline

        3. Lacrimal nerve

            a. Enters the orbit through the superior orbital fissure, superior to the common annular tendon, and courses anteriorly, between the periorbita and retrobulbar space, superior to the lateral rectus; receives a branch from the zygomaticotemporal nerve containing postganglionic parasympathetic secretomotor fibers from the pterygopalatine ganglion for the lacrimal gland

b. After supplying the lacrimal gland with postganglionic parasympathetic secretomotor fibers, the lacrimal nerve emerges from the orbit to provide cutaneous innervation to the lateral part of the upper eyelid

4. Nasociliary nerve

   a. Enters the retrobulbar space through the superior orbital fissure and common annular tendon; its branches are noted below

   b. Long ciliary nerves: given off as the nasociliary nerve courses medially, superior to the optic nerve; they enter the sclera near the optic nerve and provide general sensory innervation to the eye

   c. Posterior ethmoidal nerve: arises as the nasociliary nerve courses anteriorly between the superior oblique and medial rectus; enters the posterior ethmoidal foramen and provides sensory innervation to the sphenoidal sinus and posterior ethmoidal air cells

   d. Anterior ethmoidal nerve (terminal branch): enters the anterior ethmoidal foramen and provides sensory innervation to the anterior and middle ethmoidal air cells; it then emerges above the cribriform plate, descends through it into the nasal cavity, and divides into the internal and external nasal nerves

      1. Internal nasal nerve: provides sensory innervation to the anterosuperior parts of the lateral nasal wall and nasal septum

      2. External nasal nerve: emerges from the nasal cavity inferior to the nasal bone and provides cutaneous innervation to the dorsum and tip of the nose

   e. Infratrochlear nerve (terminal branch): emerges from the orbit inferior to the trochlea and provides cutaneous innervation to the medial part of the upper eyelid

B. Maxillary nerve

   1. Emerges from foramen rotundum into the pterygopalatine fossa and breaks up into the sensory branches noted below (suspended from the maxillary nerve within the pterygopalatine fossa is the pterygopalatine ganglion, which gives rise to postganglionic parasympathetic secretomotor fibers that are distributed to the nasal, palatal, and lacrimal glands via branches of the maxillary nerve)

   2. Posterior superior lateral nasal nerves: enter the nasal cavity through the sphenopalatine foramen and supply the posterosuperior lateral nasal wall

3. Posterior superior medial nasal nerves and their largest branch, the nasopalatine nerve

   a. Enter the nasal cavity through the sphenopalatine foramen and supply the posterosuperior, posteroinferior, and anteroinferior parts of the nasal septum

   b. The nasopalatine nerve descends anteriorly on the nasal septum, and then passes through the incisive canal and incisive fossa to provide sensory innervation to the hard palate posterior to the upper incisors

4. Greater palatine nerve

   a. Descends in the greater palatine canal and emerges from the greater palatine foramen; it then courses anteriorly, supplying the hard palate up to the incisor teeth

   b. As it descends in the inferior part of the greater palatine canal, it gives off posterior inferior lateral nasal nerves that supply the posteroinferior part of the lateral nasal wall

5. Lesser palatine nerves: descend in the greater palatine canal and emerge through the lesser palatine foramina to supply the soft palate

6. Posterior superior alveolar nerve: its branches enter the alveolar foramina on the infratemporal surface of the maxilla and supply the upper molars

7. Infraorbital nerve

   a. Enters the orbit through the inferior orbital fissure and courses forward in the infraorbital groove; as it continues forward in the infraorbital canal, it gives off the middle superior alveolar and anterior superior alveolar nerves

      1. Middle superior alveolar nerve: descends within the lateral wall of the maxillary sinus and supplies the upper premolars

      2. Anterior superior alveolar nerve: arises from the infraorbital nerve just before it emerges from the infraorbital foramen; descends within the anterior wall of the maxillary sinus and supplies the upper canine and incisors

   b. Emerges onto the face through the infraorbital foramen to supply the lower eyelid, side of the nose, upper lip, and the skin overlying the anterior surface of the maxilla

8. Zygomatic nerve

   a. Enters the orbit through the inferior orbital fissure and divides into the zygomaticofacial and zygomaticotemporal nerves

   b. Zygomaticofacial nerve: enters a zygomatico-orbital foramen and emerges from the zygomaticofacial foramen to supply the skin overlying the lateral surface of the zygomatic bone

   c. Zygomaticotemporal nerve: gives off a branch containing postganglionic parasympathetic secretomotor fibers from the pterygopalatine ganglion to the lacrimal nerve; it then enters a zygomatico-orbital foramen and emerges from the zygomaticotemporal foramen to supply the skin of the anterior part of the temple

9. Pharyngeal branch: courses posteriorly through the palatovaginal canal and provides sensory innervation to the mucosa of the nasopharynx

C. Mandibular nerve

   1. Emerges through foramen ovale, deep to the lateral pterygoid, and breaks up into the sensory and motor branches noted below

   2. Nerve to the medial pterygoid: gives rise to the nerve to the tensor tympani and the nerve to the tensor veli palatini, and then penetrates the deep surface of the medial pterygoid, innervating it

   3. Masseteric nerve: emerges superior to the lateral pterygoid and then passes laterally through the mandibular notch to supply the masseter

   4. Deep temporal nerves: the anterior deep temporal and posterior deep temporal nerves emerge between the two heads of the lateral pterygoid and superior to the lateral pterygoid, respectively; they ascend in the temporal fossa and innervate the temporalis

   5. Nerve to the lateral pterygoid: penetrates the deep surface of the lateral pterygoid, innervating it

   6. Buccal nerve: emerges between the two heads of the lateral pterygoid; some branches supply the skin of the cheek and others penetrate the buccinator to provide sensory innervation to the mucosa of the cheek

   7. Auriculotemporal nerve

      a. Courses posteriorly, deep to the lateral pterygoid; emerges posterior to the neck of the mandible and gives off postganglionic parasympathetic secretomotor fibers from the otic ganglion to the facial nerve

b. Ascends between the auricle and superficial temporal artery and provides sensory innervation to the auricle, external acoustic meatus, tympanic membrane, and posterior part of the temple

8. Lingual nerve

a. Descends deep to the lateral pterygoid and appears along its inferior border; it subsequently courses anteriorly on the lateral surfaces of the medial pterygoid and hyoglossus, and provides general sensory innervation to the anterior two-thirds of the tongue

b. Proximally, it is joined by the chorda tympani nerve, which contains taste fibers for the anterior two-thirds of the tongue and preganglionic parasympathetic fibers for synapse in the submandibular ganglion; the submandibular ganglion is suspended from the lingual nerve opposite the third lower molar and its postganglionic parasympathetic secretomotor fibers supply the adjacent submandibular and sublingual glands

9. Inferior alveolar nerve

a. Descends deep to the lateral pterygoid and appears along its inferior border, posterior to the lingual nerve; it then courses toward the mandibular foramen on the lateral surface of the medial pterygoid, inferior to the lingual nerve

b. Before entering the mandibular foramen, the inferior alveolar nerve gives off the nerve to the mylohyoid, which runs in the mylohyoid groove and then on the inferior surface of the mylohyoid muscle; the nerve to the mylohyoid innervates the mylohyoid and anterior belly of the digastric

c. Within the mandibular canal the inferior alveolar nerve provides sensory innervation to the lower teeth and gums; at the second premolar it gives off the mental nerve, which emerges from the mental foramen and provides cutaneous innervation to the lower lip and chin

VI. Abducens Nerve

A. Traverses the cavernous sinus and enters the retrobulbar space through the superior orbital fissure and common annular tendon

B. Courses anteriorly on the medial surface of the lateral rectus, innervating it

VII. Facial Nerve

A. Courses laterally within the internal acoustic meatus and, at its blind lateral end, enters the facial canal within the petrous part of the temporal bone; it then continues laterally within the facial canal along the roof of the vestibule of the inner ear and, as it approaches the medial wall of the tympanic cavity, it expands at the geniculate ganglion, which contains the cell bodies of taste fibers that course within the chorda tympani nerve

B. The greater petrosal nerve courses anteriorly from the geniculate ganglion and contains preganglionic parasympathetic fibers

    1. It emerges from the hiatus for the greater petrosal nerve in the middle cranial fossa and continues anteriorly in the sulcus for the greater petrosal nerve

    2. As the greater petrosal nerve passes horizontally across foramen lacerum, it is joined by the deep petrosal nerve from the internal carotid plexus, and becomes the nerve of the pterygoid canal; the nerve of the pterygoid canal traverses the pterygoid canal and, when it emerges into the pterygopalatine fossa, its preganglionic parasympathetic fibers synapse in the pterygopalatine ganglion

    3. From the pterygopalatine ganglion, postganglionic parasympathetic secretomotor fibers are distributed to the nasal, palatal, and lacrimal glands via branches of the maxillary nerve

C. The facial nerve continues posteriorly from the geniculate ganglion, producing the prominence of the facial canal on the medial wall of the tympanic cavity; it then descends within the posterior wall of the tympanic cavity toward the stylomastoid foramen and gives rise to the nerve to the stapedius, which innervates the stapedius, and then the chorda tympani nerve

    1. The chorda tympani nerve enters the tympanic cavity through a posterior canaliculus, courses anteriorly on the medial surface of the superior part of the manubrium, superior to the insertion of tensor tympani, and exits the tympanic cavity through an anterior canaliculus; it then emerges from the skull through the petrotympanic fissure and joins the lingual nerve

    2. The chorda tympani nerve contains taste fibers for the anterior two-thirds of the tongue and preganglionic parasympathetic fibers for synapse in the submandibular ganglion

D. The facial nerve emerges from the skull through the stylomastoid foramen and gives off its posterior auricular branch, which ascends behind the auricle to supply the auricularis posterior and occipitalis muscles; here, it also gives off branches to the posterior belly of the digastric and stylohyoid, and receives postganglionic parasympathetic secretomotor fibers for the parotid gland from the otic ganglion via the auriculotemporal nerve

E. It next enters the parotid gland, supplying it with postganglionic parasympathetic secretomotor fibers as it forms a plexus within its substance; its temporal, zygomatic, buccal, marginal mandibular, and cervical branches emerge along the borders of the parotid gland and innervate the facial muscles

VIII. Vestibulocochlear Nerve

A. Fibers of its vestibular division are associated with the utricle, saccule, and semicircular ducts, and are concerned with balance; they penetrate foramina within the medial wall of the vestibule and enter the internal acoustic meatus

B. Fibers of its cochlear division are associated with the organ of Corti within the cochlear duct and are concerned with hearing; they penetrate foramina within the region of the cochlea facing the internal acoustic meatus, join the fibers of the vestibular division, and together they course medially within the internal acoustic meatus as the vestibulocochlear nerve

IX. Glossopharyngeal Nerve

A. Exits the jugular foramen anterior to the internal jugular vein; its branches are noted below

B. Tympanic branch

1. Enters the external opening of the tympanic canaliculus on the ridge of bone between the jugular foramen and carotid canal; traverses the tympanic canaliculus, emerges through its internal opening on the floor of the tympanic cavity, and gives rise to general sensory fibers for the tympanic membrane and tympanic cavity as well as preganglionic parasympathetic fibers which join the caroticotympanic nerves from the internal carotid plexus on the promontory to form the tympanic plexus

2. The tympanic plexus gives rise to the lesser petrosal nerve, which traverses a small canal near the semicanal for the tensor tympani, emerges into the middle cranial fossa through the hiatus for the lesser petrosal nerve, continues anteriorly in the sulcus for the lesser petrosal nerve, and exits the skull through foramen ovale to reach the subjacent otic ganglion; preganglionic parasympathetic fibers within the lesser petrosal nerve synapse in the otic ganglion and postganglionic parasympathetic secretomotor fibers from the otic ganglion are distributed to the parotid gland via the auriculotemporal and facial nerves

C. Pharyngeal branches contribute to the pharyngeal plexus and provide sensory innervation to the mucosa of the oropharynx

D. The carotid sinus branch provides sensory innervation to the carotid sinus as well as the carotid body

E. As the glossopharyngeal nerve descends lateral to the stylopharyngeus, it supplies the stylopharyngeus with its only motor branch; it then accompanies the stylopharyngeus through the gap in the lateral pharyngeal wall between the superior and middle pharyngeal constrictors

F. The glossopharyngeal nerve subsequently courses anteriorly, between the palatine tonsil and hyoglossus, and provides sensory innervation, including taste, to the posterior one-third of the tongue

X. Vagus Nerve

A. Emerges from the jugular foramen posterior to the internal jugular vein and descends within the carotid sheath, behind and between the internal jugular vein and internal/common carotid artery; its branches are noted below

B. Auricular branch: enters the mastoid canaliculus on the lateral wall of the jugular foramen; its branches provide general sensory innervation to the auricle, external acoustic meatus, and tympanic membrane

C. Pharyngeal branch: contributes to the pharyngeal plexus and provides motor innervation to the muscles of the pharynx and palate, except for the stylopharyngeus and tensor veli palatini, which are innervated by the glossopharyngeal nerve and the nerve to the tensor veli palatini, respectively

D. Superior laryngeal nerve

1. Descends lateral to the pharynx and divides into the internal and external laryngeal nerves, posterosuperior to the tip of the greater cornu of the hyoid

2. Internal laryngeal nerve: penetrates the thyrohyoid membrane and provides general sensory innervation to the mucosa of the larynx superior to the vocal folds as well as to the mucosa of the superior part of the laryngopharynx; it also provides general sensory and taste innervation to the very posterior part of the tongue and epiglottis

3. External laryngeal nerve: descends inferior to the oblique line of the thyroid cartilage, deep to the sternothyroid and superficial to the inferior pharyngeal constrictor; innervates the cricothyroid and part of the inferior pharyngeal constrictor

E. Branches to the carotid body: provide sensory innervation to the carotid body

F. Recurrent laryngeal nerves

1. The right and left recurrent laryngeal nerves loop posteriorly around the right subclavian artery and aortic arch, respectively, and ascend in the grooves between the trachea and esophagus on their respective sides

2. As they ascend posterior to the lobes of the thyroid gland, they enter the larynx posterior to the cricothyroid articulation, between the inferior pharyngeal constrictor and esophagus; they innervate all the muscles of the larynx, except the cricothyroids (which are innervated by the external laryngeal nerves), and provide general sensory innervation to the mucosa of the larynx inferior to the vocal folds as well as to the mucosa of the inferior part of the laryngopharynx

XI. Accessory Nerve

A. Exits the jugular foramen lateral to the vagus nerve and descends posteriorly on the deep surface of the sternocleidomastoid, innervating it

B. It subsequently passes across the posterior triangle of the neck on levator scapulae, and then descends on the deep surface of trapezius, innervating it

XII. Hypoglossal Nerve

A. Exits the hypoglossal canal medial to the vagus nerve and then passes laterally, posterior to the vagus nerve, adhering to it

B. Descends anteriorly in the neck and emerges along the inferior border of the posterior belly of the digastric; here, it hooks around the sternocleidomastoid branch of the occipital artery, gives off the superior root of the ansa cervicalis, and then the branch of the ansa cervicalis to the thyrohyoid

C. It subsequently courses anteriorly, deep to the posterior belly of the digastric, and then between the mylohyoid and hyoglossus; innervates all the muscles of the tongue, except palatoglossus, which is innervated by the vagus nerve via the pharyngeal plexus

part **VI**

The
Upper
Limb

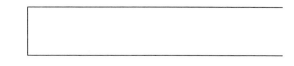

Bones and Bony Landmarks

I. Pectoral Girdle

   A. Clavicle

      1. Acromial end: flat, lateral extremity

      2. Acromial articular surface: oval facet at the acromial end; faces inferiorly and laterally

      3. Sternal end: round, medial extremity

      4. Sternal articular surface: oval facet at the sternal end

      5. Shaft: central portion that forms an S-shaped curve; medially, it is convex anteriorly, and laterally, it is convex posteriorly

      6. Groove for the subclavius muscle: depression on the inferior surface near midshaft

      7. Conoid tubercle: posterior eminence near the acromial end

      8. Trapezoid line: ridge on the inferior surface; extends laterally from the conoid tubercle

      9. Impression for the costoclavicular ligament: roughened depression on the inferior surface near the sternal end

     10. Clinical note: the clavicle is fractured more than any other bone in the body

B. Scapula

    1. Subscapular fossa: concave, anterior (costal) surface

    2. Posterior surface

        a. Spine of the scapula: posteriorly projecting, shelflike plate

        b. Base of the spine of the scapula: smooth, triangular area at the medial end of the spine of the scapula

        c. Supraspinous (supraspinatous) fossa: depression superior to the spine of the scapula

        d. Infraspinous (infraspinatous) fossa: depression inferior to the spine of the scapula

    3. Acromion

        a. Lateral extension of the spine of the scapula; overhangs the shoulder joint

        b. Acromial angle: palpable prominence where the posterior border of the acromion turns sharply anteriorly

        c. Clavicular articular surface: oval facet near the tip of the acromion; faces superiorly and medially (the clavicle overrides the acromion)

    4. Borders

        a. Superior: horizontal margin

        b. Medial (vertebral): vertical margin

        c. Lateral (axillary): oblique margin

    5. Angles

        a. Superior: site of junction of the superior and medial borders

        b. Inferior: site of junction of the medial and lateral borders

        c. Lateral: site of the junction of the superior and lateral borders

    6. Coracoid process: fingerlike process extending forward from the lateral part of the superior border; it can be palpated inferior to the acromial end of the clavicle

7. Scapular (suprascapular) notch: indentation medial to the coracoid process; converted into a foramen by the transverse scapular ligament

8. Glenoid cavity: shallow, circular depression at the lateral angle

9. Supraglenoid tubercle: roughened elevation superior to the glenoid cavity

10. Infraglenoid tubercle: roughened elevation inferior to the glenoid cavity

11. Neck: constricted region medial to the glenoid cavity

II. Humerus

A. Head: medially projecting hemisphere at the proximal end

B. Anatomical neck: groove encircling the head

C. Surgical neck: tapering proximal portion of the shaft

D. Greater tubercle: lateral, bony eminence at the proximal end

E. Lesser tubercle: anterior, bony eminence near the proximal end

F. Crest of the greater tubercle: ridge extending inferiorly from the anterior part of the greater tubercle

G. Crest of the lesser tubercle: ridge extending inferiorly from the lesser tubercle

H. Intertubercular sulcus (bicipital groove): furrow between the greater and lesser tubercles and their crests

I. Shaft: central, cylindrical portion

J. Deltoid tuberosity: roughened area on the anterolateral aspect of the humerus near midshaft

K. Radial groove: smooth, shallow furrow descending laterally on the posterior surface near midshaft; may be indistinct

L. Lateral epicondyle: lateral projection at the distal end

M. Lateral supracondylar crest: ridge extending superiorly from the lateral epicondyle

N. Medial epicondyle: prominent, medial projection at the distal end

O. Medial supracondylar crest: ridge extending superiorly from the medial epicondyle

P. Sulcus for the ulnar nerve: groove posterior to the medial epicondyle

Q. Capitulum: rounded elevation on the anterolateral aspect of the distal end

R. Radial fossa: depression above the capitulum

S. Trochlea: grooved, pulleylike, medial portion of the distal end

T. Coronoid fossa: depression above the trochlea on the anterior aspect of the distal end

U. Olecranon fossa: depression above the trochlea on the posterior aspect of the distal end

III. Bones of the Forearm

A. Radius

1. Head

a. Disclike, proximal end; its bony landmarks are noted below

b. Articular fovea: shallow, circular depression forming the proximal surface of the head

c. Articular circumference: broad rim of the head

2. Neck: constricted region distal to the head

3. Shaft

a. Central portion; its bony landmarks are noted below

b. Radial tuberosity: oblong projection distal to the anteromedial part of the neck

c. Pronator tuberosity: roughened area on the lateral surface near midshaft

d. Oblique line: slight ridge extending across the anterior surface from the radial tuberosity to the pronator tuberosity

e. Interosseous border: sharp, medial ridge

4. Styloid process: pointed prominence on the lateral side of the distal end

5. Dorsal radial tubercle: eminence on the posterior surface of the distal end

6. Ulnar notch: indentation on the medial side of the distal end

7. Carpal articular surface: concave, distal end

B. Ulna

1. Olecranon: curved protuberance forming the proximal end

2. Trochlear notch: anterior concavity between the olecranon and coronoid process

3. Coronoid process: ridgelike projection distal to the trochlear notch

4. Ulnar tuberosity: elevated, roughened area distal to the coronoid process

5. Radial notch: concavity on the lateral side of the coronoid process

6. Shaft

   a. Central portion; its bony landmarks are noted below

   b. Supinator crest: ridge extending distally from the posterior margin of the radial notch

   c. Interosseous border: sharp, lateral ridge

   d. Subcutaneous posterior border: palpable ridge extending from the olecranon to the styloid process

7. Styloid process: conical projection on the posteromedial aspect of the distal end

8. Head: rounded, distal end

IV. Bones of the Hand

A. Carpals

1. Proximal row (from lateral to medial)

   a. Scaphoid: its tubercle is the rounded elevation on the lateral part of the palmar surface

b. Lunate: crescent-moon shaped

   c. Triquetrum: pyramid-shaped

   d. Pisiform: pea-shaped; lies anterior to the triquetrum

2. Distal row (from lateral to medial)

   a. Trapezium: its tubercle is the ridge on the lateral side of the palmar surface

   b. Trapezoid: wedge-shaped

   c. Capitate: exhibits a proximal, rounded head

   d. Hamate: its hook (hamulus) is the curved process emerging from the palmar surface

3. Carpal sulcus: groove formed by the palmar surfaces of the carpals

B. Metacarpals I, II, III, IV, and V

1. Base: angular, proximal end

2. Shaft: central portion

3. Head: rounded, distal end

C. Phalanges: proximal, middle, and distal (there is no middle phalanx in the thumb)

1. Base: broad, proximal end

2. Shaft: central portion

3. Head: narrow, distal end

V. Other Bones and Bony Landmarks

A. Skull

1. External occipital protuberance: midline, rounded eminence on the posterior aspect of the skull

2. Superior nuchal line: ridge extending laterally from the external occipital protuberance

B. Vertebra

1. Spinous process: posterior projection

2. Transverse processes: lateral projections

C. Pelvic bone: the iliac crest is its convex, superior border

The Scapular Region

I. Fasciae

    A. Superficial fascia: fibrous and tough

    B. Deep fascia: covers the scapular muscles, being particularly thick on the superficial surfaces of the infraspinatus and teres minor

II. Muscles

    A. Trapezius

        1. Origin: medial part of the superior nuchal line, external occipital protuberance, ligamentum nuchae, and spinous processes of thoracic vertebrae

        2. Insertion: superior fibers—lateral clavicle; middle fibers—acromion and spine of the scapula; inferior fibers—base of the spine of the scapula

        3. Action: superior fibers—extension of the head and neck and upward rotation, retraction, and elevation of the scapula; middle fibers—retraction of the scapula; inferior fibers—upward rotation, retraction, and depression of the scapula (movements of the scapula are described on p. 304)

        4. Innervation: accessory nerve

        5. Clinical note: since the trapezius is the only muscle capable of elevating the tips of the shoulders (shrugging the shoulders), the integrity of the accessory nerves can be assessed by having the patient perform this action

B. Latissimus dorsi

    1. Origin: spinous processes of the inferior six thoracic vertebrae, spinous processes of lumbar vertebrae, and the iliac crest

    2. Insertion: its tendon twists around the inferior border of the teres major to insert in the intertubercular sulcus of the humerus

    3. Action: adduction, medial rotation, and extension of the shoulder (movements of the shoulder are described on p. 315)

    4. Innervation: thoracodorsal (middle subscapular) nerve

C. Levator scapulae

    1. Origin: transverse processes of the atlas and axis and the posterior tubercles of the transverse processes of vertebrae C3 and C4

    2. Insertion: medial border of the scapula, superior to the base of the spine

    3. Action: downward rotation, retraction, and elevation of the scapula

    4. Innervation: ventral rami of spinal nerves C3 and C4, and a branch from the dorsal scapular nerve

D. Rhomboideus minor

    1. Origin: inferior part of the ligamentum nuchae and the spinous process of T1

    2. Insertion: medial border of the scapula, at the base of the spine

    3. Action: downward rotation, retraction, and elevation of the scapula

    4. Innervation: dorsal scapular nerve

    5. May be fused with rhomboideus major

E. Rhomboideus major

    1. Origin: spinous processes of vertebrae T2 to T5

    2. Insertion: medial border of the scapula, inferior to the base of the spine

    3. Action: downward rotation, retraction, and elevation of the scapula

    4. Innervation: dorsal scapular nerve

5. Clinical note: the medial border of rhomboideus major, the superior border of latissimus dorsi, and the inferior border of trapezius form the triangle of auscultation; heart and lung sounds can be heard more clearly through this thinner region of the thoracic wall

F. Deltoid

1. Origin: lateral clavicle, acromion, and spine of the scapula

2. Insertion: deltoid tuberosity

3. Action: abduction of the shoulder; medial rotation and flexion of the shoulder (anterior fibers) and lateral rotation and extension of the shoulder (posterior fibers)

4. Innervation: axillary nerve

G. Supraspinatus

1. Origin: supraspinous fossa

2. Insertion: its tendon courses laterally, superior to the shoulder joint, and inserts on the superior aspect of the greater tubercle of the humerus

3. Action: abduction of the shoulder

4. Innervation: suprascapular nerve

H. Infraspinatus

1. Origin: infraspinous fossa

2. Insertion: posterosuperior aspect of the greater tubercle of the humerus

3. Action: lateral rotation of the shoulder

4. Innervation: suprascapular nerve

I. Teres minor

1. Origin: dorsal surface of the scapula, along the upper part of the axillary border

2. Insertion: its tendon courses laterally, posterior to the long head of the triceps brachii, and inserts on the posteroinferior aspect of the greater tubercle of the humerus

3. Action: lateral rotation and adduction of the shoulder

4. Innervation: axillary nerve

J. Teres major

1. Origin: dorsal surface of the scapula, along the lower part of the axillary border

2. Insertion: its tendon courses laterally, anterior to the long head of the triceps brachii, and inserts on the crest of the lesser tubercle of the humerus

3. Action: adduction, medial rotation, and extension of the shoulder

4. Innervation: lower subscapular nerve

K. Subscapularis

1. Origin: subscapular fossa

2. Insertion: lesser tubercle of the humerus

3. Action: medial rotation of the shoulder

4. Innervation: upper and lower subscapular nerves

III. Nerves

A. Accessory nerve: descends on the deep surface of trapezius, innervating it

B. Dorsal scapular nerve (C5): thin nerve descending on the deep surfaces of levator scapulae, rhomboideus minor, and rhomboideus major, near the medial border of the scapula; innervates part of levator scapulae, rhomboideus minor, and rhomboideus major

C. Suprascapular nerve (C5, 6): arises from the superior trunk of the brachial plexus and courses laterally, posterior to the clavicle; traverses the scapular notch (below the transverse scapular ligament) and descends on the posterior surface of the scapula, innervating supraspinatus and infraspinatus

D. Axillary nerve (C5, 6): arises from the posterior cord of the brachial plexus, courses posteriorly through the quadrangular space, and innervates the deltoid and teres minor; the quadrangular space is bounded superiorly by the teres minor, laterally by the surgical neck of the humerus, inferiorly by the teres major, and medially by the long head of the triceps brachii

E. Upper, middle, and lower subscapular nerves (C5, 6; C6, 7, 8; C5, 6, respectively): arise from the posterior cord of the brachial plexus; the upper subscapular nerve innervates the upper part of subscapularis, the middle subscapular or thoracodorsal nerve innervates latissimus dorsi, and the lower subscapular nerve innervates the lower part of subscapularis and teres major

IV. Vessels

A. Transverse cervical artery

1. Branch of the thyrocervical trunk, a branch of the proximal part of the subclavian artery; courses posteriorly toward the anterior border of trapezius and divides into a superficial and deep branch

2. Superficial branch: descends on the deep surface of trapezius with the accessory nerve

3. Deep branch: descends deep to levator scapulae, rhomboideus minor, and rhomboideus major with the dorsal scapular nerve; may arise directly from the subclavian artery, in which case it is then called the dorsal scapular artery, and the remaining artery is referred to as the superficial cervical artery

B. Suprascapular artery

1. Branch of the thyrocervical trunk; courses laterally, inferior to the transverse cervical artery

2. Passes above the transverse scapular ligament and descends on the posterior surface of the scapula with the suprascapular nerve

C. Posterior circumflex humeral artery: branch of the axillary artery; courses posteriorly through the quadrangular space with the axillary nerve

D. Circumflex scapular artery: branch of the subscapular artery, a branch of the axillary artery; reaches the posterior surface of the scapula by penetrating the origin of teres minor (some of its branches traverse the triangular space, which is bounded superiorly by the teres minor, inferiorly by the teres major, and laterally by the long head of the triceps brachii)

E. Veins: accompany their corresponding arteries

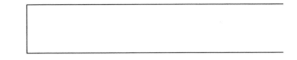

The Pectoral Region

I. Superficial Fascia

    A. Superiorly, it contains the inferior part of a thin, sheetlike muscle in the neck, the platysma

    B. Cutaneous nerves

        1. Intercostal nerves: lateral and anterior cutaneous branches of the upper six intercostal nerves (ventral rami of spinal nerves T1 to T6) supply the pectoral region; the lateral cutaneous branch of the second intercostal nerve may also supply the skin of the upper medial arm and is then called the intercostobrachial nerve

        2. Supraclavicular nerves: derived from ventral rami of spinal nerves C3 and C4; descend deep to the platysma to supplement the innervation to the superior part of the pectoral region

    C. Cephalic vein: ascends along the anterolateral aspect of the arm; passes through the deltopectoral triangle between the deltoid, pectoralis major, and clavicle, and then courses deep to pectoralis major to drain into the axillary vein

    D. Breast

        1. Glandular tissue

            a. Embedded in the fat and connective tissue of the superficial fascia of the pectoral region

            b. Extends from the second to the sixth rib and from the sternum to the midaxillary line; a portion of the glandular tissue extends toward the armpit or axilla and is called the axillary tail

    c. Composed of about 15 lobes; each lobe drains into an expanded lactiferous sinus whose associated lactiferous duct opens on the nipple

    d. Clinical note: after menopause, the glandular tissue decreases or disappears and is replaced by fat and connective tissue

2. The superficial fascia of the breast has a deep membranous layer

    a. Between the deep membranous layer of the superficial fascia and the deep fascia covering pectoralis major lies a retromammary space filled with loose connective tissue; this loose connective tissue provides for significant mobility of the breast on the anterior thoracic wall

    b. Clinical note: loss of mobility or fixation of the breast may result following extension of carcinoma of the breast into the retromammary space and underlying muscles

3. Suspensory ligaments (of Cooper)

    a. Supportive connective tissue bands within the superficial fascia; they extend from the membranous layer of the superficial fascia to the skin of the breast

    b. Clinical note: carcinoma of the breast may produce fibrosis and shortening of the suspensory ligaments; this, in turn, may produce a characteristic orange-peel dimpling of the skin of the breast

4. Nipple: cylindrical projection at the level of the fourth intercostal space in the male and more inferiorly in the female; the areola is the pigmented skin surrounding the nipple

5. Vessels

    a. Perforating branches of the internal thoracic artery, anterior and posterior intercostal arteries, and the lateral thoracic artery supply the breast; veins accompany their corresponding arteries

    b. Most lymphatic drainage is to lymph nodes within the axilla; some lymphatics follow the perforating branches of the internal thoracic artery and drain to parasternal nodes along the internal thoracic artery (some lymphatics may cross the midline)

    c. Clinical note: anastomoses between the posterior intercostal veins and vertebral venous plexuses provide a route for metastasis of carcinoma of the breast to the vertebrae, spinal cord, and brain; carcinoma of the breast also metastasizes by way of lymphatics

II. Deep Fascia

    A. Envelops the muscles of the pectoral region, covering their superficial and deep surfaces

    B. Clavipectoral fascia

        1. Deep fascia ensheathing pectoralis minor

        2. Extends from the medial border of pectoralis minor to the clavicle, enclosing the subclavius muscle; pierced superiorly by the cephalic vein, lateral pectoral nerve, and thoracoacromial vessels

        3. Extends from the lateral border of pectoralis minor to the deep fascia forming the floor of the axilla; this portion of the clavipectoral fascia produces the hollow of the armpit when the arm is abducted and is sometimes called the suspensory ligament of the axilla

III. Muscles

    A. Pectoralis major

        1. Origin: medial clavicle, sternum, and the upper six costal cartilages

        2. Insertion: crest of the greater tubercle of the humerus

        3. Action: medial rotation, adduction, flexion (clavicular part), and extension (sternocostal part) of the shoulder

        4. Innervation: medial and lateral pectoral nerves

    B. Pectoralis minor

        1. Origin: third to fifth ribs, near their costochondral junctions

        2. Insertion: coracoid process

        3. Action: downward rotation, protraction, and depression of the scapula

        4. Innervation: medial and lateral pectoral nerves

C. Subclavius

  1. Origin: first rib, near its costochondral junction

  2. Insertion: groove for the subclavius muscle on the inferior surface of the clavicle near midshaft

  3. Action: helps prevent upward dislocation of the sternoclavicular joint

  4. Innervation: nerve to the subclavius

  5. Clinical note: the subclavius may protect the subjacent subclavian vessels and brachial plexus from the sharp, splintered ends of a fractured clavicle

D. Serratus anterior

  1. Origin: upper nine ribs

  2. Insertion: costal surface of the scapula, along the medial border

  3. Action: upward rotation, protraction, and depression (lower fibers only) of the scapula

  4. Innervation: long thoracic nerve

  5. Clinical note: paralysis of the serratus anterior, perhaps following injury to the long thoracic nerve while excising axillary lymph nodes during a mastectomy, is characterized by winging of the scapula, where the medial border stands away from the thoracic wall

E. Scapulothoracic joint

  1. Functional, nonbony joint between the costal surface of the scapula and posterior thoracic wall; its movements are described below

  2. Movement of the lateral angle of the scapula superiorly is upward rotation of the scapula; the opposite movement is downward rotation of the scapula

  3. Movement of the scapula laterally and anteriorly around the thoracic wall is protraction of the scapula; the opposite movement is retraction of the scapula

  4. Movement of the superior border of the scapula superiorly is elevation of the scapula; the opposite movement is depression of the scapula

5. Movements at the scapulothoracic joint greatly increase the range of motion of the upper limb as a whole, for example, without upward rotation of the scapula the arm cannot be abducted above the horizontal; muscles that move the scapula can also stabilize it so that it affords a firm base upon which the upper limb can perform forceful movements

IV. Nerves

    A. Lateral pectoral nerve (C5, 6, 7): branches from the lateral cord of the brachial plexus, hence its name, notwithstanding its medial position on the anterior thoracic wall relative to the medial pectoral nerve; sends a branch to pectoralis minor, penetrates the clavipectoral fascia medial to pectoralis minor, and ends in pectoralis major

    B. Medial pectoral nerve (C8, T1): branches from the medial cord of the brachial plexus, hence its name; supplies pectoralis minor as it pierces it and then ends in pectoralis major

    C. Nerve to the subclavius (C5, 6): branches from the superior trunk of the brachial plexus; innervates subclavius

    D. Long thoracic nerve (C5, 6, 7): descends on serratus anterior, innervating it

V. Vessels

    A. Superior (supreme) thoracic artery: small branch from the proximal part of the axillary artery; supplies the superior part of the pectoral region

    B. Thoracoacromial artery

        1. Arises from the axillary artery posterior to pectoralis minor; emerges through the clavipectoral fascia medial to pectoralis minor and, deep to pectoralis major, gives rise to the four branches noted below

        2. Clavicular branch—courses medially, inferior to the clavicle; pectoral branch—descends on the deep surface of pectoralis major; deltoid branch—courses laterally and emerges from the deltopectoral triangle; acromial branch—courses toward the acromion, deep to the deltoid

    C. Lateral thoracic artery: arises from the axillary artery posterior to pectoralis minor, distal to the origin of the thoracoacromial artery; descends on the lateral thoracic wall near the lateral border of pectoralis minor

    D. Veins: course with their respective arteries and drain into the axillary vein

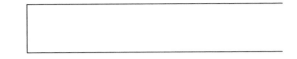

The Axilla

I. General Remarks

  A. Pyramidal space between the proximal arm and lateral thoracic wall; structures comprising its walls are noted below

    1. Anterior wall: pectoralis major and pectoralis minor (the pectoralis major forms the palpable, anterior axillary fold)

    2. Posterior wall: latissimus dorsi, teres major, and subscapularis (the latissimus dorsi and teres major form the palpable, posterior axillary fold)

    3. Medial wall: serratus anterior

    4. Lateral wall: intertubercular sulcus

    5. Base (floor): deep (axillary) fascia

    6. Apex: triangular opening between the clavicle, superior border of the scapula, and first rib; serves as the gateway for nerves and vessels passing from the neck into the upper limb

  B. Contents: axillary artery, axillary vein, axillary lymph nodes, brachial plexus, biceps brachii, and coracobrachialis; the axillary sheath, a connective tissue investment derived from the prevertebral fascia, encloses the axillary artery, axillary vein, and brachial plexus

II. Vessels

  A. Axillary artery

    1. Continuous proximally with the subclavian artery and distally with the

brachial artery; extends from the outer border of the first rib to the inferior border of teres major

2. Divided into a first part between the outer border of the first rib and medial border of pectoralis minor, a second part posterior to pectoralis minor, and a third part between the lateral border of pectoralis minor and inferior border of teres major; the first, second, and third parts of the axillary artery give rise to one, two, and three branches, respectively, as noted below

3. First part—superior thoracic artery (see p. 305)

4. Second part—thoracoacromial and lateral thoracic arteries (see p. 305)

5. Third part

   a. Subscapular artery

      1. Descends along the lateral border of the scapula and divides into the thoracodorsal and circumflex scapular arteries

         a. Thoracodorsal artery: descends with the thoracodorsal nerve to latissimus dorsi

         b. Circumflex scapular artery: winds around the lateral border of the scapula, penetrates the origin of teres minor, and anastomoses with the suprascapular artery and the superficial and deep branches of the transverse cervical artery on the posterior aspect of the scapula

      2. Clinical note: if the axillary artery is ligated proximal to the origin of the subscapular artery, the anastomoses between the circumflex scapular artery, suprascapular artery, and the deep and superficial branches of the transverse cervical artery on the posterior aspect of the scapula usually provide for adequate blood flow in the reverse direction in the subscapular artery to nourish the distal portions of the upper limb

   b. Anterior circumflex humeral artery: small branch; courses laterally, anterior to the surgical neck of the humerus, deep to the coracobrachialis and biceps brachii

   c. Posterior circumflex humeral artery: passes posteriorly through the quadrangular space and winds around the surgical neck of the humerus accompanied by the axillary nerve

B. Axillary vein

　　1. Lies medial to the axillary artery; continuous proximally with the subclavian vein and distally with the basilic vein

　　2. Receives tributaries corresponding to branches of the axillary artery as well as the cephalic vein

C. Lymphatics

　　1. Axillary lymph nodes usually number from 20 to 30; they receive lymphatic drainage from the scapular region, pectoral region (including most of the breast), and upper limb

　　2. Subgroups

　　　　a. Apical nodes: surround the first part of the axillary vessels; receive lymphatics from the other subgroups and drain into the subclavian lymphatic trunk

　　　　b. Central nodes: surround the second part of the axillary vessels; receive lymphatics from the subgroups noted below

　　　　c. Subscapular nodes: lie along the subscapular vessels; receive lymphatics from the scapular region

　　　　d. Pectoral nodes: lie along the lateral thoracic vessels; receive lymphatics from the pectoral region, including most of the breast

　　　　e. Lateral nodes: surround the third part of the axillary vessels; receive lymphatics from the upper limb

III. Brachial Plexus

A. Roots, trunks, and divisions

　　1. Roots

　　　　a. Composed of ventral rami of spinal nerves C5 to T1

　　　　b. Nerves derived from roots

　　　　　　1. Long thoracic nerve: formed by contributions from ventral rami C5, 6, and 7; descends posterior to the brachial plexus and then on serratus anterior, innervating it

2. Dorsal scapular nerve: thin nerve arising from the ventral ramus of C5; passes deep to levator scapulae, to which it sends a branch, and then descends along the medial border of the scapula on the deep surfaces of rhomboideus minor and rhomboideus major, innervating them

2. Trunks

   a. Formed by the roots of the brachial plexus after they emerge from between scalenus anterior and scalenus medius

   b. Superior trunk

      1. Formed by the union of ventral rami C5 and C6

      2. Nerves derived from the superior trunk

         a. Suprascapular nerve: courses laterally, posterior to the clavicle, and then through the scapular notch below the transverse scapular ligament; descends on the posterior surface of the scapula and innervates supraspinatus and infraspinatus

         b. Nerve to the subclavius: descends anterior to the brachial plexus and innervates subclavius

   c. Middle trunk: represents the distal continuation of ventral ramus C7

   d. Inferior trunk: formed by the union of ventral rami C8 and T1

3. Divisions

   a. Near the first rib, each trunk divides into an anterior and a posterior division

   b. Anterior divisions

      1. The anterior divisions of the superior and middle trunks unite to form the lateral cord, lateral to the axillary artery

      2. The anterior division of the inferior trunk continues distally as the medial cord, medial to the axillary artery

   c. Posterior divisions: the posterior divisions of the superior, middle, and inferior trunks unite to form the posterior cord, posterior to the axillary artery

B. Cords and branches

1. Lateral cord: gives rise to the lateral pectoral nerve and then divides into its terminal branches, the musculocutaneous nerve and the lateral root of the median nerve

2. Medial cord

   a. Gives rise to the medial pectoral, medial brachial cutaneous, and medial antebrachial cutaneous nerves, and then divides into its terminal branches, the ulnar nerve and the medial root of the median nerve

   b. The medial root of the median nerve courses laterally, anterior to the axillary artery, and merges with the lateral root of the median nerve to form the median nerve

   c. The roots of the median nerve resemble the two oblique, central portions of the letter M; the musculocutaneous and ulnar nerves form the lateral and medial vertical portions, respectively

3. Posterior cord

   a. The posterior cord gives off three subscapular nerves; the upper subscapular nerve innervates the upper part of subscapularis, the middle subscapular or thoracodorsal nerve innervates latissimus dorsi, and the lower subscapular nerve innervates the lower part of subscapularis and teres major

   b. Near the inferior border of subscapularis, the posterior cord divides into its terminal branches, the axillary and radial nerves

      1. Axillary nerve

         a. Courses posteriorly through the quadrangular space, inferior to the shoulder joint; winds around the posterior aspect of the surgical neck of the humerus and innervates the deltoid and teres minor

         b. Gives rise to the superior lateral brachial cutaneous nerve that emerges along the posterior border of the deltoid to supply the skin of the upper lateral arm

         c. Clinical note: an inferior dislocation of the humeral head from the glenoid fossa may compress the axillary nerve as it passes posteriorly through the quadrangular space, inferior to the shoulder joint; this may result in paralysis of the deltoid and teres minor and anesthesia of the skin of the upper lateral arm

2. Radial nerve

   a. Courses posteriorly, inferior to the tendon of latissimus dorsi, and descends laterally in the radial groove on the posterior aspect of the humerus

   b. Clinical note: the radial nerve is subject to compression, perhaps by crutches placed too far posteriorly, as it courses posteriorly, inferior to the tendon of latissimus dorsi

4. Since the medial and lateral cords are composed of anterior divisions, their branches generally innervate anterior musculature; the posterior cord is composed of posterior divisions and, generally, its branches innervate posterior musculature

C. Clinical notes: brachial plexus injuries

1. Erb's paralysis: results from injury to the superior trunk of the brachial plexus, perhaps as the result of extreme, contralateral lateral flexion of the head and neck during a breech delivery; muscles and skin innervated by ventral rami C5 and C6 may exhibit varying degrees of paralysis and anesthesia

2. Klumpke's paralysis: results from injury to the inferior trunk, perhaps as a result of traction as it overrides a cervical rib; muscles and skin innervated by ventral rami C8 and T1 may demonstrate varying degrees of paralysis and anesthesia

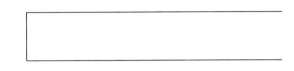

The Shoulder or Glenohumeral Joint

I. Articular Components

    A. Bony components: head of the humerus and glenoid cavity of the scapula; the glenoid cavity is widened and deepened slightly by a lip of fibrocartilage, the glenoid labrum

    B. Fibrous capsule

        1. Proximally, the fibrous capsule attaches to the circumference of the glenoid cavity; distally, it attaches to the anatomical neck of the humerus, except medially, where the attachment descends for a short distance on the shaft of the humerus

        2. It is so thin and lax that it is not strong enough by itself to keep the head of the humerus in the glenoid cavity; this function is subserved by the rotator cuff muscles

        3. Rotator cuff muscles

            a. The tendons of insertion of the subscapularis, supraspinatus, infraspinatus, and teres minor are intimately related to the fibrous capsule, forming a rotator cuff around the shoulder joint (it is deficient inferiorly); the tendons of subscapularis and supraspinatus are actually incorporated within the fibrous capsule

            b. Because of this intimate relationship, rotator cuff muscles not only serve to produce movement at the shoulder joint, but also serve to maintain the functional integrity of the shoulder joint by keeping the head of the humerus within the glenoid cavity

c. Clinical note: tears of rotator cuff tendons, especially the supraspinatus tendon, are common

4. The tendon of the long head of the biceps brachii enters an opening in the fibrous capsule at the upper end of the intertubercular sulcus, courses over the head of the humerus, and attaches to the supraglenoid tubercle

II. Ligaments

A. Superior, middle, and inferior glenohumeral ligaments

1. Attach proximally near the supraglenoid tubercle; distally, they attach along the superior, middle, and inferior regions of the anterior part of the anatomical neck of the humerus, respectively

2. They reinforce the anterior part of the fibrous capsule and help prevent anterior dislocation of the humeral head

B. Coracohumeral ligament: extends from the coracoid process to the superior part of the anatomical neck of the humerus; reinforces the superior part of the fibrous capsule and helps prevent superior dislocation of the humeral head

C. Coracoacromial ligament: extends from the coracoid process to the acromion, forming a fibrous arch above the shoulder joint; helps prevent superior dislocation of the humeral head

III. Bursae

A. Sacs lined by synovial membrane and containing synovial fluid; they serve to reduce friction between apposed surfaces

B. Subscapular bursa: interposed between the subscapularis tendon and neck of the scapula; it is continuous with the synovial cavity of the shoulder joint between the superior and middle glenohumeral ligaments

C. Subacromial bursa

1. Located between the acromion and fibrous capsule of the shoulder joint; it may occur as two separate bursae, a medial subacromial and a lateral subdeltoid bursa

2. Clinical note: the subacromial bursa is a common site of inflammation (bursitis) and source of shoulder pain

D. As the tendon of the long head of the biceps brachii courses within the shoulder joint, it is enclosed in a bursalike synovial tendon sheath formed by the synovial membrane of the shoulder joint; part of the synovial tendon sheath emerges from the fibrous capsule and descends in the intertubercular sulcus

IV. Movements of the Shoulder Joint

A. A ventral movement of the arm in a sagittal plane is flexion of the shoulder; the opposite movement is extension of the shoulder

B. Movement of the arm away from the midline in a coronal plane is abduction of the shoulder; the opposite movement is adduction of the shoulder

C. Rotation of the humerus around its longitudinal axis such that the anterior surface of the humerus turns medially is medial rotation of the shoulder; the opposite movement is lateral rotation of the shoulder

The Arm

I. Superficial Fascia

    A. Cutaneous nerves

        1. Superior lateral brachial cutaneous nerve: arises from the axillary nerve; emerges along the posterior border of the deltoid to supply the upper lateral arm

        2. Inferior lateral brachial cutaneous nerve: arises from the radial nerve; emerges from the lateral head of the triceps brachii to supply the lower lateral arm

        3. Posterior brachial cutaneous nerve: arises from the radial nerve; emerges in the proximal arm, medial to the long head of the triceps brachii, and descends to supply the posterior arm

        4. Intercostobrachial nerve (inconstant): name given to the lateral cutaneous branch of the second intercostal nerve when it supplies the upper medial arm

        5. Medial brachial cutaneous nerve: branch of the medial cord of the brachial plexus; supplies the upper medial arm

        6. Medial antebrachial cutaneous nerve: branch of the medial cord of the brachial plexus; emerges through the deep fascia on the medial aspect of the arm and supplies the anterior and lower medial arm before continuing into the forearm

    B. Superficial veins

        1. Cephalic vein: ascends along the anterolateral aspect of the arm

2. Basilic vein: ascends along the medial aspect of the arm; at about midarm, it penetrates the deep fascia adjacent to the medial antebrachial cutaneous nerve, enters the anterior compartment of the arm, and, at the inferior border of teres major, becomes the axillary vein

II. Deep (Brachial) Fascia

A. Continuous proximally with the axillary fascia and the deep fascia covering the deltoid; at the elbow, it attaches posteriorly to the olecranon and humeral epicondyles and, anteriorly, is continuous with the antebrachial fascia

B. Intermuscular septa

1. The medial and lateral intermuscular septa are inward, sheetlike extensions of the brachial fascia on the medial and lateral aspects of the arm, respectively; they attach to the humerus and divide the arm into an anterior or flexor compartment and a posterior or extensor compartment

2. The medial intermuscular septum extends from the crest of the lesser tubercle to the medial epicondyle; the lateral intermuscular septum extends from the deltoid tuberosity to the lateral epicondyle

III. Muscles

A. Flexors

1. Biceps brachii

a. Origin: long head—supraglenoid tubercle; short head—coracoid process

b. Insertion: radial tuberosity

c. Action: flexion of the elbow and shoulder; supination of the forearm, that is, lateral rotation of the radius so as to turn the palm of the hand anteriorly (in the supinated forearm, the radius and ulna are parallel)

d. Innervation: musculocutaneous nerve

e. Clinical note: the transverse humeral ligament extends from the crest of the greater tubercle to the lesser tubercle and retains the tendon of the long head of the biceps brachii in the intertubercular sulcus; dislocation of the tendon from the intertubercular sulcus may occur if the transverse humeral ligament is torn

2. Coracobrachialis

    a. Origin: coracoid process; it is fused to the short head of the biceps brachii

    b. Insertion: medial surface of the humerus at midshaft

    c. Action: adduction and flexion of the shoulder

    d. Innervation: musculocutaneous nerve

3. Brachialis

    a. Origin: distal half of the anterior surface of the humerus

    b. Insertion: ulnar tuberosity

    c. Action: flexion of the elbow

    d. Innervation: musculocutaneous nerve

B. Extensors

1. Triceps brachii

    a. Origin: long head—infraglenoid tubercle; lateral head—posterior surface of the humerus, superior to the radial groove; medial head—distal half of the posterior surface of the humerus, inferior to the radial groove

    b. Insertion: olecranon

    c. Action: extension of the elbow; adduction and extension of the shoulder (long head)

    d. Innervation: radial nerve

2. Anconeus

    a. Origin: lateral epicondyle of the humerus

    b. Insertion: lateral aspect of the olecranon and the bone immediately distal to it

    c. Action: extension of the elbow

    d. Innervation: radial nerve

IV. Nerves

    A. Musculocutaneous nerve (C5, 6, 7)

        1. Arises from the lateral cord and courses laterally, anterior to the shoulder joint; penetrates the coracobrachialis, innervating it, and then descends between biceps brachii and brachialis, innervating them

        2. Penetrates the deep fascia lateral to the tendon of the biceps brachii and continues into the forearm as the lateral antebrachial cutaneous nerve, which supplies the skin of the anterolateral forearm

        3. Clinical note: an anterior dislocation of the head of the humerus may injure the musculocutaneous nerve as it courses laterally, anterior to the shoulder joint; this may result in paralysis of the coracobrachialis, biceps brachii, and brachialis, and anesthesia of the skin of the anterolateral forearm

    B. Ulnar nerve (C8, T1)

        1. Arises from the medial cord and descends in the anterior compartment of the arm, medial to the brachial artery; at midarm, it penetrates the medial intermuscular septum, enters the posterior compartment of the arm, and descends on the anterior surface of the medial head of the triceps brachii

        2. At the elbow, it descends within the sulcus for the ulnar nerve posterior to the medial epicondyle; it has no branches in the arm

        3. Clinical note: posterior to the medial epicondyle, the ulnar nerve lies superficially; here, it is often compressed against the medial epicondyle, producing a radiating sensation that has earned this portion of the humerus the designation "funny bone"

    C. Median nerve (C6, 7, 8, T1)

        1. Descends in the anterior compartment of the arm adjacent to the brachial artery; from proximal to distal, it passes from a lateral to an anterior and then to a medial position in relation to the brachial artery

        2. It has no branches in the arm

    D. Radial nerve (C5, 6, 7, 8)

        1. Descends laterally in the radial groove between the lateral and medial heads of the triceps brachii; distally, it penetrates the lateral intermuscular septum, enters the anterior compartment of the arm, and de-

scends anterior to the lateral epicondyle between the brachialis and brachioradialis

2. Innervates triceps brachii and anconeus, and supplies the skin of the arm through its posterior brachial cutaneous and inferior lateral brachial cutaneous nerves

V. Vessels

A. Brachial artery

1. Distal continuation of the axillary artery at the inferior border of teres major; descends in the anterior compartment on the medial side of the arm and gives rise to the branches noted below

2. Profunda brachii artery

a. Arises below the inferior border of teres major and passes posteriorly to descend laterally in the radial groove with the radial nerve; distally, it terminates by dividing into the radial collateral and middle collateral arteries

1. Radial collateral artery: penetrates the lateral intermuscular septum with the radial nerve and descends with it, anterior to the lateral epicondyle

2. Middle collateral artery: descends within the medial head of the triceps brachii to the posterior aspect of the lateral epicondyle

b. May arise from or give rise to the posterior circumflex humeral artery

3. Superior ulnar collateral artery: arises near midarm; penetrates the medial intermuscular septum with the ulnar nerve and descends with it, posterior to the medial epicondyle

4. Inferior ulnar collateral artery: arises just proximal to the elbow and descends anterior to the medial epicondyle

5. Distal to the elbow joint, at the level of the neck of the radius, the brachial artery divides into its terminal branches, the ulnar and radial arteries

B. Veins: parallel their corresponding arteries; the brachial veins drain into the axillary vein, the proximal continuation of the basilic vein at the inferior border of teres major

VI. Cubital Fossa

A. Triangular depression anterior to the elbow joint

B. Boundaries

1. Lateral: proximal, medial border of the brachioradialis

2. Medial: proximal, lateral border of the pronator teres

3. Proximal: an imaginary line between the medial and lateral epicondyles of the humerus

4. Floor: brachialis (medially) and supinator (laterally)

5. Roof: antebrachial fascia; reinforced medially by the bicipital aponeurosis, a fan-shaped, fibrous expansion arising from the medial side of the tendon of the biceps brachii

C. Contents: from medial to lateral, the cubital fossa contains the median nerve, brachial artery, and tendon of the biceps brachii

The Elbow Joint

I. Articular Components

   A. Bony and ligamentous components

      1. Complex joint composed of the three articulations noted below

      2. Humeroulnar joint (sometimes referred to as the "true" elbow joint): between the trochlea of the humerus and trochlear notch of the ulna

      3. Humeroradial joint: between the capitulum of the humerus and articular fovea of the head of the radius

      4. Proximal radioulnar joint: between the articular circumference of the head of the radius and the radial notch of the ulna and annular ligament

      5. Flexion and extension of the elbow occur at the humeroulnar joint; pronation and supination of the forearm occur at the humeroradial and proximal radioulnar joints

   B. Fibrous capsule: attaches near the margins of the articular surfaces; surrounds the three component articulations, defining a single joint cavity

II. Ligaments

   A. Radial collateral ligament: triangular thickening of the lateral part of the fibrous capsule; fans out from the lateral epicondyle and attaches to the annular ligament

   B. Annular ligament

1. Internally grooved band forming about three-fourths of a circle; attaches to the anterior and posterior margins of the radial notch of the ulna and encloses the articular circumference of the head of the radius

2. Clinical note: in children, the diameter of the head of the radius is occasionally narrow enough to allow dislocation of the head of the radius from the elbow joint without tearing the annular ligament

C. Ulnar collateral ligament

1. Triangular thickening of the medial part of the fibrous capsule; its band-like parts are noted below

2. Anterior band—extends from the medial epicondyle to the coronoid process; posterior band—extends from the medial epicondyle to the olecranon; middle triangular band—fans out from the medial epicondyle to attach along the medial margin of the trochlear notch; transverse band—extends from the olecranon to the coronoid process, overlapping the distal part of the middle triangular band

D. Quadrate ligament: represents a thickening of that portion of the fibrous capsule between the radius and ulna

E. Oblique cord: ligament extending from the ulnar tuberosity to the shaft of the radius, distal to the radial tuberosity

The Forearm

I. Superficial Fascia

    A. Cutaneous nerves

        1. Lateral antebrachial cutaneous nerve: distal continuation of the musculo-cutaneous nerve; supplies the anterolateral forearm

        2. Medial antebrachial cutaneous nerve: branch of the medial cord of the brachial plexus; supplies the anteromedial forearm

        3. Posterior antebrachial cutaneous nerve: branch of the radial nerve; emerges from the lateral head of the triceps brachii proximal to the elbow and courses distally to supply the posterior forearm

    B. Superficial veins

        1. Basilic vein: arises from the medial side of the dorsal venous network on the dorsum of the hand and passes anteriorly around the medial side of the distal forearm; courses proximally on the anteromedial aspect of the forearm

        2. Cephalic vein: arises from the lateral side of the dorsal venous network on the dorsum of the hand and passes anteriorly around the lateral side of the distal forearm; courses proximally on the anterolateral aspect of the forearm

        3. Median cubital vein

            a. Communicating vein between the cephalic and basilic veins; courses superficial to the cubital fossa

b. Clinical note: the median cubital vein is frequently used for veni-puncture; penetration of the deep fascia with an exploring needle may injure the median nerve or pierce the brachial artery

II. Deep (Antebrachial) Fascia

A. Ensheaths the forearm musculature; local thickenings of the deep fascia form the common flexor tendon, common extensor tendon, and extensor reti-naculum

B. The common flexor and common extensor tendons attach proximally to the medial and lateral epicondyles, respectively; from their proximal attach-ments, they fan out and cover the superficial and contiguous surfaces of the muscles associated with their respective epicondyles

C. Extensor retinaculum

1. Transverse thickening of the deep fascia on the dorsal aspect of the dis-tal forearm and wrist; extends inferomedially from the distal part of the radius to the styloid process of the ulna, triquetrum, and pisiform

2. The space deep to the extensor retinaculum is divided by fibrous septa into compartments which contain, from lateral to medial, the tendons and synovial tendon sheaths of the abductor pollicis longus, extensor pollicis brevis, extensor carpi radialis longus, extensor carpi radialis brevis, extensor pollicis longus, extensor digitorum, extensor indicis, extensor digiti minimi, and extensor carpi ulnaris; synovial tendon sheaths are elongated bursae that ensheath tendons and function to re-duce friction between tendons and their apposed surfaces

III. Muscles

A. Superficial flexors

1. Pronator teres

a. Origin: humeral head—medial supracondylar crest and the medial epicondyle via the common flexor tendon; ulnar head—coronoid process

b. Insertion: pronator tuberosity

c. Action: pronation of the forearm, that is, medial rotation of the radius so as to turn the palm of the hand posteriorly (in the pronated fore-arm, the radius and ulna are crossed); flexion of the elbow

d. Innervation: median nerve

2. Flexor carpi radialis

   a. Origin: medial epicondyle via the common flexor tendon

   b. Insertion: at the wrist, its tendon passes through a special com-
      partment in the lateral part of the flexor retinaculum and then in-
      serts on the palmar surfaces of the bases of the second and third
      metacarpals

   c. Action: flexion and abduction of the wrist

   d. Innervation: median nerve

3. Palmaris longus

   a. Origin: medial epicondyle via the common flexor tendon

   b. Insertion: flexor retinaculum and palmar aponeurosis, thickenings
      of the deep fascia on the ventral aspect of the wrist and within the
      palm of the hand, respectively

   c. Action: flexion of the wrist

   d. Innervation: median nerve

   e. Absent in about 10 percent of individuals

4. Flexor carpi ulnaris

   a. Origin: humeral head—medial epicondyle via the common flexor ten-
      don; ulnar head—medial aspect of the olecranon and the subcutane-
      ous posterior border of the ulna

   b. Insertion: pisiform bone

   c. Action: flexion and adduction of the wrist

   d. Innervation: ulnar nerve

5. Flexor digitorum superficialis

   a. Origin: humeroulnar head—medial epicondyle via the common flexor
      tendon and coronoid process; radial head—oblique line, that is, the
      slight ridge extending from the radial tuberosity to the pronator
      tuberosity (the humeroulnar and radial heads are connected proxi-
      mally by a fibrous arch)

   b. Insertion: its four tendons pass into the palm of the hand through the carpal tunnel, an osseofibrous passageway bounded by the carpal sulcus and flexor retinaculum; they bifurcate before inserting onto the sides of the middle phalanges of digits 2, 3, 4, and 5

c. Action: flexion of the proximal interphalangeal and metacarpophalangeal joints of digits 2, 3, 4, and 5; flexion of the wrist

d. Innervation: median nerve

B. Deep flexors

1. Flexor pollicis longus

a. Origin: anterior surface of the radius, distal to the oblique line, and the adjacent interosseous membrane

b. Insertion: its tendon passes through the carpal tunnel and inserts on the palmar surface of the base of the distal phalanx of the thumb

c. Action: flexion of the interphalangeal, metacarpophalangeal, and carpometacarpal joints of the thumb; flexion of the wrist

d. Innervation: anterior interosseous nerve, a branch of the median nerve

2. Flexor digitorum profundus

a. Origin: anterior surface of the ulna and the adjacent interosseous membrane

b. Insertion: its four tendons pass through the carpal tunnel as well as the bifurcated tendons of flexor digitorum superficialis; they insert on the palmar surfaces of the bases of the distal phalanges of digits 2, 3, 4, and 5

c. Action: flexion of the distal interphalangeal, proximal interphalangeal, and metacarpophalangeal joints of digits 2, 3, 4, and 5; flexion of the wrist

d. Innervation: lateral half—anterior interosseous nerve, a branch of the median nerve; medial half—ulnar nerve

3. Pronator quadratus

a. Origin: anterior surface of the distal ulna

b. Insertion: fibers course inferolaterally to the anterior surface of the distal radius

c. Action: pronation of the forearm

d. Innervation: anterior interosseous nerve, a branch of the median nerve

C. Superficial extensors

1. Brachioradialis

    a. Origin: superior part of the lateral supracondylar crest

    b. Insertion: styloid process of the radius

    c. Action: flexion of the elbow

    d. Innervation: radial nerve; although functionally a flexor, the brachioradialis is included with the extensors because it is embryologically derived from extensor musculature and innervated by the radial nerve

2. Extensor carpi radialis longus

    a. Origin: inferior part of the lateral supracondylar crest

    b. Insertion: dorsal surface of the base of the second metacarpal

    c. Action: extension and abduction of the wrist; flexion of the elbow

    d. Innervation: radial nerve

3. Extensor carpi radialis brevis

    a. Origin: lateral epicondyle via the common extensor tendon

    b. Insertion: dorsal surface of the base of the third metacarpal

    c. Action: extension and abduction of the wrist

    d. Innervation: deep branch of the radial nerve

4. Extensor digitorum

    a. Origin: lateral epicondyle via the common extensor tendon

    b. Insertion: each of its four tendons inserts by way of a central band on the dorsal surfaces of the bases of the middle phalanges of digits 2, 3, 4, and 5, and, by way of two lateral bands on the dorsal surfaces of the bases of the distal phalanges of digits 2, 3, 4, and 5

c. Action: extension of the metacarpophalangeal and interphalangeal joints of digits 2, 3, 4, and 5; extension of the wrist

d. Innervation: posterior interosseous nerve, a branch of the radial nerve

e. On the dorsum of the hand, the tendons of extensor digitorum are joined together by fibrous bands called intertendinous connections

5. Extensor digiti minimi

   a. Origin: lateral epicondyle via the common extensor tendon

   b. Insertion: the tendon of extensor digitorum to the little finger

   c. Action: extension of the metacarpophalangeal and interphalangeal joints of the little finger; extension of the wrist

   d. Innervation: posterior interosseous nerve, a branch of the radial nerve

6. Extensor carpi ulnaris

   a. Origin: lateral epicondyle via the common extensor tendon and the subcutaneous posterior border of the ulna

   b. Insertion: dorsal surface of the base of the fifth metacarpal

   c. Action: extension and adduction of the wrist

   d. Innervation: posterior interosseous nerve, a branch of the radial nerve

   e. The extensor carpi ulnaris, extensor carpi radialis longus, and extensor carpi radialis brevis play an important role in fixing the wrist in extension, and thereby elongating the flexor digitorum superficialis, flexor digitorum profundus, and flexor pollicis longus muscles; in an elongated state, these muscles are capable of producing a more powerful contraction, and thus a more forceful grip of the hand

D. Deep extensors

   1. Supinator

      a. Origin: lateral epicondyle of the humerus, supinator crest of the ulna, and the radial collateral and annular ligaments

      b. Insertion: lateral surface of the proximal radius, as far distally as the pronator tuberosity

c. Action: supination of the forearm, that is, lateral rotation of the radius so as to turn the palm of the hand anteriorly

d. Innervation: deep branch of the radial nerve

2. Abductor pollicis longus

   a. Origin: proximal, posterior surfaces of the radius and ulna and the intervening interosseous membrane

   b. Insertion: emerges from between extensor carpi radialis brevis and extensor digitorum and inserts on the lateral side of the base of the first metacarpal

   c. Action: abduction, extension, and lateral rotation of the carpometacarpal joint of the thumb; abduction and flexion of the wrist

   d. Innervation: posterior interosseous nerve, a branch of the radial nerve

   e. The bony components of the carpometacarpal joint of the thumb are the base of the first metacarpal and the trapezium; they articulate in a saddle-shaped configuration that permits the movements described below

      1. Abduction of the carpometacarpal joint of the thumb is a ventral movement of the thumb in a sagittal plane away from the plane of the palm; adduction is a dorsal movement in a sagittal plane toward the plane of the palm

      2. Flexion of the carpometacarpal joint of the thumb is a medial movement of the thumb in a coronal plane across the surface of the palm; extension is a lateral movement in a coronal plane parallel to the plane of the palm

      3. During medial rotation of the carpometacarpal joint of the thumb, the anterior surface of the first metacarpal turns medially; during lateral rotation, the anterior surface of the first metacarpal turns laterally

3. Extensor pollicis brevis

   a. Origin: distal, posterior surface of the radius and the adjacent interosseous membrane

   b. Insertion: emerges adjacent to abductor pollicis longus and inserts on the dorsal surface of the base of the proximal phalanx of the thumb

c. Action: extension of the metacarpophalangeal and carpometacarpal joints of the thumb

d. Innervation: posterior interosseous nerve, a branch of the radial nerve

e. The tendons of abductor pollicis longus and extensor pollicis brevis form the anterior ridge of the anatomical snuff box, a triangular depression on the lateral side of the wrist at the base of the extended thumb (the posterior ridge of the anatomical snuff box is formed by the tendon of extensor pollicis longus)

4. Extensor pollicis longus

a. Origin: distal, posterior surface of the ulna and the adjacent interosseous membrane

b. Insertion: its tendon bends around the medial side of the dorsal radial tubercle, forms the posterior ridge of the anatomical snuff box, and inserts on the dorsal surface of the base of the distal phalanx of the thumb

c. Action: extension of the interphalangeal, metacarpophalangeal, and carpometacarpal joints of the thumb

d. Innervation: posterior interosseous nerve, a branch of the radial nerve

5. Extensor indicis

a. Origin: distal, posterior surface of the ulna, distal to the origin of extensor pollicis longus, and the adjacent interosseous membrane

b. Insertion: the tendon of extensor digitorum to the index finger

c. Action: extension of the metacarpophalangeal and interphalangeal joints of the index finger; extension of the wrist

d. Innervation: posterior interosseous nerve, a branch of the radial nerve

IV. Nerves

A. Radial nerve (C5, 6, 7, 8)

1. Descends anterior to the lateral epicondyle between the brachialis and brachioradialis; after innervating the brachioradialis and extensor carpi radialis longus, it divides into its terminal branches, the superficial and deep branches of the radial nerve

2. Superficial branch of the radial nerve: courses distally, deep to the brachioradialis; it has no branches in the forearm

3. Deep branch of the radial nerve: innervates extensor carpi radialis brevis and the supinator, and then penetrates the supinator lateral to the radius

4. Posterior interosseous nerve: when the deep branch of the radial nerve emerges from the supinator on the posterior aspect of the forearm, it is called the posterior interosseous nerve; the posterior interosseous nerve descends between the superficial and deep extensors and innervates extensor digitorum, extensor digiti minimi, extensor carpi ulnaris, abductor pollicis longus, extensor pollicis brevis, extensor pollicis longus, and extensor indicis

5. Clinical note: wrist drop

   a. The radial nerve lies directly on the humerus as it descends in the radial groove; sharp, splintered ends of a fractured humerus may injure the radial nerve and result in loss of the ability to fix the wrist in extension because of paralysis of extensor carpi radialis longus, extensor carpi radialis brevis, and extensor carpi ulnaris

   b. Without the ability to fix the wrist in extension, the flexor digitorum superficialis, flexor digitorum profundus, and flexor pollicis longus cannot be elongated and, therefore, the hand cannot forcefully grip objects; since the hand appears pendulous when the forearm is outstretched, the condition is known as wrist drop

B. Median nerve (C6, 7, 8, T1)

   1. Exits the cubital fossa between the humeral and ulnar heads of pronator teres, passes posterior to the fibrous arch connecting the humeroulnar and radial heads of flexor digitorum superficialis, and gives off the anterior interosseous nerve

   2. The anterior interosseous nerve descends on the interosseous membrane between flexor pollicis longus and flexor digitorum profundus; it innervates flexor pollicis longus, the lateral half of flexor digitorum profundus, and pronator quadratus

   3. After giving off the anterior interosseous nerve, the median nerve continues distally deep to flexor digitorum superficialis; at the wrist it lies superficially, lateral to the palmaris longus tendon and the tendons of flexor digitorum superficialis

   4. The median nerve innervates pronator teres, flexor carpi radialis, palmaris longus, and flexor digitorum superficialis; it also innervates

flexor pollicis longus, the lateral half of flexor digitorum profundus, and pronator quadratus through the anterior interosseous nerve

C. Ulnar nerve (C8, T1)

1. Passes into the forearm between the humeral and ulnar heads of flexor carpi ulnaris and courses distally between flexor carpi ulnaris and flexor digitorum profundus; at the wrist it lies superficially, lateral to the tendon of flexor carpi ulnaris

2. Innervates flexor carpi ulnaris and the medial half of flexor digitorum profundus

V. Vessels

A. Ulnar artery

1. Descends deep to pronator teres, and then, accompanied by the median nerve, passes posterior to the fibrous arch connecting the humeroulnar and radial heads of flexor digitorum superficialis; the ulnar artery soon leaves the median nerve to join the ulnar nerve between flexor carpi ulnaris and flexor digitorum profundus and, at the wrist, lies lateral to the ulnar nerve

2. The branches noted below arise in close succession from the proximal part of the ulnar artery

3. Anterior ulnar recurrent artery: courses proximally, anterior to the medial epicondyle, and anastomoses with the inferior ulnar collateral artery

4. Posterior ulnar recurrent artery: courses proximally, posterior to the medial epicondyle, and anastomoses with the superior ulnar collateral artery

5. Common interosseous artery

a. Bifurcates almost immediately into the anterior and posterior interosseous arteries

b. Anterior interosseous artery: descends on the interosseous membrane with the anterior interosseous nerve

c. Posterior interosseous artery: courses posteriorly, above the superior border of the interosseous membrane, and emerges from deep to the supinator in the posterior forearm adjacent to the posterior interosseous nerve; here, it gives off the interosseous recurrent artery, which courses proximally, posterior to the lateral epicondyle, to anastomose with the middle collateral artery, and then descends with the posterior interosseous nerve between the superficial and deep extensors

B. Radial artery

1. Courses laterally, anterior to the tendon of the biceps brachii, and gives off the radial recurrent artery, which courses proximally, anterior to the lateral epicondyle, to anastomose with the radial collateral artery

2. The radial artery continues distally, deep to the brachioradialis, with the superficial branch of the radial nerve; at the wrist it lies superficially, between the tendons of flexor carpi radialis and brachioradialis

C. The arterial anastomoses around the elbow allow blood to flow to the forearm and hand when the elbow joint is maximally flexed and the brachial artery compressed

D. Veins: parallel their corresponding arteries

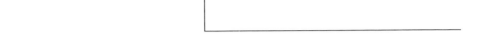

The Wrist or Radiocarpal Joint

I. Articular Components

   A. Bony and fibrocartilaginous components: the concave, carpal articular surface of the radius and concave, inferior surface of the articular disc of the ulna articulate with the reciprocally convex, proximal articular surfaces of the scaphoid, lunate, and triquetrum; the oblong shape of the wrist joint permits flexion, extension, abduction, and adduction, but not rotation

   B. Fibrous capsule: attaches near the margins of the articular surfaces; reinforced by the ligaments noted below

II. Ligaments

   A. Collateral ligaments

      1. Radial collateral ligament: extends from the styloid process of the radius to the scaphoid and trapezium

      2. Ulnar collateral ligament: extends from the styloid process of the ulna to the triquetrum and pisiform

   B. Palmar ligaments

      1. Palmar radiocarpal ligament: extends from the anterior margin of the carpal articular surface of the radius to the palmar surfaces of the scaphoid, lunate, and triquetrum

2. Palmar ulnocarpal ligament: extends from the styloid process of the ulna and anterior margin of the articular disc of the ulna to the palmar surfaces of the lunate and triquetrum

C. Dorsal ligament: the dorsal radiocarpal ligament extends from the posterior margin of the carpal articular surface of the radius to the dorsal surfaces of the scaphoid, lunate, and triquetrum

The Hand

I. Superficial Fascia

    A. Palmar side of the hand

        1. Tough and fibrous; anchors the skin to the deep fascia

        2. Cutaneous nerves

            a. Palmar branch of the median nerve: arises from the median nerve proximal to the wrist; supplies the midpalm and thenar eminence, the circular mound at the base of the thumb

            b. Palmar branch of the ulnar nerve: arises from the ulnar nerve proximal to the wrist; supplies the hypothenar eminence, the oblong mound at the base of the little finger

            c. Digital branches of the median nerve: arise from the median nerve as it emerges from the carpal tunnel; a proper palmar digital nerve supplies the lateral side of the thumb and three common palmar digital nerves bifurcate into proper palmar digital nerves for the medial side of the thumb, both sides of the index and middle fingers, and the lateral side of the ring finger

            d. Digital branches of the ulnar nerve: arise from the superficial branch of the ulnar nerve lateral to the pisiform; a proper palmar digital nerve supplies the medial side of the little finger and a common palmar digital nerve bifurcates into proper palmar digital nerves for the lateral side of the little finger and the medial side of the ring finger

e. The relatively large size of the cutaneous nerves to the palmar side of the hand is a reflection of the exquisite sensitivity of the skin of this region

3. Superficial veins: drain to the dorsal venous network on the dorsum of the hand

4. Muscle: palmaris brevis

  a. Origin: palmar aponeurosis

  b. Insertion: courses medially within the superficial fascia to insert into the skin on the medial border of the hand

  c. Action: increases the power of the grip by elevating and tensing the hypothenar eminence

  d. Innervation: superficial branch of the ulnar nerve

5. Clinical note: because of the tough, fibrous nature of the superficial fascia, infections within the palm tend to spread to the loose, more expansile, superficial fascia on the dorsum of the hand

B. Dorsum of the hand

  1. Loose; provides mobility to the skin

  2. Cutaneous nerves

    a. Superficial branch of the radial nerve

      1. Emerges posterior to the tendon of the brachioradialis and courses posteriorly around the lateral side of the wrist

      2. Gives rise to dorsal digital nerves that supply the lateral side of the hand and the proximal portions of the lateral three and one-half digits; proper palmar digital nerves from the median nerve supply the distal portions of the lateral three and one-half digits

    b. Dorsal branch of the ulnar nerve

      1. Emerges posterior to the tendon of the flexor carpi ulnaris and courses posteriorly around the medial side of the wrist

      2. Gives rise to dorsal digital nerves that supply the medial side of the hand and the proximal portions of the medial one and one-half digits; proper palmar digital nerves from the superficial

branch of the ulnar nerve supply the distal portions of the medial one and one-half digits

3. Dorsal venous network

    a. Assumes a highly variable pattern; the basilic and cephalic veins arise from the medial and lateral sides of the dorsal venous network, respectively

    b. Clinical note: the dorsal venous network is a frequent site for the infusion of intravenous fluids

II. Deep Fascia

A. Palmar side of the hand

  1. Thenar and hypothenar fasciae: ensheath the muscles within the thenar and hypothenar eminences, respectively

  2. Flexor retinaculum (transverse carpal ligament)

    a. Transverse thickening of the deep fascia attaching medially to the pisiform and hook of the hamate and laterally to the tubercles of the scaphoid and trapezium; spans the carpal sulcus, the groove formed by the palmar surfaces of the carpals, converting it into the carpal tunnel

    b. The carpal tunnel transmits the median nerve and the tendons and synovial tendon sheaths of flexor digitorum superficialis, flexor digitorum profundus, and flexor pollicis longus

  3. Palmar aponeurosis: central thickening of the deep fascia within the palm; attaches proximally to the flexor retinaculum and distally, via four slips, to the fibrous tendon sheaths of digits 2, 3, 4, and 5

  4. Fibrous tendon sheaths: elongated, fibrous tunnels derived from the deep fascia; they extend from the heads of the metacarpals to the distal phalanges and bind down the tendons and synovial tendon sheaths of flexor digitorum superficialis, flexor digitorum profundus, and flexor pollicis longus

B. Dorsum of the hand

  1. The deep fascia overlies the tendons of the extensor muscles and contributes to the formation of the extensor expansions

2. Extensor expansions

   a. Mobile, triangular aponeuroses covering the dorsal aspects of the proximal phalanges of digits 2, 3, 4, and 5 (the bases of the extensor expansions face proximally)

   b. Centrally, they are thickened by an extensor digitorum tendon; their lateral and medial edges are thickened by the insertions of the lumbricals, palmar interossei, and dorsal interossei

III. Muscles

   A. Thenar muscles

      1. Abductor pollicis brevis

         a. Origin: flexor retinaculum and the tubercles of the scaphoid and trapezium

         b. Insertion: lateral side of the base of the proximal phalanx of the thumb

         c. Action: abduction and flexion of the carpometacarpal joint of the thumb (the movements of the carpometacarpal joint of the thumb are described on p. 331); flexion of the metacarpophalangeal joint of the thumb

         d. Innervation: recurrent branch of the median nerve

      2. Flexor pollicis brevis

         a. Origin: superficial head—flexor retinaculum and tubercle of the trapezium; deep head—palmar surfaces of the trapezoid and capitate

         b. Insertion: superficial head—passes superficial to the tendon of flexor pollicis longus and inserts on the lateral side of the base of the proximal phalanx of the thumb; deep head—passes deep to the tendon of flexor pollicis longus to join the insertion of the superficial head

         c. Action: flexion of the carpometacarpal and metacarpophalangeal joints of the thumb

         d. Innervation: superficial head—recurrent branch of the median nerve; deep head—deep branch of the ulnar nerve

      3. Opponens pollicis

         a. Origin: flexor retinaculum and tubercle of the trapezium

b. Insertion: lateral side of the shaft of the first metacarpal

c. Action: medial rotation and flexion of the carpometacarpal joint of the thumb; simultaneous performance of these actions allows the tip of the thumb to contact the tip of digit 2, 3, 4, or 5, a movement referred to as opposition of the thumb (the reverse movement is called reposition of the thumb)

d. Innervation: recurrent branch of the median nerve

B. Hypothenar muscles

1. Abductor digiti minimi

a. Origin: pisiform bone

b. Insertion: medial side of the base of the proximal phalanx of the little finger

c. Action: flexion and abduction of the metacarpophalangeal joint of digit 5 (abduction of the metacarpophalangeal joints of digits 2, 3, 4, and 5 is defined as movement in the plane of the palm away from an imaginary longitudinal axis through the center of the middle finger— the opposite movement is adduction)

d. Innervation: deep branch of the ulnar nerve

2. Flexor digiti minimi brevis

a. Origin: flexor retinaculum and hook of the hamate

b. Insertion: medial side of the base of the proximal phalanx of the little finger

c. Action: flexion of the metacarpophalangeal joint of the little finger

d. Innervation: deep branch of the ulnar nerve

3. Opponens digiti minimi

a. Origin: flexor retinaculum and hook of the hamate

b. Insertion: medial side of the shaft of the fifth metacarpal

c. Action: lateral rotation and flexion of the carpometacarpal joint of the little finger; simultaneous performance of these actions cups the hand and increases the power of the grip

d. Innervation: deep branch of the ulnar nerve

C. Adductor pollicis

   1. Origin: oblique head—palmar surfaces of the capitate and bases of the second and third metacarpals; transverse head—palmar surface of the shaft of the third metacarpal

   2. Insertion: medial side of the base of the proximal phalanx of the thumb

   3. Action: adduction and flexion of the carpometacarpal joint of the thumb; flexion of the metacarpophalangeal joint of the thumb

   4. Innervation: deep branch of the ulnar nerve

D. Lumbricals and interossei

   1. Lumbricals (four)

      a. Origin: first lumbrical—lateral side of the flexor digitorum profundus tendon to the index finger; second lumbrical—lateral side of the flexor digitorum profundus tendon to the middle finger; third lumbrical —adjacent sides of the flexor digitorum profundus tendons to the middle and ring fingers; fourth lumbrical—adjacent sides of the flexor digitorum profundus tendons to the ring and little fingers

      b. Insertion: the tendons of the first, second, third, and fourth lumbricals insert into the lateral sides of the bases of the extensor expansions of digits 2, 3, 4, and 5, respectively

      c. Action: extension of the interphalangeal joints and flexion of the metacarpophalangeal joints of digits 2, 3, 4, and 5

      d. Innervation: first and second lumbricals—digital branches of the median nerve; third and fourth lumbricals—deep branch of the ulnar nerve

   2. Palmar interossei (three)

      a. Origin: first palmar interosseus—medial side of the shaft of the second metacarpal; second palmar interosseus—lateral side of the shaft of the fourth metacarpal; third palmar interosseus—lateral side of the shaft of the fifth metacarpal

      b. Insertion: first palmar interosseous—medial sides of the bases of the proximal phalanx and extensor expansion of digit 2; second palmar interosseous—lateral sides of the bases of the proximal phalanx and extensor expansion of digit 4; third palmar interosseous—lateral sides of the bases of the proximal phalanx and extensor expansion of digit 5

c. Action: adduction of the metacarpophalangeal joints of digits 2, 4, and 5 toward an imaginary longitudinal axis through the center of the middle finger; flexion of the metacarpophalangeal joints and extension of the interphalangeal joints of digits 2, 4, and 5

d. Innervation: deep branch of the ulnar nerve

3. Dorsal interossei (four)

a. Origin: first dorsal interosseous—adjacent sides of the first and second metacarpals; second dorsal interosseous—adjacent sides of the second and third metacarpals; third dorsal interosseous—adjacent sides of the third and fourth metacarpals; fourth dorsal interosseous —adjacent sides of the fourth and fifth metacarpals

b. Insertion: first dorsal interosseous—lateral sides of the bases of the proximal phalanx and extensor expansion of digit 2; second dorsal interosseous—lateral sides of the bases of the proximal phalanx and extensor expansion of digit 3; third dorsal interosseous—medial sides of the bases of the proximal phalanx and extensor expansion of digit 3; fourth dorsal interosseous—medial sides of the bases of the proximal phalanx and extensor expansion of digit 4

c. Action: abduction of the metacarpophalangeal joints of digits 2, 3, and 4 away from an imaginary longitudinal axis through the center of the middle finger; flexion of the metacarpophalangeal joints and extension of the interphalangeal joints of digits 2, 3, and 4

d. Innervation: deep branch of the ulnar nerve

IV. Nerves

A. Median nerve (C6, 7, 8, T1)

1. Traverses the carpal tunnel between the flexor retinaculum and the tendons and synovial tendon sheaths of flexor digitorum superficialis; at the distal border of the flexor retinaculum, the median nerve divides into digital branches (see p. 339) and the recurrent branch of the median nerve

2. The recurrent branch of the median nerve turns proximally over the distal border of the flexor retinaculum and innervates abductor pollicis brevis, the superficial head of flexor pollicis brevis, and opponens pollicis

3. Clinical note: carpal tunnel syndrome

a. Results from compression of the median nerve within the carpal tunnel; may be caused by inflammation and swelling of the tendons and synovial tendon sheaths of flexor digitorum superficialis, flexor digitorum profundus, and flexor pollicis longus, a condition known as tenosynovitis

b. Compression of the median nerve may result in paralysis of abductor pollicis brevis, the superficial head of flexor pollicis brevis, opponens pollicis, and the first and second lumbricals, as well as anesthesia of the skin on the lateral three and one-half digits (the skin of the midpalm and thenar eminence is usually spared, since the palmar branch of the median nerve arises proximal to the carpal tunnel); the compression is sometimes relieved surgically by severing the flexor retinaculum

B. Ulnar nerve (C8, T1)

1. Descends anterior to the flexor retinaculum and lateral to the pisiform; here, it divides into its terminal branches, the superficial and deep branches of the ulnar nerve

   a. Superficial branch of the ulnar nerve: gives rise to digital branches and innervates palmaris brevis (see pp. 339 and 340)

   b. Deep branch of the ulnar nerve

      1. Disappears into the hypothenar musculature between abductor digiti minimi and flexor digiti minimi brevis; after piercing opponens digiti minimi, it courses laterally in the deep palm on the anterior surfaces of the palmar and dorsal interossei

      2. Innervates abductor digiti minimi, flexor digiti minimi brevis, opponens digiti minimi, the third and fourth lumbricals, adductor pollicis, and the palmar and dorsal interossei

2. Clinical note: claw hand

   a. The ulnar nerve is particularly susceptible to injury where it lies superficially, lateral to the pisiform; injury here may result in paralysis of abductor digiti minimi, flexor digiti minimi brevis, opponens digiti minimi, the third and fourth lumbricals, adductor pollicis, and the palmar and dorsal interossei, as well as anesthesia of the skin on the medial one and one-half digits (the skin of the hypothenar eminence may be spared, since the palmar branch of the ulnar nerve arises proximal to the wrist)

   b. Paralysis of the palmar and dorsal interossei and loss of their function as flexors of the metacarpophalangeal joints of digits 2, 3, 4, and 5, may result in these joints being pulled into extension by extensor

digitorum; this, in turn, produces increased flexion of the interphalangeal joints of digits 2, 3, 4, and 5

   c. Paralysis of adductor pollicis, and loss of its function as an adductor
of the carpometacarpal joint of the thumb, may result in the carpometacarpal joint of the thumb being pulled into abduction by abductor pollicis longus and abductor pollicis brevis

   d. If the positions described above are assumed by the digits, the hand
appears clawlike, and thus the condition is called claw hand

V. Vessels

A. Ulnar artery

1. Descends anterior to the flexor retinaculum and lateral to the ulnar
nerve; here, it divides into its terminal branches, the superficial palmar
arch and deep palmar branch

2. Superficial palmar arch

   a. Courses laterally, between the palmar aponeurosis and tendons of
flexor digitorum superficialis; it is completed laterally by the superficial palmar branch of the radial artery

   b. Gives rise to a proper palmar digital artery for the medial side of the
little finger and three common palmar digital arteries that bifurcate
into proper palmar digital arteries for the lateral side of the little
finger, both sides of the ring and middle fingers, and the medial side
of the index finger

3. Deep palmar branch: accompanies the deep branch of the ulnar nerve
between abductor digiti minimi and flexor digiti minimi brevis; after
piercing opponens digiti minimi, it completes the deep palmar arch
medially

B. Radial artery

1. Proximal to the wrist, as the radial artery descends between the tendons
of flexor carpi radialis and brachioradialis, it gives off a superficial palmar branch, which penetrates the thenar musculature and completes the
superficial palmar arch laterally; the radial artery then winds around the
lateral side of the wrist between the radial collateral ligament and the tendons of abductor pollicis longus and extensor pollicis brevis

2. It subsequently traverses the anatomical snuff box, passes deep to the

tendon of extensor pollicis longus, penetrates the first dorsal interosseous, and enters the deep palm posterior to adductor pollicis; here, it divides into its terminal branches, the deep palmar arch and princeps pollicis artery

3. Deep palmar arch: courses medially on the anterior surfaces of the palmar and dorsal interossei, paralleling the deep branch of the ulnar nerve, and is completed medially by the deep palmar branch of the ulnar artery; gives rise to palmar metacarpal arteries that anastomose with the common palmar digital arteries from the superficial palmar arch

4. Princeps pollicis artery: gives rise to the radialis indicis artery for the lateral side of the index finger and then bifurcates into proper palmar digital arteries for each side of the thumb

C. Veins: accompany their corresponding arteries

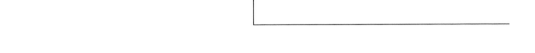

Other Joints of the Upper Limb

I. The Sternoclavicular Joint

    A. Articular components

        1. Bony components: sternal articular surface of the clavicle and the clavicular notch of the manubrium and costal cartilage of the first rib

        2. Fibrous capsule: attaches near the margins of the articular surfaces

    B. Ligaments

        1. Anterior and posterior sternoclavicular ligaments: reinforce the anterior and posterior aspects of the fibrous capsule, respectively

        2. Interclavicular ligament: spans the jugular notch, uniting the sternal ends of the clavicles

        3. Costoclavicular ligament: extends from the costochondral junction of the first rib to the impression for the costoclavicular ligament on the inferior surface of the clavicle near the sternal end; helps prevent upward displacement of the clavicle and dislocation of the sternoclavicular joint

    C. Articular disc: oval, fibrocartilaginous plate dividing the sternoclavicular joint into two synovial cavities

II. The Acromioclavicular Joint

    A. Articular components

        1. Bony components: acromial articular surface of the clavicle and the clavicular articular surface of the acromion

2. Fibrous capsule: attaches near the margins of the articular surfaces

B. Ligaments

1. Acromioclavicular ligament: reinforces the superior aspect of the fibrous capsule

2. Coracoclavicular ligament

a. Its medial part, or conoid ligament, is shaped like an inverted cone, whose base attaches superiorly to the conoid tubercle of the clavicle and whose apex attaches inferiorly to the coracoid process; its lateral part, or trapezoid ligament, is quadrilateral and attaches superiorly to the trapezoid line of the clavicle and inferiorly to the coracoid process

b. Helps prevent upward displacement of the clavicle and dislocation of the acromioclavicular joint

C. Clinical note: dislocation of the acromioclavicular joint is commonly referred to as a shoulder separation even though the shoulder joint is not involved

III. The Antebrachial Interosseous Membrane

A. Fibrous joint uniting the interosseous borders of the radius and ulna; the connective tissue fibers of the interosseous membrane course medially and inferiorly, and thus help distribute longitudinal forces along the radius to the ulna

B. Separates the anterior (flexor) and posterior (extensor) compartments of the forearm and provides attachment for muscles

IV. The Distal Radioulnar Joint

A. Bony and fibrocartilaginous components

1. Symphysial portion: the medial margin of the carpal articular surface of the radius and the styloid process of the ulna are united by the triangular, fibrocartilaginous articular disc of the ulna (its base attaches laterally to the radius)

2. Synovial portion: L-shaped; its horizontal part lies between the head of the ulna and superior surface of the articular disc of the ulna, and its vertical part lies between the head of the ulna and ulnar notch of the radius

B. Fibrous capsule: attaches near the margins of the articular surfaces

part **VII**

The
Lower
Limb

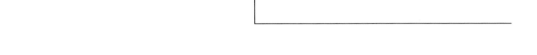

Bones and Bony Landmarks

I. Pelvic (Hip) Bone

    A. Composed of three bones, the ilium, ischium, and pubis; they meet in the acetabulum (a cup-shaped cavity that receives the head of the femur) and fuse at about age 16

    B. Ilium

        1. Ala

            a. Upper, flat, expanded, winglike part; its bony landmarks are noted below

            b. Auricular surface: medial, ear-shaped, articular region; forms a synovial sacroiliac joint with an auricular surface of the sacrum

            c. Iliac fossa: anterior, shallow concavity

            d. Iliac crest: convex, superior border; its highest point is on a level with the spinous process of vertebra L4

            e. Tubercle of the iliac crest: lateral projection of the iliac crest about 5 centimeters posterior to the anterior superior iliac spine; it is on a level with the spinous process of vertebra L5

            f. Anterior superior iliac spine: prominence at the anterior end of the iliac crest; palpable at the junction of the anterolateral abdominal wall and thigh

            g. Anterior inferior iliac spine: prominence between the anterior superior iliac spine and acetabulum

h. Posterior superior iliac spine: prominence at the posterior end of the iliac crest; its location is usually indicated on the surface of the body by a dimple

i. Posterior inferior iliac spine: projection inferior to the posterior superior iliac spine

j. Greater sciatic notch: concavity inferior to the posterior inferior iliac spine; converted into the greater sciatic foramen by the sacrospinous ligament, which extends from the sacrum to the ischial spine

k. Gluteal (posterior) surface

  1. Posterior gluteal line: slight ridge extending from the posterior part of the iliac crest to the greater sciatic notch

  2. Anterior gluteal line: slight ridge extending from the tubercle of the iliac crest to the greater sciatic notch

  3. Inferior gluteal line: slight ridge extending from the anterior inferior iliac spine to the greater sciatic notch

2. Body: lower, bulky portion that forms the superior part of the acetabulum; medially, it is divided from the ala by a ridge, the arcuate line

C. Ischium

1. Body: bulky, superior portion that forms the posteroinferior part of the acetabulum; medially, it exhibits a pointed projection, the ischial spine

2. Ramus: inferior, curved part that exhibits a posterior, bony mass, the ischial tuberosity

3. Lesser sciatic notch: concavity between the ischial tuberosity and ischial spine; converted into the lesser sciatic foramen by the sacrospinous and sacrotuberous ligaments (the sacrospinous and sacrotuberous ligaments extend from the sacrum to the ischial spine and ischial tuberosity, respectively)

D. Pubis

1. Body

  a. Wide, medial part; its bony landmarks are noted below

  b. Pubic crest: superior border

    c. Pubic tubercle: rounded projection at the lateral end of the pubic crest

    d. Symphysial surface: oval, medial surface

  2. Superior ramus

    a. Upper part that bounds the obturator foramen superiorly and forms the anteroinferior part of the acetabulum; its bony landmarks are noted below

    b. Pecten pubis: ridge extending posteriorly from the pubic tubercle; continuous anteriorly and posteriorly with the pubic crest and arcuate line, respectively

    c. Iliopubic eminence: rounded elevation between the superior ramus of the pubis and iliac fossa

    d. Obturator crest: ridge extending from the pubic tubercle to the inferior part of the acetabulum; the obturator canal is formed by a gap in the obturator membrane medial to the obturator crest (the obturator membrane is a dense connective tissue sheet closing the obturator foramen, except superiorly where it forms the obturator canal)

  3. Inferior ramus: flat, lower part; with the ramus of the ischium, it bounds the obturator foramen inferiorly

II. Sacrum: triangular bone formed by the fusion of the five sacral vertebrae

III. Coccyx: small, triangular bone formed by three to five rudimentary coccygeal vertebrae; may occur in two or three separate parts

IV. Femur

  A. Head: medially projecting sphere at the proximal end

  B. Fovea of the head of the femur: roughened pit near the center of the head

  C. Neck: constricted region between the head and shaft; forms an angle of about 125° with the shaft

  D. Greater trochanter: large, lateral prominence extending superiorly at the junction of the neck and shaft

E. Trochanteric fossa: deep pit on the medial aspect of the greater trochanter

F. Lesser trochanter: rounded, medial projection at the junction of the neck and shaft

G. Intertrochanteric line: slight ridge between the greater and lesser trochanters anteriorly

H. Intertrochanteric crest: prominent ridge between the greater and lesser trochanters posteriorly

I. Quadrate tubercle: rounded elevation near the middle of the intertrochanteric crest

J. Gluteal tuberosity: vertical, roughened ridge inferior to the intertrochanteric crest

K. Shaft: central, cylindrical portion

L. Linea aspera: ridge on the posterior aspect of the shaft

M. Medial and lateral lips of the linea aspera: medial and lateral margins of the linea aspera, respectively

N. Medial condyle: convex, bony mass forming the medial part of the distal end

O. Medial epicondyle: prominence on the medial aspect of the medial condyle

P. Adductor tubercle: small projection on the superior surface of the medial condyle

Q. Lateral condyle: convex, bony mass forming the lateral part of the distal end

R. Lateral epicondyle: prominence on the lateral aspect of the lateral condyle

S. Intercondylar fossa: depression between the medial and lateral condyles

T. Intercondylar line: ridge between the posterior surface of the femur and intercondylar fossa

U. Patellar surface: smooth, grooved surface between the medial and lateral condyles anteriorly

V. Patella

    A. Apex: pointed, distal end

    B. Base: superior border

    C. Articular surface: smooth, posterior face

    D. Anterior surface: convex, roughened face

VI. Bones of the Leg

    A. Tibia

       1. Medial and lateral condyles: bony masses forming the medial and lateral parts of the proximal end; their superior articular surfaces are flat and smooth

       2. Intercondylar eminence: elevation between the superior articular surfaces of the medial and lateral condyles; exhibits a medial and a lateral intercondylar tubercle

       3. Anterior and posterior intercondylar areas: flat regions anterior and posterior to the intercondylar eminence, respectively

       4. Fibular articular surface: round facet on the posteroinferior aspect of the lateral condyle

       5. Tibial tuberosity: anterior, roughened protuberance at the proximal end

       6. Shaft: central portion; triangular in cross-section

       7. Subcutaneous anterior border: palpable ridge extending from the tibial tuberosity to the distal end

       8. Medial subcutaneous surface: broad, palpable surface medial to the subcutaneous anterior border

       9. Lateral and posterior surfaces: form the nonpalpable lateral and posterior faces of the shaft; provide attachment for muscles

      10. Soleal line: slight ridge descending medially across the posterior surface of the proximal tibia

      11. Interosseous border: ridge between the lateral and posterior surfaces

12. Medial malleolus: inferiorly projecting process on the medial side of the distal end; forms the prominent, palpable eminence at the medial side of the ankle

13. Fibular notch: indentation on the lateral side of the distal end

14. Inferior articular surface: concave, distal end

B. Fibula

1. Head: blunt, proximal end; forms a palpable eminence below the knee on the lateral side of the proximal leg

2. Neck: constricted region inferior to the head

3. Shaft: central portion

4. Posterior, medial, and lateral surfaces: provide attachment for muscles

5. Interosseous border: ridge on the medial surface of the shaft

6. Lateral malleolus: flattened, pointed, distal end; forms the prominent, palpable eminence at the lateral side of the ankle

VII. Bones of the Foot

A. Tarsals

1. Talus

a. Head: convex, distal end

b. Neck: constricted region proximal to the head

c. Trochlea tali: smooth, convex, superior articular surface; it is wider anteriorly

d. Anterior and middle calcanean articular surfaces: smooth, contiguous facets adjacent to the head on the plantar surface

e. Posterior calcanean articular surface: concave facet on the posterior portion of the plantar surface

f. Sulcus tali: groove between the contiguous anterior and middle calcanean articular surfaces and the posterior calcanean articular surface

2. Calcaneus

  a. Cuboid articular surface: smooth, anterior end

  b. Sustentaculum tali: medial, shelflike projection; exhibits a groove for the flexor hallucis longus tendon on its inferior surface

  c. Anterior and middle talar articular surfaces: smooth, contiguous facets on the superior surface of the sustentaculum tali and the adjacent bone

  d. Posterior talar articular surface: smooth, convex facet near the middle of the dorsal surface

  e. Sulcus calcanei: groove between the contiguous anterior and middle talar articular surfaces and the posterior talar articular surface

  f. Sinus tarsi: canal formed by the apposed sulcus calcanei and sulcus tali

3. Navicular: its tuberosity is the rounded eminence on its inferomedial surface; its talar articular surface is the concave, proximal face

4. Medial cuneiform: lies anterior to the medial part of the navicular

5. Intermediate cuneiform: lies anterior to the central part of the navicular

6. Lateral cuneiform: lies anterior to the lateral part of the navicular

7. Cuboid

  a. Calcanean articular surface: smooth, proximal face

  b. Groove for the peroneus longus tendon: transverse gutter along the distal, plantar surface

  c. Tuberosity: prominence posterior to the lateral end of the groove for the peroneus longus tendon

B. Metatarsals I, II, III, IV, and V

  1. Base: angular, proximal end

  2. Shaft: central portion

  3. Head: rounded, distal end

4. Tuberosity of the fifth metatarsal: posteriorly projecting process on the lateral side of its base

C. Phalanges: proximal, middle, and distal (there is no middle phalanx of the hallux)

1. Base: wide, proximal end

2. Shaft: central portion

3. Head: narrow, distal end

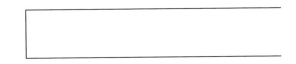

The Gluteal Region

I. Superficial Fascia

    A. Thick, fatty, cushionlike pad

    B. Cutaneous nerves

        1. Superior clunial nerves: branches of dorsal rami of spinal nerves L1, 2, and 3; descend over the iliac crest to supply the superior buttock

        2. Middle clunial nerves: branches of dorsal rami of spinal nerves S1, 2, and 3; supply the medial buttock

        3. Inferior clunial nerves: branches of the posterior femoral cutaneous nerve; hook around the inferior border of gluteus maximus to supply the inferior buttock

        4. Lateral cutaneous branch of the iliohypogastric nerve: descends over the iliac crest to supply the lateral buttock

II. Deep Fascia

    A. Ensheaths the gluteus maximus; superolateral to the gluteus maximus, it covers the gluteus medius

    B. Attaches superiorly to the iliac crest and medially to the sacrum; inferiorly and laterally, it is continuous with the deep fascia of the thigh or fascia lata

III. Muscles

    A. Gluteal muscles

        1. Gluteus maximus

            a. Origin: gluteal surface of the ilium, posterior to the posterior gluteal line, and the sacrum, coccyx, and sacrotuberous ligament

            b. Insertion: iliotibial tract, a bandlike thickening of the fascia lata extending from the tubercle of the iliac crest to the anterior aspect of the lateral tibial condyle, and the gluteal tuberosity (anteroinferior fibers)

            c. Action: extension, lateral rotation, and adduction of the hip; its insertion into the iliotibial tract helps maintain the knee in its fully extended and locked position

            d. Innervation: inferior gluteal nerve

            e. The trochanteric bursa, the largest bursa in the body, lies between the gluteus maximus and greater trochanter

        2. Gluteus medius

            a. Origin: gluteal surface of the ilium, between the anterior and posterior gluteal lines, and the deep fascia covering the muscle

            b. Insertion: posterior aspect of the greater trochanter

            c. Action: extension, lateral rotation, and abduction of the hip; its role as an abductor of the hip includes preventing the opposite side of the pelvis from sagging when supporting the body on the lower limb of the same side

            d. Innervation: superior gluteal nerve

        3. Gluteus minimus

            a. Origin: gluteal surface of the ilium, between the anterior and inferior gluteal lines

            b. Insertion: anterior aspect of the greater trochanter

            c. Action: flexion, medial rotation, and abduction of the hip; its role as an abductor of the hip includes preventing the opposite side of the pelvis from sagging when supporting the body on the lower limb of the same side

d. Innervation: superior gluteal nerve

e. Clinical note: if the gluteus medius and gluteus minimus muscles are weakened, perhaps from poliomyelitis, the individual walks with a waddling gait characterized by a sagging of the pelvis on the opposite side when the weight of the body is supported on one lower limb; such a gait is sometimes referred to as the Trendelenburg sign

4. Tensor fasciae latae

a. Origin: iliac crest, just posterior to the anterior superior iliac spine

b. Insertion: iliotibial tract

c. Action: flexion, medial rotation, and abduction of the hip, and lateral rotation and extension of the knee; its insertion into the iliotibial tract helps maintain the knee in its fully extended and locked position

d. Innervation: superior gluteal nerve

B. Lateral rotators

1. Piriformis

a. Origin: ventral surface of the sacrum

b. Insertion: emerges from the pelvis into the gluteal region through the greater sciatic foramen and inserts on the medial aspect of the greater trochanter

c. Action: lateral rotation of the hip

d. Innervation: nerve to the piriformis

e. Nerves and vessels passing from the pelvis into the gluteal region traverse the greater sciatic foramen and emerge either along the superior or inferior border of the piriformis

2. Obturator internus

a. Origin: internal surface of the obturator membrane and the surrounding bone

b. Insertion: emerges into the gluteal region through the lesser sciatic foramen, turns at an acute angle over the ischium, and inserts on the medial aspect of the greater trochanter

c. Action: lateral rotation of the hip

d. Innervation: nerve to the obturator internus

3. Superior gemellus

   a. Origin: ischial spine

   b. Insertion: obturator internus tendon

   c. Action: lateral rotation of the hip

   d. Innervation: nerve to the obturator internus

4. Inferior gemellus

   a. Origin: ischial tuberosity

   b. Insertion: obturator internus tendon

   c. Action: lateral rotation of the hip

   d. Innervation: nerve to the quadratus femoris

5. Quadratus femoris

   a. Origin: ischial tuberosity, inferior to the inferior gemellus

   b. Insertion: quadrate tubercle and the bone inferior to it

   c. Action: lateral rotation of the hip

   d. Innervation: nerve to the quadratus femoris

   e. Located deeply, between the quadratus femoris and inferior gemellus, the obturator externus tendon courses toward its insertion within the trochanteric fossa

IV. Nerves

   A. Superior gluteal nerve (L4, 5, S1): emerges from the greater sciatic foramen superior to the piriformis and courses forward between gluteus medius and gluteus minimus; innervates gluteus medius, gluteus minimus, and tensor fasciae latae

   B. Inferior gluteal nerve (L5, S1, 2): emerges from the greater sciatic foramen inferior to the piriformis and ramifies on the deep surface of the gluteus maximus, innervating it

C. Sciatic nerve (L4, 5, S1, 2, 3)

    1. Broadest nerve in the body; it is actually two nerves, the tibial and common peroneal nerves, bound together by connective tissue

    2. Emerges from the greater sciatic foramen inferior to the piriformis and descends posterior to the quadratus femoris between the ischial tuberosity and greater trochanter; in about 10 percent of individuals the common peroneal nerve emerges through or superior to the piriformis

    3. Has no branches in the gluteal region; supplies skin and muscles of the lower limb

D. Posterior femoral cutaneous nerve (S1, 2, 3): emerges from the greater sciatic foramen inferior to the piriformis and medial to the sciatic nerve; gives rise to the inferior clunial nerves and then supplies the skin of the posterior thigh

E. Nerve to the obturator internus (L5, S1, 2): emerges from the greater sciatic foramen inferior to the piriformis and descends on the posterior surface of the superior gemellus, innervating it; it then enters the lesser sciatic foramen and innervates obturator internus

F. Nerve to the quadratus femoris (L4, 5, S1): emerges from the greater sciatic foramen inferior to the piriformis and descends deep to the superior gemellus, the obturator internus tendon, inferior gemellus, and quadratus femoris; innervates the inferior gemellus and quadratus femoris

G. Pudendal nerve (S2, 3, 4)

    1. Emerges from the greater sciatic foramen inferior to the piriformis and descends posterior to the ischial spine; it then enters the lesser sciatic foramen and passes into the pudendal canal deep to the sacrotuberous ligament (the pudendal canal is a passageway within the obturator fascia covering the obturator internus muscle)

    2. Has no branches in the gluteal region; supplies skin and muscles of the perineum

V. Vessels

A. Superior gluteal artery

    1. Emerges from the greater sciatic foramen superior to the piriformis and divides into a deep and a superficial branch

2. The deep branch courses forward between gluteus medius and gluteus minimus with the superior gluteal nerve; the superficial branch courses forward between gluteus medius and gluteus maximus without an accompanying nerve

B. Inferior gluteal artery: emerges from the greater sciatic foramen inferior to the piriformis and courses with the inferior gluteal nerve on the deep surface of the gluteus maximus

C. Internal pudendal artery

1. Emerges from the greater sciatic foramen inferior to the piriformis; descends posterior to the ischial spine, lateral to the pudendal nerve and medial to the nerve to the obturator internus

2. Enters the lesser sciatic foramen and passes into the pudendal canal with the pudendal nerve; has no branches in the gluteal region

D. Veins: accompany their corresponding arteries

VI. Clinical Note: Intramuscular Injections

A. The gluteal region is a common site for intramuscular injections

B. For this purpose the gluteal region is often divided into four quadrants: upper medial, upper lateral, lower medial, and lower lateral

1. Injections into the lower quadrants may injure the sciatic nerve and other nerves and vessels emerging into the gluteal region along the inferior border of the piriformis; injections into the upper medial quadrant and the medial half of the upper lateral quadrant may injure the superior gluteal nerve and vessels, which emerge into the gluteal region along the superior border of the piriformis (the common peroneal nerve may also be subject to injury here, if it enters the gluteal region through or superior to the piriformis)

2. Injections into the lateral half of the upper lateral quadrant are relatively free of risk, because branches of the superior gluteal nerve and vessels are quite small in this region

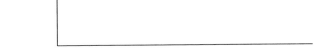

The Hip Joint

I. Articular Components

  A. Bony components

    1. Head of the femur: covered with articular cartilage, except at a central, roughened pit, the fovea of the head of the femur

    2. Acetabulum

      a. Cup-shaped cavity on the external surface of the hip bone; the acetabular notch is the gap in its inferior wall

      b. The head of the femur articulates at the bottom of the acetabulum with the horseshoe-shaped lunate surface, which surrounds a central, fat-filled depression, the acetabular fossa

      c. The acetabular labrum is the fibrocartilaginous lip along the rim of the acetabulum; the part of the acetabular labrum that spans the acetabular notch is termed the transverse acetabular ligament

  B. Fibrous capsule

    1. Attaches proximally to the external surface of the acetabulum and transverse acetabular ligament; attaches distally to the medial aspect of the greater trochanter, the intertrochanteric line, the medial aspect of the base of the neck, and halfway along the posterior aspect of the neck

    2. Reinforced by the iliofemoral, pubofemoral, and ischiofemoral ligaments

II. Ligaments

    A. Iliofemoral ligament

        1. Strong, triangular ligament; its apex attaches to the anterior inferior iliac spine, its base attaches along the intertrochanteric line, and its medial and lateral edges are thickened

        2. Resists extension and medial rotation of the hip; with slight extension of the hip, the tautness developed in the iliofemoral ligaments can balance the trunk on the femoral heads with minimal activity of the iliopsoas

    B. Pubofemoral ligament: narrow band extending from the obturator crest to the medial aspect of the base of the neck; resists extension, medial rotation, and abduction of the hip

    C. Ischiofemoral ligament: wide band extending forward from the posterior and inferior aspects of the acetabulum to the medial aspect of the greater trochanter; resists extension and medial rotation of the hip

    D. Ligament of the head of the femur: flattened band extending from the fovea of the head of the femur to the transverse acetabular ligament and the bone on either side of the acetabular notch; resists adduction of the hip

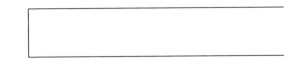

The Thigh

I. Superficial Fascia

  A. Cutaneous nerves

    1. Genital branch of the genitofemoral nerve and the ilioinguinal nerve: emerge from the superficial inguinal ring and supply the proximal, medial thigh

    2. Cutaneous branch of the obturator nerve: arises from the anterior branch of the obturator nerve and supplies the medial midthigh

    3. Medial cutaneous nerve of the thigh: branch of the femoral nerve; supplies the distal, medial thigh

    4. Femoral branch of the genitofemoral nerve: descends deep to the inguinal ligament with the femoral artery; supplies the proximal, anterior thigh

    5. Intermediate cutaneous nerve of the thigh: branch of the femoral nerve; supplies the distal, anterior thigh

    6. Lateral femoral cutaneous nerve: descends deep to or through the inguinal ligament, just medial to the anterior superior iliac spine; supplies the lateral thigh

    7. Posterior femoral cutaneous nerve: descends in the posterior thigh deep to the deep fascia; supplies the posterior thigh

  B. Superficial vessels

    1. Four arteries, as noted below, arise from the proximal part of the femoral artery and emerge into the superficial fascia through the deep fascia

or saphenous hiatus, an oval aperture in the deep fascia inferolateral to the pubic tubercle; the superficial epigastric artery ascends on the anterior abdominal wall, the superficial circumflex iliac artery courses laterally toward the anterior superior iliac spine, the superficial external pudendal artery courses medially, superficial to the spermatic cord/round ligament, and the deep external pudendal artery courses medially, deep to the spermatic cord/round ligament (corresponding veins drain into the great saphenous vein)

2. Great saphenous vein: ascends in the superficial fascia on the medial aspect of the thigh; passes through the saphenous hiatus and drains into the femoral vein

3. Lymphatics: superficial lymphatics of the lower limb drain to superficial inguinal nodes along the inguinal ligament and superior end of the great saphenous vein; superficial inguinal nodes drain through the saphenous hiatus to deep inguinal and external iliac nodes, which parallel the femoral and external iliac vessels, respectively

II. Deep Fascia (Fascia Lata)

A. Thick, fibrous, dense connective tissue stocking ensheathing the thigh; inward, sheetlike extensions of the fascia lata, the medial and lateral intermuscular septa, attach to the linea aspera and separate the anterior compartment of the thigh from the medial and posterior compartments, respectively (there is no intermuscular septum between the medial and posterior compartments; there is no lateral compartment)

B. Iliotibial tract: bandlike thickening of the fascia lata along the lateral aspect of the thigh; extends from the tubercle of the iliac crest to the anterior aspect of the lateral tibial condyle

III. Muscles

A. Anterior compartment

1. Sartorius

a. Origin: anterior superior iliac spine

b. Insertion: shaft of the tibia, inferior to the medial tibial condyle, via the pes anserinus; from anterior to posterior, the tendons of sartorius, gracilis, and semitendinosus fuse and insert together via the three-pronged pes anserinus or "goose foot" tendon

c. Action: flexion, lateral rotation, and abduction of the hip; flexion and medial rotation of the knee

d. Innervation: femoral nerve

2. Rectus femoris

a. Origin: straight head—anterior inferior iliac spine; reflected head—body of the ilium, superior to the acetabulum

b. Insertion: patella

c. Action: extension of the knee; flexion of the hip

d. Innervation: femoral nerve

3. Vastus lateralis

a. Origin: lateral lip of the linea aspera

b. Insertion: patella

c. Action: extension of the knee

d. Innervation: femoral nerve

4. Vastus medialis

a. Origin: medial lip of the linea aspera

b. Insertion: patella

c. Action: extension of the knee

d. Innervation: nerve to the vastus medialis, a branch of the femoral nerve

5. Vastus intermedius

a. Origin: anterior, medial, and lateral surfaces of the shaft of the femur

b. Insertion: patella

c. Action: extension of the knee

d. Innervation: femoral nerve

e. The rectus femoris, vastus lateralis, vastus medialis, and vastus intermedius comprise the four heads of the quadriceps femoris muscle; all four heads converge distally and insert on the patella via the quadriceps tendon, which continues from the patella to the tibial tuberosity as the patellar ligament

6. Articularis genus

   a. Origin: anterior surface of the distal femur

   b. Insertion: synovial membrane of the suprapatellar bursa, an extension of the synovial cavity of the knee joint superior to the patella

   c. Action: draws the suprapatellar bursa proximally during extension of the knee, thereby preventing its interposition, and possible injury, between the patella and femur

   d. Innervation: femoral nerve

7. Iliopsoas

   a. Origin: iliacus—iliac fossa; psoas major—bodies and transverse processes of lumbar vertebrae

   b. Insertion: descends deep to the lateral part of the inguinal ligament and inserts on the lesser trochanter

   c. Action: flexion of the hip; flexion of the lumbar vertebrae (psoas major only)

   d. Innervation: iliacus—femoral nerve; psoas major—ventral rami L1, 2, and 3

B. Medial compartment

1. Pectineus

   a. Origin: pecten pubis

   b. Insertion: shaft of the femur, from the lesser trochanter to the linea aspera

   c. Action: adduction and flexion of the hip

   d. Innervation: femoral nerve; receives an occasional branch from the obturator nerve and a branch from the accessory obturator nerve, when it is present

e. Because the pectineus is often solely innervated by the femoral nerve, it may be considered an anterior compartment muscle

2. Adductor longus

    a. Origin: body of the pubis

    b. Insertion: upper part of the medial lip of the linea aspera, inferior to the attachment of pectineus and posterior to the attachment of vastus medialis

    c. Action: adduction and flexion of the hip

    d. Innervation: anterior branch of the obturator nerve

3. Adductor brevis

    a. Origin: body and inferior ramus of the pubis

    b. Insertion: upper part of the medial lip of the linea aspera, posterior to the attachment of adductor longus and anterior to the attachment of adductor magnus

    c. Action: adduction and flexion of the hip

    d. Innervation: anterior and posterior branches of the obturator nerve

4. Adductor magnus

    a. Origin: superior fibers—inferior ramus of the pubis; inferior fibers— ramus and tuberosity of the ischium

    b. Insertion: superior fibers—upper part of the medial lip of the linea aspera; inferior fibers—lower part of the medial lip of the linea aspera and adductor tubercle

    c. Action: superior fibers—adduction and flexion of the hip; inferior fibers—adduction and extension of the hip

    d. Innervation: superior fibers—posterior branch of the obturator nerve; inferior fibers—tibial division of the sciatic nerve

5. Gracilis

    a. Origin: body and inferior ramus of the pubis

    b. Insertion: shaft of the tibia, inferior to the medial tibial condyle, via the pes anserinus

c. Action: adduction of the hip; flexion and medial rotation of the knee

d. Innervation: anterior branch of the obturator nerve

6. Obturator externus

    a. Origin: external surface of the obturator membrane and the surrounding bone

    b. Insertion: trochanteric fossa

    c. Action: lateral rotation of the hip

    d. Innervation: posterior branch of the obturator nerve

C. Posterior compartment

1. Biceps femoris

    a. Origin: long head—ischial tuberosity; short head—lower part of the lateral lip of the linea aspera, posterior to the attachment of the vastus lateralis

    b. Insertion: head of the fibula

    c. Action: flexion and lateral rotation of the knee; extension of the hip (long head)

    d. Innervation: long head—tibial division of the sciatic nerve; short head—common peroneal division of the sciatic nerve

2. Semitendinosus

    a. Origin: ischial tuberosity; it is fused to the long head of the biceps femoris

    b. Insertion: its long, cordlike tendon inserts on the shaft of the tibia, inferior to the medial tibial condyle, via the pes anserinus

    c. Action: flexion and medial rotation of the knee; extension of the hip

    d. Innervation: tibial division of the sciatic nerve

3. Semimembranosus

    a. Origin: ischial tuberosity via a long, membranelike tendon

b. Insertion: posterior aspect of the medial tibial condyle

c. Action: flexion and medial rotation of the knee; extension of the hip

d. Innervation: tibial division of the sciatic nerve

4. The biceps femoris, semitendinosus, and semimembranosus are sometimes referred to as the hamstrings

D. When standing on one lower limb, the extensors, flexors, adductors, and abductors of the hip act like guy wires in steadying and balancing the body on the head of the femur

IV. Nerves

A. Femoral nerve (L2, 3, 4)

1. Descends into the anterior compartment of the thigh deep to the inguinal ligament, about midway along its length; breaks up immediately into the sensory and motor branches noted below

2. Sensory branches: the medial and intermediate cutaneous nerves of the thigh supply the skin of the distal medial and distal anterior thigh, respectively; the saphenous nerve emerges at the knee between the sartorius and gracilis and descends on the medial aspect of the leg and foot to supply the skin of the leg and foot

3. Motor branches: innervate sartorius, rectus femoris, vastus lateralis, vastus medialis, vastus intermedius, articularis genus, and pectineus (in the pelvis, the femoral nerve innervates the iliacus)

4. Clinical note: the femoral nerve is liable to injury where it lies superficially just below the inguinal ligament; injury may result in anesthesia of the skin and paralysis of the muscles supplied by its sensory and motor branches, respectively

B. Obturator nerve (L2, 3, 4)

1. Divides into an anterior and a posterior branch within the obturator canal

2. Anterior branch: enters the medial compartment of the thigh above obturator externus and descends between adductor longus and adductor brevis; innervates adductor longus, gracilis, part of adductor brevis, and gives off a cutaneous branch to the medial midthigh (occasionally, it innervates part of pectineus)

3. Posterior branch: pierces obturator externus and descends in the medial compartment of the thigh between adductor brevis and adductor magnus; innervates obturator externus, part of adductor brevis, and the superior fibers of adductor magnus

4. Clinical note: sectioning of the obturator nerve is sometimes carried out to relieve spasticity of the adductor muscles

C. Accessory obturator nerve (L3, 4): present in about 10 percent of individuals; descends into the thigh above the superior ramus of the pubis and innervates part of pectineus

D. Sciatic nerve (L4, 5, S1, 2, 3)

1. Descends in the posterior compartment of the thigh deep to the long head of biceps femoris; its tibial division innervates the long head of biceps femoris, semitendinosus, semimembranosus, and the inferior fibers of adductor magnus, and its common peroneal division innervates the short head of biceps femoris

2. Divides into the tibial and common peroneal nerves in the distal thigh

V. Vessels

A. Femoral artery

1. Commences deep to the inguinal ligament medial to the femoral nerve and extends as far distally as the adductor hiatus, an opening in the adductor magnus tendon superior to the adductor tubercle; continuous proximally with the external iliac artery and distally with the popliteal artery—the profunda femoris artery is its only major branch

2. Profunda femoris artery

a. Arises from the posterior side of the femoral artery just below the inguinal ligament and descends initially between adductor longus and adductor brevis, and then between adductor longus and adductor magnus; its branches are noted below

b. Lateral circumflex femoral artery: arises from the lateral aspect of the proximal portion of the profunda femoris artery and courses laterally, deep to rectus femoris (it may arise from the femoral artery)

c. Medial circumflex femoral artery: arises from the medial aspect of the proximal portion of the profunda femoris artery (it may arise from the femoral artery), and courses posteriorly, between the iliopsoas and pectineus; an acetabular branch passes deep to the transverse acetabular ligament and reaches the head of the femur along the ligament of the head of the femur

d. Perforating arteries (four): arise at regular intervals and penetrate the adductor magnus insertion to supply the posterior compartment (the proximal two perforating arteries also penetrate the adductor brevis insertion); the distal two perforating arteries are the terminal branches of the profunda femoris artery

B. Obturator artery

1. Arises within the pelvis from the internal iliac artery, emerges into the thigh through the obturator canal with the anterior and posterior branches of the obturator nerve, and encircles the obturator externus near its origin from the obturator membrane; an acetabular branch passes deep to the transverse acetabular ligament and reaches the head of the femur along the ligament of the head of the femur

2. Clinical note: the acetabular branches of the obturator and medial circumflex femoral arteries may be insufficient by themselves to prevent avascular necrosis of the head of the femur if it becomes separated from its ascending blood supply following fracture of the neck of the femur

C. Veins: accompany their corresponding arteries

VI. The Femoral Triangle, Adductor Canal, and Popliteal Fossa

A. Femoral triangle

1. Boundaries

a. Superior: inguinal ligament

b. Lateral: upper medial border of sartorius

c. Medial: medial border of adductor longus

d. Roof: fascia lata

e. Floor: iliopsoas (laterally) and pectineus (medially)

2. Contents

    a. Descending into the femoral triangle, from lateral to medial, are the femoral nerve, femoral artery, femoral vein, and femoral canal; the proximal portions of the femoral artery and vein, as well as the femoral canal, are enclosed in a connective tissue investment, the femoral sheath

    b. The femoral canal is a conical cavity containing loose connective tissue and some deep inguinal lymph nodes; its proximal end or base is the femoral ring, which is bordered anteriorly by the medial end of the inguinal ligament, medially by the lacunar ligament, posteriorly by the pectineus, and laterally by the femoral vein

3. Clinical notes

    a. In a femoral hernia, a loop of intestine passes through the femoral ring and into the femoral canal, and may protrude through the saphenous hiatus; femoral hernias occur more frequently in females, perhaps because the femoral ring is wider

    b. The superficial location of the femoral artery within the femoral triangle makes it suitable for catheterization procedures as well as for direct compression to control downstream hemorrhaging

B. Adductor canal

  1. Triangular tunnel in the middle third of the thigh; extends from the femoral triangle to the adductor hiatus

  2. Boundaries

    a. Anteromedial: sartorius

    b. Lateral: vastus medialis

    c. Posterior: adductor longus (superiorly) and adductor magnus (inferiorly)

  3. Contents

    a. In the adductor canal the femoral artery descends anterior to the femoral vein; they become the popliteal artery and vein after passing through the adductor hiatus

    b. The saphenous nerve, a branch of the femoral nerve, descends in the adductor canal, but does not traverse the adductor hiatus; it emerges at the knee between the sartorius and gracilis and descends on the medial aspect of the leg and foot to provide cutaneous innervation to the leg and foot

   c. The nerve to the vastus medialis, also a branch of the femoral nerve, descends in the proximal part of the adductor canal before innervating vastus medialis

C. Popliteal fossa

   1. Diamond-shaped depression located posteriorly, just above the knee joint

   2. Boundaries

      a. Superior: semimembranosus and semitendinosus (medially) and the biceps femoris (laterally)

      b. Inferior: medial head of the gastrocnemius (medially) and the lateral head of the gastrocnemius and plantaris (laterally)

      c. Anterior: posterior surface of the distal femur

      d. Posterior: deep (popliteal) fascia

   3. Contents

      a. Descending vertically in the middle of the popliteal fossa, from superficial to deep, are the tibial nerve, popliteal vein, and popliteal artery; the common peroneal nerve descends laterally between the tendon of the biceps femoris and the lateral head of the gastrocnemius

      b. The popliteal artery gives rise to the following branches within the popliteal fossa

         1. Medial superior genicular artery: courses deep to semimembranosus and semitendinosus

         2. Lateral superior genicular artery: courses deep to biceps femoris

         3. Middle genicular artery: pierces the posterior part of the fibrous capsule of the knee joint and supplies the cruciate ligaments of the knee

         4. Medial inferior genicular artery: courses deep to the medial head of the gastrocnemius

5. Lateral inferior genicular artery: courses deep to the lateral head of the gastrocnemius

6. Anastomoses between the genicular arteries allow blood to flow to the leg and foot when the knee is maximally flexed and the popliteal artery compressed

c. Veins

1. Corresponding genicular veins drain into the popliteal vein

2. The small saphenous vein ascends in the superficial fascia of the posterior leg and then penetrates the popliteal fascia to drain into the popliteal vein

The Knee Joint

I. Articular Components

    A. Bony components: medial and lateral condyles of the femur and tibia; patellar surface of the femur and articular surface of the patella

    B. Fibrous capsule

        1. Anterior part

            a. Superior and inferior to the patella, the fibrous capsule is formed by the quadriceps tendon and patellar ligament, respectively

            b. Medially and laterally, the anterior part of the fibrous capsule is formed by the medial and lateral patellar retinacula, respectively; the patellar retinacula are fibrous expansions of the quadriceps tendon which attach distally along the anterior margins of the articular surfaces of the tibial condyles (the lateral patellar retinaculum is reinforced by the iliotibial tract)

        2. Posterior part

            a. Attaches proximally along the intercondylar line and the adjacent articular margins of the medial and lateral femoral condyles; attaches distally posterior to the posterior intercondylar area and along the adjacent posterior margins of the articular surfaces of the tibial condyles, except where the popliteus tendon penetrates the fibrous capsule posterior to the lateral tibial condyle

            b. A thickened portion of the posterior part of the fibrous capsule, superior to the entrance of the popliteus tendon, is called the arcuate ligament; another thickened portion, the oblique popliteal ligament, is a fibrous expansion of the tendon of semimembranosus that ascends laterally from the posterior aspect of the medial tibial condyle across the posterior part of the fibrous capsule

3. Medial and lateral parts: attach along the articular margins of the femoral and tibial condyles on the medial and lateral sides of the knee, respectively; the medial part of the fibrous capsule is reinforced by the tibial collateral ligament

II. Ligaments

A. Collateral ligaments

1. Tibial collateral ligament: broad, flat band extending between the medial femoral epicondyle and medial tibial condyle; reinforces the medial part of the fibrous capsule and attaches to the medial meniscus

2. Fibular collateral ligament: round cord extending between the lateral femoral epicondyle and head of the fibula; it stands clear of the fibrous capsule

3. The tibial and fibular collateral ligaments prevent medial and lateral separation of the knee joint, respectively

B. Cruciate ligaments

1. Lie within the knee joint, inside the fibrous capsule, but outside the synovial cavity

2. Anterior cruciate ligament: arises from the anterior intercondylar area of the tibia and passes superiorly, posteriorly, and laterally to the medial surface of the lateral femoral condyle; prevents anterior displacement of the tibia on the femur (or posterior displacement of the femur on the tibia)

3. Posterior cruciate ligament: arises from the posterior intercondylar area of the tibia and passes superiorly, anteriorly, and medially to the lateral surface of the medial femoral condyle; prevents posterior displacement of the tibia on the femur (or anterior displacement of the femur on the tibia)

4. Clinical note: simultaneous forced abduction of the knee and anterior displacement of the tibia on the femur may tear the tibial collateral and anterior cruciate ligaments, as well as the medial meniscus because of

its attachment to the tibial collateral ligament; this is a common athletic injury and is sometimes referred to as the "unhappy triad"

C. The collateral and cruciate ligaments reach their maximum degree of tautness, and thus provide maximum stability to the knee, at full extension

III. Menisci

A. Structure

1. Crescentic, fibrocartilaginous wedges interposed between the femoral and tibial condyles; they are thick along their convex, outer margins, thin along their concave, inner margins, and lubricated on their superior and inferior surfaces by synovial fluid

2. The convex, outer margins of the menisci are loosely attached to the fibrous capsule, except for a posterior portion of the lateral meniscus, which is separated from the fibrous capsule by the popliteus tendon; the part of the fibrous capsule between the menisci and the tibial condyles is sometimes referred to as the coronary ligament

3. The medial and lateral menisci are C-shaped and O-shaped, respectively; their anterior and posterior pointed ends or horns attach outside the synovial cavity to the anterior and posterior intercondylar areas, respectively (the anterior horns of the menisci may be united by the transverse ligament of the knee)

B. Function: the menisci cushion compression forces and lubricate the articular surfaces of the femoral and tibial condyles by distributing synovial fluid in windshield-wiper fashion

IV. Synovial Membrane and Bursae

A. Synovial membrane

1. The synovial cavity between the femoral and tibial condyles is horseshoe-shaped (the open portion of the horseshoe faces posteriorly); however, anteriorly, the synovial membrane extends superiorly between the quadriceps femoris and femur to form the suprapatellar bursa

2. The synovial membrane lines the fibrous capsule, except for its central, posterior part; here, on each side, the synovial membrane reflects forward and leaves the fibrous capsule to attach along the articular margins of the femoral and tibial condyles on each side of the intercondylar fossa

3. Infrapatellar fat pad

    a. Mass of fat inferior to the patella, between the synovial membrane and patellar ligament

    b. A bilayered, crescentic, infrapatellar synovial fold extends from the infrapatellar fat pad to the front of the intercondylar fossa; here, its two component synovial membranes separate, cover the anterior surfaces of the cruciate ligaments, and then continue posteriorly, attaching along the articular margins of the femoral and tibial condyles on each side of the intercondylar fossa (they become continuous with the synovial membranes that reflected forward off the posterior part of the fibrous capsule)

B. Bursae

1. Anterior bursae: suprapatellar bursa—superior extension of the synovial cavity of the knee between the quadriceps femoris and femur; prepatellar bursa—between the apex of the patella and skin; superficial infrapatellar bursa—between the tibial tuberosity and skin; deep infrapatellar bursa—between the patellar ligament and tibia

2. Medial bursa: anserine bursa—between the pes anserinus and tibial collateral ligament

3. Lateral bursae (unnamed): between the tendon of the biceps femoris and fibular collateral ligament; between the popliteus tendon and lateral condyle of the femur (it communicates with the synovial cavity of the knee joint)

4. Posterior bursae (unnamed): between the fibrous capsule and lateral head of the gastrocnemius; between the fibrous capsule and medial head of the gastrocnemius; between the tendon of the semimembranosus and medial condyle of the tibia

The Leg

I. Superficial Fascia

    A. Cutaneous nerves

        1. Saphenous nerve: branch of the femoral nerve that emerges at the medial side of the knee between the sartorius and gracilis; descends on the medial aspect of the leg and supplies the medial and anterior leg

        2. Lateral sural cutaneous nerve: branch of the common peroneal nerve; emerges from the popliteal fossa and supplies the proximal, lateral leg

        3. Superficial peroneal nerve: branch of the common peroneal nerve; emerges through the deep fascia about midway along the lateral aspect of the leg and supplies the distal, lateral leg

        4. Medial sural cutaneous nerve

            a. Arises from the tibial nerve in the popliteal fossa; after being joined by a communicating branch from the common peroneal nerve, it is called the sural nerve

            b. The sural nerve emerges from the popliteal fossa in the groove between the two heads of the gastrocnemius and supplies the posterior leg

    B. Superficial veins

        1. Great saphenous vein: courses anterior to the medial malleolus and ascends on the medial aspect of the leg adjacent to the saphenous nerve

2. Small saphenous vein: courses posterior to the lateral malleolus and ascends in the middle of the posterior leg adjacent to the sural nerve; pierces the popliteal fascia and drains into the popliteal vein

3. Clinical note: in infants the great saphenous vein is sometimes used for venipuncture where it lies anterior to the medial malleolus

II. Deep (Crural) Fascia

A. General structure

1. Attaches superiorly near the articular margins of the tibial condyles, except posteriorly where it is continuous with the popliteal fascia; inferiorly, it is continuous with the deep fascia of the foot

2. Tightly invests the anterior and lateral compartments of the leg, but is loose over the posterior compartment

B. Intermuscular septa

1. Anterior intermuscular septum: inward, sheetlike extension of the crural fascia that attaches to the anterior aspect of the fibula; separates the anterior and lateral compartments of the leg

2. Posterior intermuscular septum: inward, sheetlike extension of the crural fascia that attaches to the posterior aspect of the fibula; separates the lateral and posterior compartments of the leg

3. Transverse intermuscular septum: loose connective tissue membrane extending from the posterior intermuscular septum to the crural fascia on the medial side of the leg; separates the superficial and deep parts of the posterior compartment of the leg

4. Clinical note: because of the tight investment of the anterior and lateral compartments by crural fascia and the anterior and posterior intermuscular septa, increased pressure in these compartments, perhaps due to edema, may compress and injure the enclosed structures; the pressure is sometimes relieved by incising the crural fascia, a surgical procedure known as fasciotomy

C. Retinacula

1. Local thickenings of deep fascia that bind down tendons and synovial tendon sheaths; synovial tendon sheaths are elongated bursae that ensheath tendons and function to reduce friction between tendons and their apposed surfaces

2. Extensor retinacula

    a. Superior extensor retinaculum: transverse band between the anterior aspects of the distal tibia and fibula

    b. Inferior extensor retinaculum

        1. Y-shaped band anterior to the ankle joint

        2. The stem of the Y is attached laterally to the dorsal surface of the calcaneus; medially, it splits into a superior arm which attaches to the medial malleolus and an inferior arm which merges with the deep fascia on the medial side of the foot

    c. From medial to lateral, the superior and inferior extensor retinacula bind down the tendons and synovial tendon sheaths of tibialis anterior, extensor hallucis longus, extensor digitorum longus, and peroneus tertius

3. Flexor retinaculum: descends posteriorly from the medial malleolus to the medial surface of the calcaneus; from anterior to posterior, it binds down the tendons and synovial tendon sheaths of tibialis posterior, flexor digitorum longus, and flexor hallucis longus

4. Peroneal (fibular) retinacula

    a. Superior peroneal (fibular) retinaculum: descends posteriorly from the lateral malleolus to the lateral surface of the calcaneus

    b. Inferior peroneal (fibular) retinaculum: lies anteroinferior to the superior peroneal retinaculum; extends from the lower lateral surface of the calcaneus to the upper lateral surface of the calcaneus, just short of the stem of the inferior extensor retinaculum

    c. From anterior to posterior, the superior and inferior peroneal retinacula bind down the tendons and synovial tendon sheaths of peroneus brevis and peroneus longus

III. Muscles

  A. Anterior compartment

    1. Tibialis anterior

      a. Origin: crural fascia; proximal, lateral surface of the tibia and the adjacent interosseous membrane

b. Insertion: medial surfaces of the medial cuneiform and base of the first metatarsal

c. Action: dorsiflexion of the ankle; inversion of the foot

d. Innervation: deep peroneal nerve

e. During dorsiflexion of the ankle, the dorsum of the foot moves superiorly; during plantar flexion of the ankle, the dorsum of the foot moves inferiorly

f. During inversion of the foot, the medial border of the foot is elevated; during eversion of the foot, the lateral border of the foot is elevated

2. Extensor hallucis longus

   a. Origin: medial surface of the distal fibula and the adjacent interosseous membrane

   b. Insertion: dorsal surface of the base of the distal phalanx of the hallux

   c. Action: extension of the interphalangeal and metatarsophalangeal joints of the hallux; dorsiflexion of the ankle

   d. Innervation: deep peroneal nerve

3. Extensor digitorum longus

   a. Origin: lateral condyle of the tibia, the upper anterior surface of the interosseous membrane, medial surface of the proximal two-thirds of the fibula (distally, it attaches lateral to the origin of extensor hallucis longus), anterior intermuscular septum, and crural fascia

   b. Insertion: each of its four tendons inserts by way of a central band on the dorsal surfaces of the bases of the middle phalanges of digits 2, 3, 4, and 5, and by way of two lateral bands on the dorsal surfaces of the bases of the distal phalanges of digits 2, 3, 4, and 5

   c. Action: extension of the metatarsophalangeal and interphalangeal joints of digits 2, 3, 4, and 5; dorsiflexion of the ankle

   d. Innervation: deep peroneal nerve

4. Peroneus (fibularis) tertius

   a. Origin: medial surface of the distal fibula, lateral to the origin of extensor hallucis longus (its muscle belly is usually an indistinguish-able distal continuation of the extensor digitorum longus muscle)

    b. Insertion: dorsal surface of the base of the fifth metatarsal

    c. Action: eversion of the foot; dorsiflexion of the ankle

    d. Innervation: deep peroneal nerve

B. Lateral compartment

  1. Peroneus (fibularis) longus

    a. Origin: head, neck, and proximal, lateral surface of the fibula; crural fascia and the anterior and posterior intermuscular septa

    b. Insertion: its tendon hooks around the lateral malleolus and passes forward to the lateral side of the cuboid; it then rounds the lateral side of the cuboid on its tuberosity, courses medially within the groove for the peroneus longus tendon, and inserts on the lateral surfaces of the medial cuneiform and base of the first metatarsal

    c. Action: eversion of the foot; plantar flexion of the ankle

    d. Innervation: superficial peroneal nerve

  2. Peroneus (fibularis) brevis

    a. Origin: distal, lateral surface of the fibula and the anterior and posterior intermuscular septa

    b. Insertion: its tendon hooks around the lateral malleolus and passes forward to insert on the dorsal surface of the tuberosity of the fifth metatarsal

    c. Action: eversion of the foot; plantar flexion of the ankle

    d. Innervation: superficial peroneal nerve

C. Posterior compartment: superficial muscles

  1. Gastrocnemius

    a. Origin: its medial and lateral heads originate from the posterior surface of the femur, superior to the medial and lateral femoral condyles, respectively

b. Insertion: posterior surface of the calcaneus via the tendo calcaneus (Achilles tendon)

c. Action: plantar flexion of the ankle; flexion of the knee

d. Innervation: tibial nerve

2. Soleus

a. Origin: soleal line of the tibia and the posterior surface of the proximal fibula; the tibial and fibular origins are connected superiorly by a fibrous arch

b. Insertion: its tendon fuses with the tendon of the gastrocnemius and inserts on the posterior surface of the calcaneus via the tendo calcaneus; the soleus and the two heads of the gastrocnemius may be referred to as the triceps surae

c. Action: plantar flexion of the ankle

d. Innervation: tibial nerve

3. Plantaris

a. Origin: posterior surface of the femur, superior to the origin of the lateral head of the gastrocnemius

b. Insertion: its long, thin tendon descends medially between the gastrocnemius and soleus and inserts on the posterior surface of the calcaneus, medial to the tendo calcaneus

c. Action: plantar flexion of the ankle; flexion of the knee

d. Innervation: tibial nerve

e. Absent in about 10 percent of individuals

D. Posterior compartment: deep muscles

1. Popliteus

a. Origin: lateral surface of the lateral femoral condyle, within the fibrous capsule of the knee joint

b. Insertion: emerges from the knee joint posterior to the lateral tibial condyle and inserts on the posterior surface of the tibia, superior to the soleal line

c. Action: unlocks the fully extended knee at the beginning of flexion by laterally rotating the femur; flexion and medial rotation of the knee

d. Innervation: tibial nerve

2. Flexor hallucis longus

   a. Origin: posterior surface of the fibula, distal to the origin of the soleus

   b. Insertion: just below the ankle joint, its tendon passes forward within the groove for the flexor hallucis longus tendon on the inferior surface of the sustentaculum tali; it continues forward in the sole of the foot and inserts on the plantar surface of the base of the distal phalanx of the hallux

   c. Action: flexion of the interphalangeal and metatarsophalangeal joints of the hallux; inversion of the foot and plantar flexion of the ankle

   d. Innervation: tibial nerve

3. Tibialis posterior

   a. Origin: medial surface of the fibula, posterior surface of the tibia (distal to the soleal line), and the intervening interosseous membrane

   b. Insertion: in the distal leg, its tendon courses medially, anterior to the tendon of flexor digitorum longus, and then hooks around the medial malleolus; it subsequently passes forward and inserts on the tuberosity of the navicular and the plantar surfaces of the cuneiforms and bases of metatarsals 2, 3, and 4

   c. Action: inversion of the foot; plantar flexion of the ankle

   d. Innervation: tibial nerve

4. Flexor digitorum longus

   a. Origin: posterior surface of the tibia, medial to the origin of tibialis posterior

   b. Insertion: its tendon hooks around the medial malleolus, posterior to the tendon of tibialis posterior, and enters the sole of the foot; within the sole of the foot, its tendon divides into four tendons which pass through the bifurcated tendons of flexor digitorum brevis and insert on the plantar surfaces of the bases of the distal phalanges of digits 2, 3, 4, and 5

c. Action: flexion of the distal interphalangeal, proximal interphalangeal, and metatarsophalangeal joints of digits 2, 3, 4, and 5; inversion of the foot and plantar flexion of the ankle

d. Innervation: tibial nerve

IV. Nerves

A. Tibial nerve (L4, 5, S1, 2, 3)

1. Exits the popliteal fossa and descends deep to the gastrocnemius and then deep to the fibrous arch connecting the tibial and fibular origins of the soleus; it then continues distally between the transverse intermuscular septum and tibialis posterior

2. Innervates gastrocnemius, soleus, plantaris, popliteus, flexor hallucis longus, tibialis posterior, and flexor digitorum longus

3. At the ankle, the tibial nerve courses deep to the flexor retinaculum, between the tendons of flexor digitorum longus and flexor hallucis longus; here, it gives off the medial calcanean nerve to the skin of the heel and then divides into its terminal branches, the medial and lateral plantar nerves

B. Common peroneal (fibular) nerve (L4, 5, S1, 2)

1. After leaving the popliteal fossa, it lies superficially, posterior to the head of the fibula; the common peroneal nerve then penetrates the posterior intermuscular septum and, as it passes forward in the lateral compartment between the neck of the fibula and peroneus longus, it divides into its terminal branches, the deep and superficial peroneal nerves

2. Deep peroneal (fibular) nerve

a. Penetrates the anterior intermuscular septum and descends in the anterior compartment, anterior to the interosseous membrane; descends initially between tibialis anterior and extensor digitorum longus, and subsequently between tibialis anterior and extensor hallucis longus

b. Innervates tibialis anterior, extensor hallucis longus, extensor digitorum longus, and peroneus tertius

3. Superficial peroneal (fibular) nerve: descends in the lateral compartment between peroneus longus and peroneus brevis, innervating them;

emerges into the superficial fascia about midway along the lateral aspect of the leg and supplies the skin of the distal, lateral leg

4. Clinical note: foot drop

   a. The deep peroneal nerve is subject to possible injury by the sharp, splintered ends of a fractured neck of the fibula; injury may result in loss of the ability to dorsiflex the ankle due to paralysis of tibialis anterior, extensor hallucis longus, extensor digitorum longus, and peroneus tertius

   b. Since the foot appears pendulous when the lower limb is elevated, the condition is known as foot drop

V. Vessels

A. Popliteal artery: descends deep to the gastrocnemius with the tibial nerve; at the inferior border of the popliteus, it divides into its terminal branches, the anterior and posterior tibial arteries

B. Anterior tibial artery: passes anteriorly, above the superior border of the interosseous membrane, and descends in the anterior compartment with the deep peroneal nerve; when the anterior tibial artery crosses the ankle joint, it becomes the dorsalis pedis artery

C. Posterior tibial artery

   1. Descends with the tibial nerve on the posterior surface of tibialis posterior and then deep to the flexor retinaculum; at the ankle, deep to the flexor retinaculum, the posterior tibial artery divides into its terminal branches, the medial and lateral plantar arteries

   2. Peroneal (fibular) artery

      a. Arises from the proximal part of the posterior tibial artery and descends between flexor hallucis longus and tibialis posterior; gives off branches that penetrate the posterior intermuscular septum to supply the muscles of the lateral compartment (peroneus longus and peroneus brevis)

      b. A perforating branch passes anteriorly below the inferior border of the interosseous membrane onto the dorsum of the foot; it may be the source of the dorsalis pedis artery

D. Veins: accompany their corresponding arteries

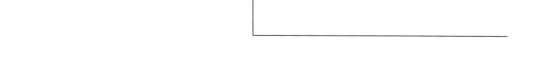

The Ankle or Talocrural Joint

I. Articular Components

    A. Bony components: the inferior articular surface of the tibia, lateral surface of the medial malleolus, and medial surface of the lateral malleolus articulate with the trochlea tali; since the trochlea tali is wider anteriorly, the ankle joint is more stable in dorsiflexion

    B. Fibrous capsule: attaches near the margins of the articular surfaces; reinforced by the ligaments noted below

II. Ligaments

    A. Medial or deltoid ligament

        1. Triangular; its apex attaches superiorly to the medial malleolus

        2. Inferiorly, it separates into four parts; the tibionavicular part attaches to the tuberosity of the navicular, the anterior tibiotalar part attaches anteriorly to the medial surface of the talus, the tibiocalcanean part attaches to the sustentaculum tali, and the posterior tibiotalar part attaches posteriorly to the medial surface of the talus

        3. Resists eversion of the foot

        4. Clinical note: the deltoid ligament is so strong that extreme eversion will often fracture the medial malleolus rather than tear the deltoid ligament

B. Lateral ligament

    1. Composed of three separate ligaments; superiorly, they attach to the lateral malleolus

    2. Inferiorly, the anterior talofibular ligament attaches to the lateral surface of the neck of the talus, the calcaneofibular ligament attaches to the lateral surface of the calcaneus, and the posterior talofibular ligament attaches to the posterior surface of the talus

    3. Resists inversion of the foot

    4. Clinical note: the anterior talofibular ligament is commonly torn by extreme inversion of the foot

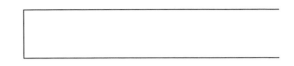

The Foot

I. Dorsum

    A. Superficial fascia

        1. Loose; provides mobility to the skin

        2. Cutaneous nerves

            a. After providing cutaneous innervation to the dorsum of the foot, the superficial peroneal nerve gives rise to dorsal digital nerves for the skin of the digits, except for the adjacent sides of digits 1 and 2, which are supplied by dorsal digital nerves from the deep peroneal nerve

            b. The saphenous and sural nerves supply the medial and lateral borders of the foot, respectively

        3. Dorsal venous arch: spans the metatarsals; the great and small saphenous veins arise from the medial and lateral sides of the dorsal venous arch, respectively

    B. Deep fascia

        1. Overlies the tendons and muscles on the dorsum of the foot and contributes to the formation of the extensor expansions

        2. Extensor expansions

            a. Mobile, triangular aponeuroses covering the dorsal aspects of the proximal phalanges of digits 2, 3, 4, and 5 (the bases of the extensor expansions face proximally)

b. Centrally, they are thickened by an extensor digitorum longus tendon; their lateral and medial edges are thickened by the insertions of the lumbricals, plantar interossei, and dorsal interossei

C. Muscles

1. Extensor digitorum brevis

    a. Origin: dorsal surface of the calcaneus

    b. Insertion: its three tendons insert into the tendons of extensor digitorum longus to digits 2, 3, and 4

    c. Action: extension of the metatarsophalangeal and interphalangeal joints of digits 2, 3, and 4

    d. Innervation: deep peroneal nerve

2. Extensor hallucis brevis

    a. Origin: dorsal surface of the calcaneus; it is fused to the extensor digitorum brevis

    b. Insertion: dorsal surface of the base of the proximal phalanx of the hallux

    c. Action: extension of the metatarsophalangeal joint of the hallux

    d. Innervation: deep peroneal nerve

D. Deep peroneal nerve: courses forward on the dorsum of the foot between the tendons of extensor hallucis longus and extensor digitorum longus; innervates extensor digitorum brevis and extensor hallucis brevis and then bifurcates into the dorsal digital nerves for the skin on the adjacent sides of digits 1 and 2

E. Dorsalis pedis artery: courses forward on the dorsum of the foot with the deep peroneal nerve; penetrates the first dorsal interosseous muscle and enters the sole of the foot to complete the plantar arch medially

II. Plantar Aspect

A. Superficial fascia

1. Tough, thick, fibrous padding; anchors the skin to the deep fascia

2. Cutaneous nerves: arise from the tibial nerve deep to the flexor retinaculum; the medial calcanean nerve supplies the heel, the medial plantar nerve supplies the medial side of the foot and the medial three and one-half digits, and the lateral plantar nerve supplies the lateral side of the foot and the lateral one and one-half digits

3. Superficial veins: drain to the dorsal venous arch

B. Deep fascia

   1. Medially and laterally, it ensheaths muscles of the hallux and little toe, respectively

   2. Plantar aponeurosis: central thickening of the deep fascia within the sole of the foot; attaches proximally to the calcaneus and distally, via five slips, to the fibrous tendon sheaths of the digits

   3. Fibrous tendon sheaths: elongated, fibrous tunnels derived from the deep fascia; they extend from the heads of the metatarsals to the distal phalanges and bind down the tendons and synovial tendon sheaths of flexor digitorum brevis, flexor digitorum longus, and flexor hallucis longus

C. Muscles

   1. First layer

      a. Abductor hallucis

         1. Origin: flexor retinaculum, calcaneus, and plantar aponeurosis

         2. Insertion: medial side of the base of the proximal phalanx of the hallux and the adjacent sesamoid bone

         3. Action: abduction and flexion of the metatarsophalangeal joint of the hallux (abduction of the metatarsophalangeal joints is defined as movement in the plane of the foot away from an imaginary longitudinal axis through the center of the second digit—the opposite movement is adduction)

         4. Innervation: medial plantar nerve

      b. Flexor digitorum brevis

         1. Origin: calcaneus and plantar aponeurosis

         2. Insertion: its four tendons bifurcate before inserting onto the sides of the middle phalanges of digits 2, 3, 4, and 5

3. Action: flexion of the proximal interphalangeal and metatarso-phalangeal joints of digits 2, 3, 4, and 5

4. Innervation: medial plantar nerve

c. Abductor digiti minimi

1. Origin: calcaneus

2. Insertion: lateral side of the base of the proximal phalanx of the little toe

3. Action: abduction and flexion of the metatarsophalangeal joint of the little toe

4. Innervation: lateral plantar nerve

2. Second layer

a. Tendon of flexor digitorum longus: courses laterally, crossing superficial to the tendon of flexor hallucis longus; divides into four tendons that pass through the bifurcated tendons of flexor digitorum brevis and insert on the plantar surfaces of the bases of the distal phalanges of digits 2, 3, 4, and 5

b. Tendon of flexor hallucis longus: courses forward in the sole of the foot; at the base of the proximal phalanx of the hallux, it passes between the insertions of the medial and lateral heads of flexor hallucis brevis, and their associated sesamoid bones, before inserting on the plantar surface of the base of the distal phalanx of the hallux

c. Quadratus plantae (flexor accessorius)

1. Origin: calcaneus

2. Insertion: lateral side of the tendon of flexor digitorum longus

3. Action: corrects the medial pull of the flexor digitorum longus tendon on digits 2, 3, 4, and 5, rendering it more in line with the longitudinal axis of the foot

4. Innervation: lateral plantar nerve

d. Lumbricals (four)

1. Origin: first lumbrical—medial side of the flexor digitorum longus

tendon to digit 2; second lumbrical—adjacent sides of the flexor digitorum longus tendons to digits 2 and 3; third lumbrical—adjacent sides of the flexor digitorum longus tendons to digits 3 and 4; fourth lumbrical—adjacent sides of the flexor digitorum longus tendons to digits 4 and 5

2. Insertion: the tendons of the first, second, third, and fourth lumbricals insert into the medial sides of the bases of the extensor expansions of digits 2, 3, 4, and 5, respectively

3. Action: extension of the interphalangeal joints and flexion of the metatarsophalangeal joints of digits 2, 3, 4, and 5

4. Innervation: first lumbrical—medial plantar nerve; second, third, and fourth lumbricals—lateral plantar nerve

3. Third layer

   a. Flexor hallucis brevis

      1. Origin: plantar surfaces of the cuboid and lateral cuneiform; distally, it divides into a medial and a lateral head

      2. Insertion: medial head—medial side of the base of the proximal phalanx of the hallux and the adjacent sesamoid bone; lateral head—lateral side of the base of the proximal phalanx of the hallux and the adjacent sesamoid bone

      3. Action: flexion of the metatarsophalangeal joint of the hallux

      4. Innervation: medial plantar nerve

   b. Adductor hallucis

      1. Origin: oblique head—plantar surfaces of the bases of the second, third, and fourth metatarsals; transverse head—plantar surfaces of the fibrous capsules of the metatarsophalangeal joints of digits 2, 3, 4, and 5

      2. Insertion: lateral side of the base of the proximal phalanx of the hallux and the adjacent sesamoid bone

      3. Action: adduction and flexion of the metatarsophalangeal joint of the hallux

      4. Innervation: lateral plantar nerve

c. Flexor digiti minimi brevis

   1. Origin: plantar surface of the base of the fifth metatarsal

   2. Insertion: lateral side of the base of the proximal phalanx of the little toe

   3. Action: flexion of the metatarsophalangeal joint of the little toe

   4. Innervation: lateral plantar nerve

4. Fourth layer

   a. Plantar interossei (three)

      1. Origin: first plantar interosseous—medial side of the shaft of the third metatarsal; second plantar interosseous—medial side of the shaft of the fourth metatarsal; third plantar interosseous—medial side of the shaft of the fifth metatarsal

      2. Insertion: first plantar interosseous—medial sides of the bases of the proximal phalanx and extensor expansion of digit 3; second plantar interosseous—medial sides of the bases of the proximal phalanx and extensor expansion of digit 4; third plantar interosseous—medial sides of the bases of the proximal phalanx and extensor expansion of digit 5

      3. Action: adduction of the metatarsophalangeal joints of digits 3, 4, and 5 toward an imaginary longitudinal axis through the center of the second digit; flexion of the metatarsophalangeal joints and extension of the interphalangeal joints of digits 3, 4, and 5

      4. Innervation: lateral plantar nerve

   b. Dorsal interossei (four)

      1. Origin: first dorsal interosseous—adjacent sides of the first and second metatarsals; second dorsal interosseous—adjacent sides of the second and third metatarsals; third dorsal interosseous— adjacent sides of the third and fourth metatarsals; fourth dorsal interosseous—adjacent sides of the fourth and fifth metatarsals

      2. Insertion: first dorsal interosseous—medial sides of the bases of the proximal phalanx and extensor expansion of digit 2; second dorsal interosseous—lateral sides of the bases of the proximal phalanx and extensor expansion of digit 2; third dorsal interosseous—lateral sides of the bases of the proximal phalanx and

extensor expansion of digit 3; fourth dorsal interosseous—lateral sides of the bases of the proximal phalanx and extensor expansion of digit 4

   3. Action: abduction of the metatarsophalangeal joints of digits 2, 3, and 4 away from an imaginary longitudinal axis through the center of the second digit; flexion of the metatarsophalangeal joints and extension of the interphalangeal joints of digits 2, 3, and 4

   4. Innervation: lateral plantar nerve

D. Nerves

   1. The medial and lateral plantar nerves are the terminal branches of the tibial nerve; they arise deep to the flexor retinaculum and enter the sole of the foot deep to abductor hallucis

   2. Medial plantar nerve

      a. Initially, it courses forward, deep to abductor hallucis, and supplies abductor hallucis, flexor hallucis brevis, flexor digitorum brevis, and the first lumbrical, as well as the skin on the medial side of the foot

      b. It then emerges from between abductor hallucis and flexor digitorum brevis and gives rise to plantar digital nerves for the skin of the medial three and one-half digits

   3. Lateral plantar nerve

      a. Courses laterally, between flexor digitorum brevis and quadratus plantae; upon reaching the fifth metatarsal, it reverses direction, and courses medially on the inferior surfaces of the plantar and dorsal interossei

      b. Innervates quadratus plantae, abductor digiti minimi, flexor digiti minimi brevis, the second, third, and fourth lumbricals, adductor hallucis, and the plantar and dorsal interossei; it also supplies the skin on the lateral side of the foot and gives rise to plantar digital nerves for the skin of the lateral one and one-half digits

E. Vessels

   1. The medial and lateral plantar arteries are the terminal branches of the posterior tibial artery; they arise deep to the flexor retinaculum and enter the sole of the foot with the medial and lateral plantar nerves, deep to abductor hallucis

2. Medial plantar artery: courses with the medial plantar nerve; gives rise to the plantar digital artery for the medial side of the hallux as well as branches that anastomose with the plantar metatarsal arteries

3. Lateral plantar artery

   a. Courses with the lateral plantar nerve; as it courses medially on the inferior surfaces of the plantar and dorsal interossei, it is referred to as the plantar arch, which is completed medially by the dorsalis pedis artery

   b. The plantar arch gives rise to plantar metatarsal arteries that, in turn, give rise to plantar digital arteries for the lateral four and one-half digits

4. Veins: accompany their corresponding arteries

Other Joints
of the Lower Limb

I. The Proximal Tibiofibular Joint: the bony components are the fibular articular surface of the tibia and the head of the fibula; the fibrous capsule attaches near the margins of the articular surfaces and is reinforced anteriorly and posteriorly by the anterior and posterior ligaments of the head of the fibula, respectively

II. The Crural Interosseous Membrane: fibrous joint between the interosseous borders of the tibia and fibula; separates the anterior and posterior compartments of the leg and provides attachment for muscles

III. The Distal Tibiofibular Joint

    A. Fibrous joint uniting the fibular notch of the tibia and the medial surface of the distal fibula

    B. Component ligaments

        1. The interosseous ligament binds the apposed surfaces of the tibia and fibula; it is continuous superiorly with the crural interosseous membrane

        2. The anterior and posterior tibiofibular ligaments bind the distal tibia and fibula anteriorly and posteriorly, respectively

IV. The Subtalar or Talocalcanean Joint

    A. Articular components

1. Bony components: posterior calcanean articular surface on the plantar surface of the talus and the posterior talar articular surface on the dorsal surface of the calcaneus

2. Fibrous capsule: attaches near the margins of the articular surfaces

B. Ligaments

1. The interosseous talocalcanean ligament lies within the sinus tarsi, extending from the sulcus tali to the sulcus calcanei; the cervical ligament lies lateral to the sinus tarsi and extends from the lateral surface of the neck of the talus to the dorsal surface of the calcaneus

2. Medial and lateral talocalcanean ligaments extend from the medial and lateral surfaces of the talus to the sustentaculum tali and lateral surface of the calcaneus, respectively

V. The Talocalcaneonavicular Joint

A. Articular components

1. Bony and ligamentous components

a. The head of the talus articulates with the talar articular surface of the navicular and the superior surface of the plantar calcaneonavicular or spring ligament

b. The anterior and middle calcanean articular surfaces adjacent to the head on the plantar surface of the talus articulate with the anterior and middle talar articular surfaces on the superior surface of the sustentaculum tali and the adjacent bone

2. Fibrous capsule: attaches near the margins of the articular surfaces; surrounds the component articulations, defining a single joint cavity

B. Ligaments

1. The plantar calcaneonavicular or spring ligament is a broad, thick band extending from the sustentaculum tali to the plantar surface of the navicular; its superior surface articulates with the head of the talus

2. The talonavicular ligament extends from the dorsal surface of the neck of the talus to the dorsal surface of the navicular; the calcaneonavicular part of the bifurcate ligament extends from the dorsal surface of the calcaneus to the lateral surface of the navicular

VI. The Calcaneocuboid Joint

   A. Articular components

      1. Bony components: cuboidal articular surface of the calcaneus and the calcanean articular surface of the cuboid

      2. Fibrous capsule: attaches near the margins of the articular surfaces

   B. Ligaments

      1. The calcaneocuboid part of the bifurcate ligament extends from the dorsal surface of the calcaneus to the dorsal surface of the cuboid

      2. The long plantar ligament extends from the plantar surface of the calcaneus to the plantar surface of the cuboid, along the bony ridge proximal to the groove for the peroneus longus tendon; some fibers may continue forward to the bases of metatarsals 2, 3, 4, and 5, and convert the groove for the peroneus longus tendon into an osseofibrous tunnel

      3. The short plantar or plantar calcaneocuboid ligament lies deep to the long plantar ligament, extending from the plantar surface of the calcaneus to the plantar surface of the cuboid

   C. Inversion and eversion occur primarily at the subtalar, talocalcaneonavicular, and calcaneocuboid joints

INDEX

Aorta (*continued*)
  ascending, 63
  coarctation of, 79
  descending, 60
  thoracic, 60
Aperture
  orbital, 162
  piriform, 162
  thoracic
    inferior, 33
    superior, 33
Apex
  of heart, 51
  of petrous part of temporal bone, 167, 172
  of prostate, 148
Aponeurosis
  bicipital, 322
  of external abdominal oblique, 76
  of internal abdominal oblique, 76
  palmar, 341
  plantar, 399
  of transversus abdominis, 76
Appendices epiploicae, 106
Appendix, 106
Aqueduct
  of cochlea, 269
  vestibular, 173, 267
Arachnoid
  of brain, 190
  of spinal cord, 25–26
Arcades, 108
Arch
  aortic, 63
  costal, 32
  of cricoid cartilage, 254
  dental, 170, 174
  dorsal venous, of foot, 397
  fibrous
    of flexor digitorum superficialis, 327
    of soleus, 390
  jugular venous, 206
  palatoglossal, 235
  palatopharyngeal, 235
  palmar
    deep, 348
    superficial, 347
  plantar, 404
  pubic, 125
  superciliary, 163
  tendinous, 145
  vertebral, 11
  zygomatic, 165

Arcus tendineus, 145
Area
  bare, of liver, 90, 98
  intercondylar, 357
Areola, 35, 302
Arm, 317–22
Arteries
  alveolar
    anterior superior, 229
    inferior, 229
    posterior superior, 229
  angular, 185
  aorta. *See* Aorta
  appendicular, 108
  auricular
    deep, 228–29
    posterior, 188, 218
  axillary, 307–8
  brachial, 321
  brachiocephalic trunk, 63
  bronchial, 46, 60
  buccal, 186, 229
  of bulb, 138
  carotid
    common, 63, 216–17
    external, 217–18, 223–24
    internal, 217
  cecal, 108
  celiac trunk, 101–2
  central, of retina, 203
  cervical
    ascending, 219
    deep, 219
    superficial, 219, 299
    transverse, 218–19, 299
  ciliary
    anterior, 203
    posterior, 203
  circumflex, 53
    anterior, humeral, 308
    deep, iliac, 78–79
    lateral, femoral, 376
    medial, femoral, 376–77
    posterior, humeral, 299, 308
    scapular, 299, 308
    superficial, iliac, 370
  colic
    left, 108
    middle, 107
    right, 107
  collateral
    inferior ulnar, 321